With contributions by

PETER GANN, M.S., M.D.

Chief, Occupational Medicine, Division of Epidemiology
and Disease Control, New Jersey State Department of
Health; Clinical Assistant Professor of Epidemiology,
Rutgers Medical School, Piscataway, New Jersey

OCCUPATIONAL EPIDEMIOLOGY

G. STEPHEN BOWEN, M.D., M.P.H.

Medical Epidemiologist, Field Services Division,
Epidemiology Program Office, Centers for Disease
Control, Atlanta, Georgia

With the collaboration of

RICHARD MORTON, M.B.B.S., M.P.H.

Albert Einstein College of Medicine, New York, New York

Second Edition

MAUSNER & BAHN
Epidemiology–
An Introductory Text

JUDITH S. MAUSNER, M.D., M.P.H.
Late Professor of Community and Preventive Medicine
(Epidemiology), The Medical College of Pennsylvania, Philadelphia

SHIRA KRAMER, Ph.D.
Epidemiologist, Children's Cancer Research Center,
Children's Hospital of Philadelphia; Assistant Professor
of Epidemiology, University of Pennsylvania School of Medicine,
Philadelphia

Philadelphia
London
Toronto
Mexico City
Rio de Janeiro
Sydney
Tokyo

W. B. SAUNDERS COMPANY

GOVERNORS STATE UNIVERSITY
UNIVERSITY PARK
IL 60466

W.B. SAUNDERS COMPANY
A Division of
Harcourt Brace & Company

The Curtis Center
Independence Square West
Philadelphia, Pennsylvania 19106

Library of Congress Cataloging in Publication Data

Mausner, Judith S.
    Epidemiology: an introductory text.
    At head of title: Mausner & Bahn.
    Includes bibliographies.

    1. Epidemiology.   I. Kramer, Shira.   II. Title.
III. Title: Mausner & Bahn.   VI. Title: Mausner and Bahn.

RA651.M33 1985   614.4   83-20292
ISBN 0–7216–6181–5

Listed here is the latest translated edition of this book together with the language of the translation and the publisher

Spanish—*First Edition*—Nueva Editorial Interamericana S.A.de C.V. Mexico 4, D.F. Mexico

Japanese—*Second Edition*—Nishimura Company Ltd., Niigata-shi, Japan

Mausner and Bahn EPIDEMIOLOGY   ISBN   0–7216–6181–5

Last digit is the print number: 18   17   16   15   14

Judith S. Mausner
1924 – 1983

The tragic and untimely death of the senior author and originator of this text was a great loss to us personally and to the epidemiological community.

Dr. Mausner worked on the preparation of this edition almost to the very end of her life, despite the handicaps resulting from a terminal illness. At the time of her death the manuscript was virtually complete and, in large part, in press.

This textbook stands as proof of the many contributions Judith Mausner made to epidemiology and particularly to the teaching of our discipline.

With affection for a valued colleague and with a profound sense of loss, we dedicate this edition to her memory.

SHIRA KRAMER

RICHARD F. MORTON

PREFACE

This text is designed to provide a background in epidemiology for an introductory course in epidemiology, community medicine, health administration, or public health. It is also intended as a review for students preparing for examinations in preventive medicine. Certain diseases are cited for purposes of illustration, but no attempt is made to present a comprehensive survey. However, the basic principles presented should provide the background for investigating the epidemiology of specific diseases.

We consider it important that all health professionals — not just those who serve as health officers or who do research in epidemiology — be familiar with epidemiologic principles and methods. Epidemiology and biostatistics, no less than physiology and pathology, are basic disciplines essential to both clinical and community medicine. They provide a way of thinking about health and disease.

In reading the medical literature, it is also important to follow critically a chain of evidence and to avoid the major pitfalls of epidemiologic inference. Epidemiologic sophistication fosters a questioning attitude; without it medical practices may be introduced and accepted even though they may lack adequate support from well-controlled studies.

Finally, health workers have an increasing role in providing preventive services and in maintaining the health of a community. It is important, then, to familiarize oneself with the methods appropriate to the epidemiologic study of acute and chronic disease, the analytic methods of demography, and the theory behind screening programs.

We hope that our text will serve, at least for some, as a stepping-stone to more advanced studies in epidemiology and preventive medicine. There is a great need for epidemiologists and other specialists in preventive medicine to participate actively in the prevention of disease and maintenance of health in population groups.

We mourn the premature death, in 1980, of Anita K. Bahn, coauthor of the first edition of this text.

In addition to those who contributed to the first edition we would like to acknowledge the contributions of Richard Morton, Donald Balaban, Richard Burian, Helen C. Chase, Samuel Greenhouse, Douglas Eubanks, Douglas Edwards, Morton Levin, Ralph M. Richart, and Ira Rosenwaike. Beth Sonnenshein contributed greatly by providing references to government publications. We want to express our appreciation to the staff of the National Center for Health Statistics for their helpfulness and efficiency in providing health data. For assistance with typing we are indebted to Vickie Taylor and Frances Seeds for their unfailing willingness and cooperation.

Finally, as was true of the first edition, all of our contacts with the publisher, W. B. Saunders Company, were helpful and pleasant. We want to thank the staff of W. B. Saunders for their skilled and friendly assistance in helping us bring this project to completion.

The debt we owe our husbands, Bernard Mausner and Leon Josowitz, for their unfailing support and encouragement is beyond measure.

JUDITH S. MAUSNER

SHIRA KRAMER

CONTENTS

8

PROPHYLACTIC AND THERAPEUTIC TRIALS: EXPERIMENTAL STUDIES... 195

9

SCREENING IN THE DETECTION OF DISEASE.......................... 214

10

POPULATION DYNAMICS AND HEALTH................................ 239

11

EPIDEMIOLOGIC ASPECTS OF INFECTIOUS DISEASE................ 263

12

OCCUPATIONAL EPIDEMIOLOGY 302

Peter Gann

13

SELECTED STATISTICAL TOPICS 329

EPIDEMIOLOGIC ORIENTATION TO HEALTH AND DISEASE

1

EPIDEMIOLOGY DEFINED

Epidemiology may be defined as **the study of the distribution and determinants of diseases and injuries in human populations.** That is, epidemiology is concerned with the *frequencies* and types of illnesses and injuries in *groups* of people and with the *factors* that influence their distribution. This implies that disease is not randomly distributed throughout a population, but rather that subgroups differ in the frequency of different diseases. Further, knowledge of this uneven distribution can be used to investigate causal factors and thus to lay the groundwork for programs of prevention and control. The contribution of epidemiology to the advance of medical science was expressed well by Frost in 1936:

Epidemiology at any given time is something more than the total of its established facts. It includes their orderly arrangement into chains of inference which extend more or less beyond the bounds of direct observation. Such of these chains as are well and truly laid guide investigation to the facts of the future; those that are ill-made fetter progress.

POPULATION MEDICINE AND EPIDEMIOLOGY

Knowledge about human health and disease is the sum of the contributions of a large number of disciplines — anatomy, microbiology, pathology, immunology, clinical medicine, radiology — the list is potentially very long. However, the various disciplines can be grouped according to their methods and underlying concepts. When this is done, three major categories emerge: one consists of the basic sciences (e.g., biochemistry, physiology, pathology), another the clinical sciences (e.g., adult medicine, neonatology, obstetrics and gynecology, urology), and the third population medicine. In different settings, population medicine is also referred to as community medicine, preventive medicine, or social medicine, or, more traditionally, as public health. This field is concerned with the study of health and disease in human populations.

The concerns of population medicine are quite different from those of the clinical disciplines. **Clinical medicine** focusses largely on the medical care of individuals. Typically, these have been sick people who have presented themselves for help; in recent years examination of apparently well people has been encouraged in order to detect disease in early stages. In **population medicine** the community replaces the individual patient as the primary focus of concern. The problem here is to evaluate the health of a defined community, including those members who would benefit from, but do not seek, medical care. This approach requires specific techniques and skills in addition to those needed for clinical practice. The principles and methods underlying population medicine form the subject matter of this book.

It is readily apparent that the basic sciences, clinical sciences, and population medicine are all highly interrelated. A physician is guided toward a correct diagnosis in an individual patient not only by the patient's history, physical findings, and laboratory data, but also by knowledge of the distribution of diseases by such factors as age, sex, ethnicity, and socioeconomic status. For example, cancer of the pancreas, which is difficult to diagnose on clinical grounds, is more probable in an elderly smoker than in an adolescent. Knowledge of the attributes of the patient can help guide the selection of diagnostic procedures.

Information about the illnesses prevalent in the community also contributes to diagnosis. For a patient with fever and respiratory disease, for example, the physician will want to know if an influenza epidemic is in progress or if there has been a recent upsurge in streptococcal isolations.

Conversely, assessment of the level of occurrence of disease in a population is dependent on the accuracy of the diagnoses made on individual patients and on the completeness with which reportable diseases are made known to public health authorities. Such reporting can lead to containment of an outbreak resulting from contamination of food or water or can show the need for an intensified immunization program against measles. In addition, the accuracy of both individual diagnoses and epidemiologic assessment is dependent on adequate laboratory support. This is particularly important for organisms that require special techniques for isolation and identification, such as *Legionella*, the agent of legionnaire's disease.

Tuberculosis, although on the wane, provides a good illustration of the three different approaches to the same disease. The basic sciences are concerned with various aspects of the tubercle bacillus — its structure and antigenic composition, growth in different media, and resistance to specified antibiotics — and with host responses, such as the extent to which tubercles become walled off by fibrous tissue. Clinical study of a case entails diagnosis, estimation of the extent and activity of disease, choice of therapy, appraisal of the patient's response, and adequate follow-up of chemotherapy.

As a community problem, the control of tuberculosis involves other considerations. Several points are at issue: (1) recognition of its high occurrence in particularly susceptible groups, such as infants, alcoholics, and recent Oriental immigrants to the United States; (2) awareness of the need to follow up household contacts of cases; and (3) the assurance of chemotherapy continuing for an adequate period. Tuberculosis used to require long periods of institutional care. Outpatient chemotherapy, by removing the need for inpatient supervision, has all but eliminated the need for beds for tuberculosis patients.

Although there is a trend toward increasing integration of the basic sciences, clinical sciences, and community medicine, each of these three approaches has its major locus of activity and specific methods. The basic sciences are primarily sited in the laboratory and use experimental techniques. Clinical activities are carried out in hospital wards, emergency rooms, ambulatory care clinics, and the offices of private physicians. Epidemiologic knowledge, largely based on observational studies, is gathered from a variety of sources by professionals called *epidemiologists* whose responsibility it is to develop a comprehensive picture of health problems in the community. In part, the information needed can be derived from the records of clinical facilities; however, these may vary in accuracy and completeness. Furthermore, since community diagnosis requires information about the health problems and needs of all segments of the population, including those not under medical supervision, it may be necessary to carry out surveys of samples of the population. On the basis of the information obtained, health services needed to supplement those already in existence may be developed.

In summary, population medicine necessitates a systematic way of studying both the patterns of occurrence of disease in a community and the patterns of delivery of medical care, since the services offered both influence and are influenced by the amount and nature of disease and by the changes in modes of therapy. Epidemiology is the discipline that provides this systematic approach.

HEALTH AND DISEASE

Although we have defined epidemiology in terms of disease, its central concern is maintenance of health through the prevention of disease. Unfortunately, it is easier to define and measure disease, disability, and death than to produce an operational definition of health.

Health is a rather elastic concept; it may be defined merely as the absence of disease and disability or it may be given a much more positive meaning, as in the Constitution of the World Health Organization (1948):

Health is a state of complete physical, mental and social well-being and not merely the absence of disease or infirmity.

In recent years, this statement has been amplified to include the ability to lead a socially and economically productive life (Mahler, 1981). The definition given may represent an unobtainable ideal, but the goal, nevertheless, is to achieve maximum well-being for all segments of the population. Perhaps a more realistic formulation is that proposed by Dubos (1968). After noting the utopian character of the WHO definition, Dubos goes on to say that health is not to be considered "an ideal state of well-being achieved through the complete elimination of disease, but as a modus vivendi enabling imperfect men to achieve a rewarding and not too painful existence while they cope with an imperfect world." Attempts by national and international committees to quantify health status have led to some promising suggestions for its measurement (Sullivan, 1966). Nevertheless, both physical and mental health are still measured mainly through their converse, disease and death. Thus, of necessity, this text also will focus primarily on measurement of morbidity and mortality even though our ultimate goal is a more positive one.

The Need for Rates

Central to the measurement of disease and identification of high-risk groups in a population is the *rate,* relating cases or events to a population base. The numerator of a rate is the number of people with the disease being counted; the denominator is the population at risk of the disease or event. Note that in a rate (1) the numerator is the number of people to whom something happens, and (2) everyone in the denominator must be at risk of entering the numerator. Rates of disease are called *morbidity* rates; rates of death, *mortality* rates.

$$Rate = \frac{Number\ of\ events,\ cases,\ or\ deaths}{Population\ in\ same\ area}\ in\ a\ time\ period$$

The fallacy of looking only at numbers of cases without relating them to the population from which the cases derive is shown by the following hypothetical data, comparing the number of deaths associated with two modes of transportation, automobiles and private aviation:

	Automobiles	Private Aviation
Number of fatalities per year	1,000	50
Number exposed to risk	100,000	1,000
Rate of fatal injury	$\frac{1,000}{100,000} = 0.01$	$\frac{50}{1,000} = 0.05$

Note that the number of deaths among drivers is twenty times that among pilots, but since the number of drivers exposed is one hundred times greater, the actual fatality rate is lower for drivers than for pilots. In summary, then, epidemiologic statements require specification of a denominator as well as a numerator.

In contrast, clinically oriented studies usually focus only on the numerator, such as the fatalities in the chart, or the number of sick persons who seek medical care.

For a further example of the difference in the two approaches, consider two reports on ulcer disease. A clinical report bore the title "Problem of the gastric ulcer reviewed: Study of 1,000 cases" (Smith et al., 1953). An epidemiologic study of gastric ulcer indicated annual incidence rates of 0.44 per 1000 persons aged 15 years and older (Bonnevie, 1975) and noted that, in contrast to earlier studies, gastric ulcer is now more common in males than in females.

Low as well as high rates of disease have provided useful clues to etiology. For example, absence of pellagra in attendants in mental hospitals at a time when it was prevalent in patients led Goldberger (1914) to reject the then popular hypothesis that pellagra is of infectious origin in favor of a hypothesis of nutritional deficiency. The virtual absence of carcinoma of the cervix among nuns (Gagnon, 1950) in contrast to the high rate among prostitutes (Røjel, 1953) suggested that sexual activity was probably an important etiologic factor. To quote a British epidemiologist (Morris, 1955):

The main function of epidemiology is to discover groups in the population with high rates of disease, and with low, so that causes of disease and of freedom from disease can be postulated. . . . The biggest promise of this method lies in relating diseases to the ways of living of different groups, and by doing so to unravel "causes" of disease about which it is possible to do something. . . .

The great advantage of this kind of approach to prevention is that it may be applicable in the early stages of our knowledge of diseases, to disrupt the pattern of causation before the intimate nature of diseases is understood. Sufficient facts may be established for this by epidemiological methods alone, or in combination with others. The opportunity may thus offer to deal with one "cause," or with various combinations of causes. . . .

THE NATURAL HISTORY OF DISEASE

The development of disease is often an irregularly evolving process, and the point at which a person should be labelled "diseased" rather than "not diseased" may be arbitrary. Many diseases — especially chronic disease, which may last years or decades — have a natural life history. By "natural history" we refer to the course of disease over time, unaffected by treatment. Like the "seven ages of man," chronic disease may be considered to extend over time through a sequence of stages. As knowledge accumulates, it has become apparent that factors favoring the development of chronic disease often are present early in life, antedating the appearance of clinical disease by many years.

Since each disease has its own life history, any general formulation is necessarily arbitrary. Nevertheless, it may be useful to develop a schematic picture of the natural history of disease as a framework within which to understand different approaches to prevention and control.

Stage of Susceptibility

In this stage, disease has not developed but the groundwork has been laid by the presence of factors that favor its occurrence. For example, fatigue and acute and chronic alcoholism heighten susceptibility to pneumonia; inadequate maternal nurturing predisposes to emotional illness; high serum cholesterol levels increase the probability that overt coronary heart disease will develop; immune suppression is believed to increase the risk of developing cancer.

Factors whose presence is associated with an increased probability that disease will develop later are called *risk factors*. The need to identify such factors is becoming more apparent with the growing awareness that chronic diseases represent our major health challenge.

Risk factors may be immutable or susceptible to change. Such factors as age, sex, race, and family history, which are not subject to change, are often major determinants of risk. However, some risk factors can be altered, as when smokers can be persuaded to give up smoking. Others are not now amenable to change, but their identification may still be useful for identifying persons who deserve close medical supervision.

It should be pointed out that even when there is a strong statistical association between a risk factor and a disease, this does not mean that *all* individuals with the risk factor will necessarily develop the disease nor that *absence* of the risk factor will ensure absence of the disease. Our inability to identify all the factors contributing to risk of disease limits our ability to predict for individuals.

Stage of Presymptomatic Disease

At this stage there is no manifest disease, but usually through the interaction of factors pathogenetic changes have started to occur. At this stage, the changes are essentially below the level of the "clinical horizon," the imaginary dividing line above which disease manifests itself through detectable signs or symptoms. Examples of presymptomatic disease are atherosclerotic changes in coronary vessels prior to any signs or symptoms of illness, and premalignant (and, unfortunately, sometimes malignant) alterations in tissue.

Stage of Clinical Disease

By this stage sufficient end-organ changes have occurred so that there are recognizable signs or symptoms of disease. It is important, whenever possible, to subdivide this stage for better management of cases and for purposes of epidemiologic study. There are several possible bases for classification. Depending on the specific disease, classification may be based on morphological subdivision or on functional or therapeutic considerations.

Different classificatory schemes are used for different diseases. Cancer is usually classified on morphological grounds that express the extent of disease, i.e., the location of the tumor and its histological type and extent. A commonly used procedure is to place each tumor into one of three categories: localized, with regional metastases, or with generalized spread.

The importance of staging for prognosis of cancer can be seen in Figure 1–1, which gives five-year relative survival rates for cancer of different organs according to whether the cancer was localized or showed regional spread at the time of diagnosis. While prognoses vary according to the different sites of cancers, it is uniformly true that at each site survival is better for localized cases than for those with regional involvement. Clearly, stage is the major influence on prognosis.

Functional and therapeutic classification is exemplified by the widely used categorization of cardiac disease of the New York Heart Association (1964). The following is adapted from their schema:

Functional Classification
Class I   No limitation of physical activity because of discomfort
Class II   Slight limitation of physical activity; patient comfortable at rest but ordinary activity produces discomfort

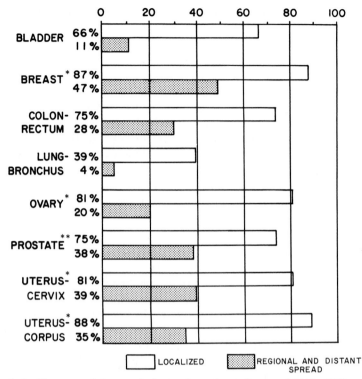

Figure 1-1 Five-year relative survival rates for patients diagnosed 1964–1973, selected sites of cancer. Relative survival is the ratio of the survival rate of an observed group to the survival of the general population similar in age, race and sex. (From Biometry Branch, National Cancer Institute, National Institutes of Health.)

　* Female only.
　** Male only.

Class III　Marked limitation of physical activity; comfortable at rest but less than ordinary activity causes discomfort
Class IV　Inability to carry out any physical activity without discomfort

Therapeutic Classification
Class A　Physical activity need not be restricted in any way
Class B　Ordinary physical activity need not be restricted, but patient is advised against severe efforts
Class C　Ordinary physical activity should be moderately restricted
Class D　Ordinary physical activity should be markedly restricted
Class E　Complete bed rest advised; patient confined to bed or chair

Note that functional and therapeutic classifications do not always parallel each other. For example, a patient with a recent heart attack or active rheumatic carditis may not have symptoms upon physical exertion, but may be advised to remain at complete rest (Class I, E).

　As suggested above, classification, or staging, of disease is of great importance for epidemiologic study. Effective grouping reduces variability, yielding relatively homogeneous subgroups. This is important for evaluation of the effect of prophylactic or therapeutic agents (see discussion of clinical trials in Chapter 8); for comparative studies of disease in different groups, i.e., international, regional, occupational, and so on; and for clinical management of patients.

At present we do not have a complete understanding of the natural history of many diseases. We do not know why an individual with a number of risk factors, for example, may not progress to clinical disease. Much research in recent years has been directed to the follow-up of large groups over time (longitudinal studies) to attempt to gain this understanding.

Stage of Disability

Some diseases run their course and then resolve completely, either spontaneously or under the influence of therapy. However, there are a number of conditions which give rise to a residual defect of short or long duration, leaving the person disabled to a greater or lesser extent. On occasion a disease that is usually self-limited may later give rise to chronic disability. For example, a small proportion of cases of measles are followed by development of subacute sclerosing panencephalitis, a progressive neurologic disorder (Brody et al., 1972).

Although disability can be defined in various ways, in community surveys it usually means any limitation of a person's activities, including his psychosocial role as parent, wage earner, and member of his community. The National Health Survey (see Chapter 4) defines disability as "any temporary or long-term reduction of a person's activity as a result of an acute or chronic condition" (1958). Note that the emphasis is on loss of function rather than on structural defect. Individuals vary widely in their reaction to physical impairment. Two persons with the same amount of tissue damage from heart disease, for example, may show marked differences in their resultant level of disability. While there is a substantial amount of disability associated with acute illness, the extent of protracted disability resulting from chronic illness is of greater significance for society.

LEVELS OF PREVENTION

Implicit in the scheme just presented is the notion that a disease evolves over time and that as this occurs pathologic changes may become fixed and irreversible. Therefore, the aim is to push back the level of detection and intervention to the precursors and risk factors of disease. This lays the emphasis squarely on preventive rather than curative medicine.

With *prevention* a dominant theme, it may be well to elaborate upon this word. In a narrow sense, prevention simply means inhibiting the development of a disease before it occurs. However, in current usage, the term has been extended to include measures that interrupt or slow the progression of disease. For this reason several levels of prevention are said to exist. *Primary* prevention (appropriate in the stage of susceptibility) is prevention of disease by altering susceptibility or reducing exposure for susceptible individuals; *secondary* prevention (applied in early disease, i.e., preclinical and clinical stages) is the early detection and treatment of disease; *tertiary* prevention (appropriate in the stage of advanced disease or disability) is the alleviation of disability resulting from disease and attempts to restore effective functioning.

Primary Prevention

Prevention of the occurrence of disease consists of measures that fall into two major categories: general health promotion and specific protective measures. *General health promotion* includes provision of conditions at home, work, and school that favor healthy living, e.g., good nutrition, adequate clothing, shelter, rest, and recreation. It also encompasses the broad area of health education, which includes not only instruction in hygiene, but also such diverse areas as sex education, anticipatory guidance for children and parents, and counselling in preparation for retirement. *Specific protective measures* include immunizations, environmental sanitation (e.g., purification of water supplies), and protection against accidents and occupational hazards.

The past successes of public health in developed countries have been accomplished largely by primary prevention of infectious disease through environmental protection and immunization. The most pressing problem in these countries today is chronic disease whose prevention requires both knowledge of new environmental hazards related to advances in technology and modification of deeply rooted individual behavior, such as dietary patterns, physical activity, and the use of alcohol and tobacco.

Information on different ill effects of some of these behavior patterns continues to accumulate. Such effects of alcoholism as cirrhosis of the liver and increased rates of certain cancers have been known for many years, but it is only since the 1970s that the fetal alcohol syndrome (FAS) has been recognized as a consequence of alcohol ingestion during pregnancy (Jones et al., 1974). The clinical features of this syndrome are varied, but the more common manifestations are mental retardation, microcephaly, deficiency in length and weight both pre- and postnatally, and a set of characteristic facial abnormalities. The amount of alcohol consumed by the pregnant woman does not have to be large to induce deleterious effects. A study of women enrolled in the Kaiser-Permanente Health Plan (Harlap and Shiono, 1980) indicated an increased risk of spontaneous abortion among women who took as little as one to two drinks daily. There are still uncertainties about clinical delineation of FAS and the full range of risk factors; these are currently being investigated further.

Another obdurate and important problem is that of deaths and injuries from accidents, especially motor vehicle crashes. Future efforts at primary prevention will probably focus both on attempts to influence individual behavior and on environmental controls (e.g., reduced exposure to asbestos in the workplace, passive restraints in cars, altered composition of dietary fats) which will in part shift health-related decisions from the individual to the social level.

Secondary Prevention

Secondary prevention refers to early detection and prompt treatment of disease. With such measures it is sometimes possible to either cure disease or slow its progression, prevent complications, limit disability, and reverse communicability of infectious diseases. On a community basis, early treatment of persons with infectious diseases (e.g., sexually transmitted infections) may protect others from acquiring the infection and thus provide at once secondary prevention for the infected individuals and primary prevention for their potential contacts. Because of our inability to prevent certain diseases, efforts at control of many chronic diseases center primarily around secondary prevention. Examples are diabetes, hypertension, in situ carcinoma of the cervix, and glaucoma.

As is true of primary prevention, secondary prevention is a responsibility of physicians both in private practice and in community posts. Health departments and other community agencies often conduct screening surveys designed to uncover asymptomatic disease and to alter the natural history of the condition detected.

Tertiary Prevention

This consists of *limitation of disability* and *rehabilitation* where disease has already occurred and left residual damage. Early physiotherapy to an affected limb to restore motion and prevent contractures exemplifies measures for the limitation of disability. Rehabilitation is the name given to attempts to restore an affected individual to a useful, satisfying, and, where possible, self-sufficient role in society. Its major theme is maximal utilization of the individual's residual capacities, with emphasis on remaining abilities rather than on losses. Since modern rehabilitation includes psychosocial and vocational as well as medical components, it calls for good teamwork from a variety of professions, as shown in Figure 1–2. It may also require extensive physical facilities (such as special vehicles and modifications of the home setting) and sufficient funding to provide a variety of services over a prolonged period of time.

Until the occurrence of death, it may be possible throughout the evolution of a disease process to apply appropriate measures to prevent continued progression and deterioration of the patient's condition. The different levels of prevention can be fully understood only in relation to the natural history of disease. Figure 1–3 shows the different levels of prevention and modes of intervention that may be applied during the different stages in the natural history of disease. The clearer our understanding of the natural history of a disease, the greater may be the opportunities for developing effective points of intervention.

The interrelations between natural history and levels of prevention will be illustrated by a specific example, stroke.

PSYCHOSOCIAL

Social Evaluation
Social Service
Psychologic Service
  Psychometrics
  Evaluation
  Counselling
Family Counselling
Psychiatric Service
Spiritual Counselling
Recreation

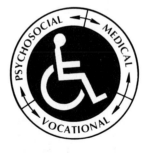

MEDICAL

Medical Diagnosis,
  Treatment and Super-
  vision of Medical
  Services

VOCATIONAL

Evaluation
  Vocational History
  Vocational Diagnostic Services
    Psychometrics and evaluation
    Prevocational interests
      and aptitude exploration
Counselling
Vocational Training
Placement
  Selective Industrial
  Transitional—Sheltered Workshop
Homebound

Figure 1–2 A schematic diagram of rehabilitation services. (Adapted from Rehabilitation Service, Hospital of the University of Pennsylvania, Philadelphia, PA.)

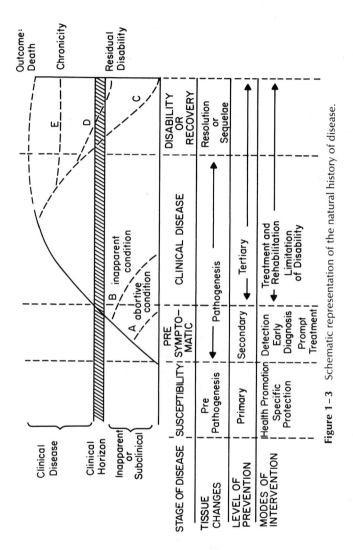

Figure 1 – 3 Schematic representation of the natural history of disease.

APPLICATION OF PREVENTION AND
NATURAL HISTORY: STROKE

Stroke, a term familiar to laymen as well as physicians, refers to a symptom complex of neurologic deficit lasting at least 24 hours, which results from damage to the brain by alteration of its blood supply. Stroke is a manifestation of cerebrovascular disease (CVD). The effects are variable and depend on the extent and location of the damage to nervous tissue; there may be impairment of speech or cerebration, or paralysis of one or more portions of the body.

Cerebrovascular disease is an important health problem. It is the third leading cause of death in the United States, resulting in some 200,000 deaths annually. It is also a major contributor to disability. The National Center for Health Statistics estimated in 1975 that there are over 300,000 noninstitutionalized people in this country paralyzed as the result of a stroke.

There are several mechanisms of stroke: large artery thrombosis, lacunae (small infarcts deep in the brain), embolism, intracranial hematoma, subarachnoid hemorrhage, and aneurysm and arteriovenous malformations (Mohr et al., 1978). Since cerebral thrombosis accounts for more than half of all strokes, the following section will focus primarily on cerebral thrombosis and its consequence, brain infarction.

Many years ago, stroke was regarded as a disease of older persons that comes on without warning and without relation to the person's health status in earlier life. Persons with markedly elevated blood pressure were known to be at high risk of hemorrhagic stroke, but infarction was regarded as an unpredictable occurrence. Since little was known about prevention, stroke was regarded fatalistically. At best there was a modest concern for rehabilitative measures.

In the past few decades, advances in different disciplines have led to better understanding and new perspectives about the problem of stroke. Among them are increased awareness of the importance of the extracranial vessels (carotids and the vertebral-basilar system) in the production of stroke, anticoagulant therapy and other pharmacologic advances, and technical achievements in vascular surgery and diagnostic radiology.

Epidemiology has also contributed to our current understanding by sharpening our picture of the natural history of stroke. We now know that stroke does not occur at random but that factors identifiable in early life influence the probability that stroke will occur years later. Much of our information about the natural history of stroke is derived from populations placed under observation many years ago, initially for the study of coronary heart disease (CHD). The information recorded at

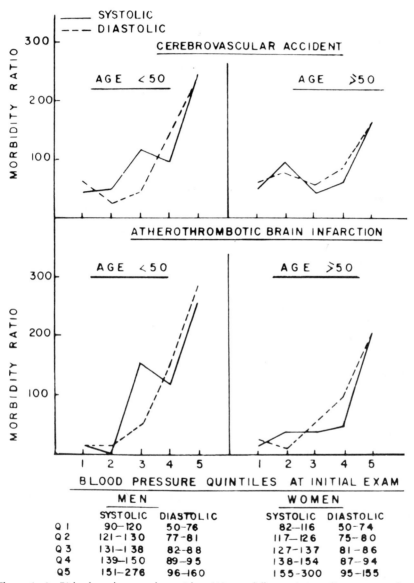

Figure 1–4 Risk of cerebrovascular accident (16-year follow-up) according to antecedent blood pressure level. Men and women 30 to 62 years of age at entry: Framingham study. (Reproduced by permission of the American Heart Association, Inc.)

entry into these studies has made it possible to identify subsequently factors related to occurrence of stroke. For example, a major study was carried out in Framingham, Massachusetts, in which a community sample of some 5200 people was followed biennially since 1948 (Kannel et al., 1970), with respect to history, physical examination, chest x-ray, EKG, and blood determinations. Several risk factors for stroke were identified, but the major finding was the overwhelming importance of hypertension as a precursor to cerebral thrombosis as well as to hemorrhage (Ostfeld, 1980).

Figure 1–4 demonstrates the clear relationship between blood pressure and subsequent stroke experience in the Framingham data. For both brain infarction and hemorrhagic stroke, the morbidity ratio is seen to be much higher for persons with hypertension than for those with normal blood pressure on initial examination.

Additional factors contributing to risk are cardiac abnormalities (i.e., left ventricular hypertrophy on electrocardiogram or cardiac enlargement on x-ray) (Wolf et al., 1973). The contribution of factors such as elevated blood lipids, glucose intolerance, obesity, and cigarette smoking is not clearly defined.

Figure 1–5 shows the risk of CVD according to blood pressure status and indicates that cardiac impairment and level of blood pressure both contribute independently to risk.

One aspect of stroke that has received increasing attention over the past quarter-century is the phenomenon of transient ischemic attacks (TIA). TIA is a focal neurologic deficit of abrupt onset and brief duration followed by complete recovery. It was hoped that TIA might prove a useful indicator of impending stroke and lead to surgical or pharmacologic intervention. Unfortunately, even though approximately 40 per cent of persons with TIA will have a stroke within five years, TIAs occur uncommonly among all stroke patients. Whisnant (1973) showed that only about 10 per cent of patients with cerebral infarction had had a TIA before their stroke.

Review of the considerations just outlined indicates that stroke may be viewed not as an isolated occurrence, but as the late or final manifestation of a long chain of events. Before facts about risk factors for stroke became available, only tertiary prevention, i.e., rehabilitation after a stroke had occurred, seemed possible. Treatment emphasized early physical therapy to prevent contractures and muscle atrophy, early ambulation to prevent thromboembolic complications, and active occupational and psychologic rehabilitation.

In the light of current knowledge, prevention of stroke is being implemented through primary and secondary prevention, especially the former. Secondary prevention through recognition and treatment of

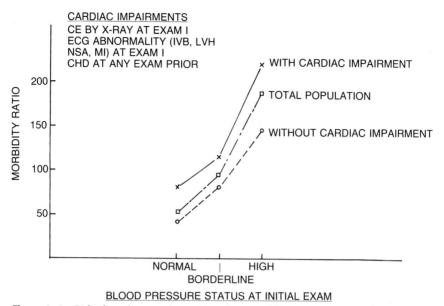

Figure 1 – 5 Risk of cerebrovascular accident (16-year follow-up) according to blood pressure status and evidence of cardiac impairment. Men and women 30 to 62 years of age at entry: Framingham study. (CE, cardiac enlargement, ECG, electrocardiogram; IVB, intraventricular block; LVH, left ventricular hypertrophy; NSA nonspecific abnormalities; MI, myocardial infarction; CHD, coronary heart disease). (From Kannel, W. B., Wolf, P. A., et al.: Epidemiologic assessment of the role of blood pressure in stroke. The Framingham Study. J.A.M.A., *214*:301. Copyright 1970, American Medical Association.)

TIA is applied when possible, but the limitations of this approach have been noted.

However, the identification of high blood pressure as a major risk factor has led to a series of intervention trials. In the first ones, the Veterans Administration (VA), using male veterans as subjects, reported that antihypertensive treatment reduced morbidity and mortality from high blood pressure (VA — 1967, 1970, 1972). The first VA trial showed beneficial results from treating patients whose diastolic blood pressure (DBP) was between 115 and 129. In subsequent trials, intervention at lower levels of blood pressure was undertaken. The results were essentially the same: Treatment led to lowered morbidity and mortality, although not all of the findings were statistically significant. As a result of these limited trials, it was decided to test the effects of antihypertensive therapy on the general population — people of both sexes, all races, and younger as well as middle-aged adults.

A number of such trials have been undertaken; two of the largest and most ambitious will be outlined briefly. The first trial, the Hypertension Detection and Follow-up Program (HDFP), screened almost 200,000 persons in 1973 and 1974. In the process of screening and rescreening this group, the investigators discovered over 10,000 persons who had a mean DBP of 90 mm Hg or above. These subjects were designated as hypertensive, were enrolled in the study, and were randomized into one of two groups: One group received a rigid course of care (stepped care, or SC); those in the other group were referred to their usual source of care (referred care, or RC). Subjects were followed for five years; the endpoint of the study was total mortality (all causes). Five-year mortality was 17 per cent lower for the SC subjects than for the RC group, and the difference was 20 per cent greater for the group with DBP of 90 to 104 mm Hg.

Another large trial carried out about the same time focussed on people at high risk for vascular disease. The purpose of the study, known as the Multiple Risk Factor Intervention Trial (MRFIT), was to select for intervention a group of people at unusually high risk for vascular disease because of multiple risk factors — high blood pressure, elevated blood lipids, and cigarette smoking.

The results of this trial (J.A.M.A., 1982) showed that both the experimental and the control groups developed a decline in risk factor levels. This may have accounted for the fact that there was a nonsignificant difference between the groups with respect to CHD mortality. The possibility that diuretic medication in high doses caused adverse effects in subgroups of patients with electrocardiographic abnormalities is being investigated further.

A promising development in recent years has been decline in the mortality from stroke (Fig. 1–6), which reflects, at least in part, a decrease in occurrence. The declining mortality in the early part of the century antedates the introduction of antihypertensive agents. But in recent years mortality has been falling faster, by about 4 to 5 per cent per year, and it seems reasonable to infer that the widespread screening of the population that was initiated in the 1970s, as well as the systematic use of antihypertensive drugs, have contributed to the accelerating drop in mortality. Work is also underway to develop auxiliary methods to understand and control the influence of stress and lifestyle on blood pressure.

This brief survey of the preventive approach to one major health problem, stroke, highlights the contribution that epidemiologic investigation and appropriate public health programming can make to the health of the population. Thus, a condition that was once considered an inevitable accompaniment to aging is now being approached through preventive efforts directed at people early in their lives and early in the development of disease. This is an exciting prospect indeed.

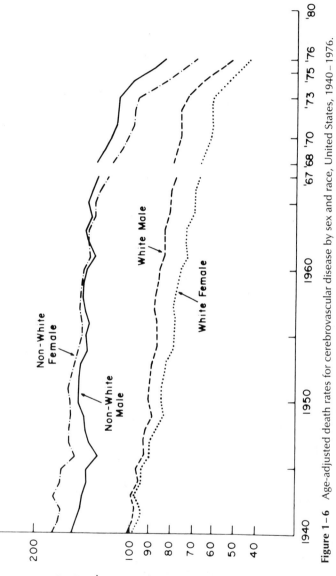

Figure 1–6 Age-adjusted death rates for cerebrovascular disease by sex and race, United States, 1940–1976.

SUMMARY

This chapter has set the stage for epidemiology within the framework of population medicine. Clinical and epidemiologic approaches to the study of disease were contrasted, as were the concepts of health and disease. Rates were presented as fundamental tools in epidemiology.

The chapter introduced a model of the natural history of disease over time, emphasizing precursors to the appearance of clinically detectable disease that increase the likelihood of disease development in the future. The term *risk factor* was introduced to identify such predisposing conditions in the individual. The importance of subdividing the stages of clinical disease on anatomic or functional grounds was stressed, as was the personal and societal impacts of the stages of disability.

The concept of levels of prevention—primary, secondary, and tertiary—was outlined and developed in relation to the natural history of disease. This was illustrated by reference to stroke. The modern approach to this disease extends beyond rehabilitation to include identification of risk factors and early detection and therapy.

In the next chapter, we will expand the definition of epidemiology, delineate its scope, and present several epidemiologic models of the causation of disease.

REFERENCES

Bonnevie, O.: The incidence of gastric ulcer in Copenhagen County. Scand. J. Gastroenterol., 10:231, 1975.

Brody, J. A., Detels, R., et al.: Measles-antibody titres in sibships of patients with subacute sclerosing panencephalitis and controls. Lancet, 1:177, 1972.

Constitution of the World Health Organization, 1948. In Basic Documents, 15th Ed. WHO, Geneva, 1964.

Dubos, R.: Determinants of Health and Disease in Man, Medicine and Environment (Chap. 4). Frederick A. Praeger, New York, 1968.

Frost, W. H.: Introduction to Snow on Cholera. Commonwealth Fund, New York, 1936. (Reprinted by Hafner Publishing Company, New York, 1965.)

Gagnon, F.: Contribution to study of etiology and prevention of cancer of cervix of uterus. Am. J. Obstet. Gynecol., 60:516, 1950.

Goldberger, J.: The cause and prevention of pellagra. Public Health Rep., 29:2354, 1914. (Reprinted in Terris, M. (Ed.): Goldberger on Pellagra. Louisiana State University Press, Baton Rouge, 1964.)

Harlap, S., and Shiono, P. H.: Alcohol, smoking and incidence of spontaneous abortions in the first and second trimesters. Lancet, 2:173, 1980.

The Hypertension Detection and Follow-up Program Cooperative Group: Five-year findings of the Hypertension Detection and Follow-up Program: Reduction in mortality in persons with high blood pressure, including mild hypertension. J.A.M.A., 242:2562, 1979.

Jones, K. L., Smith, D. W., Streissguth, A. P., et al: Outcome in offspring of chronic alcoholic women. Lancet, 1:1076, 1974.

Kannel, W. B., Wolf, P. A., et al.: Epidemiologic assessment of the role of blood pressure in stroke. The Framingham study. J.A.M.A., 214:301, 1970.

Mahler, H.: Health for all by the year 2000. World Health Stat., Feb-Mar, 1981.

Mohr, J. P., Caplan, L. R., Melski, J. W., Goldstein, R. J., Duncan, G. W., Kistler, J. P., Pessin, M. S., and Bleich, H. L.: The Harvard Cooperative Stroke Registry: A prospective registry. Neurology, 28:754, 1978.

Morris, J. N.: Uses of epidemiology. Br. Med. J., 2:395, 1955.

Multiple Risk Factor Intervention Trial Research Group: Multiple Risk Factor Intervention Trial. Risk Factor Changes and Mortality Results. J.A.M.A., 248:1465, 1982.

National Health Survey: Concepts and definitions in the Health Household-Interview Survey. USPHS Pub. No. 584-A3, U.S. Government Printing Office, Washington, D.C., 1958.

New York Heart Association, Inc.: Diseases of the Heart and Blood Vessels—Nomenclature and Criteria for Diagnosis, 6th Ed. Little, Brown and Company, Boston, 1964.

Ostfeld, A. M.: A review of stroke epidemiology. Epidemiol. Rev., 2:136, 1980.

Røjel, J.: The interrelation between uterine cancer and syphilis. Acta Pathol. Microbiol. Scand. (Suppl.), 97:3, 1953.

Smith, F. H., Boles, R. S., Jr., et al.: Problems of the gastric ulcer reviewed: Study of 1000 cases. J.A.M.A., 153:1505, 1953.

Sullivan, D. F.: Conceptual problems in developing an index of health. U.S. Dept. of Health, Education, and Welfare, USPHS Pub. No. 1000, Series 2, No. 17, U.S. Govt. Printing Office, Washington, D.C., 1966.

Veterans Administration Cooperative Study Group on Antihypertensive Agents: Effects of treatment on morbidity in hypertension: I. Results in patients with diastolic blood pressures averaging 115 through 129 mm Hg. J.A.M.A., 202:116, 1967.

Veterans Administration Cooperative Study Group on Antihypertensive Agents: Effects of treatment on morbidity in hypertension: II. Results in patients with diastolic blood pressure averaging 90 through 114 mm Hg. J.A.M.A., 213:1143, 1970.

Veterans Administration Cooperative Study Group on Antihypertensive Agents: Effects of treatment on morbidity in hypertension: III. Influence of age, diastolic pressure, and prior cardiovascular disease; further analysis of side effects. Circulation, 45:991, 1972.

Whisnant, J. P., Matsumoto, N., and Elveback, L. R.: Attacks in a community. Rochester, Minnesota, 1955 through 1969. Mayo Clin. Proc., 48:194, 1973.

Wolf, P. A., Kannel, W. B., et al.: The role of impaired cardiac function in atherosclerotic brain infarction. The Framingham study. Am. J. Public Health, 63:52, 1973.

EPIDEMIOLOGIC CONCEPTS

2

THE SCOPE OF EPIDEMIOLOGY

The definition of epidemiology given previously, **the study of the distribution and determinants of diseases and injuries in human populations,** is quite inclusive. For many years, the province of epidemiology was generally considered to be restricted to the infectious diseases. This was an understandable focus, since the major scourges of humans in the past were epidemics of communicable disease. Only after the major infectious diseases had come under some satisfactory control did investigation shift toward the chronic diseases of later life—the vascular diseases, arthritides, and malignant neoplasms.

Epidemiologic methods are now being applied to other conditions and areas of research as well—to injuries, adverse drug reactions, drug addiction, congenital defects, mental illness, family planning, and health services research. There has also been a shift to evaluation of certain exposures (e.g., to chemicals or ionizing radiation) as possible sources of disease. That is, many recent studies define groups by exposure to possible hazards rather than by the present existence of disease. (This approach is discussed further in Chapter 8, under Prospective Studies). Finally, epidemiologic principles and methods are now being applied to evaluation of the effects of new approaches to prevention as well as treatment and to the organization of health care.

Although the early history of epidemiology is largely concerned with studies of infectious disease, there are on record epidemics traced to noninfectious causes. Two outstanding examples from the eighteenth century are lead poisoning and scurvy. Colic among cider drinkers in Devonshire, England, was traced to intoxication with lead (Baker, 1767). In that era, it was the practice to transport cider in leaden jugs or to process it in lead-containing presses. The acidity of the cider caused enough lead to be leached into the liquid to cause acute lead toxicity. The occurrence of scurvy in epidemic proportions on board British ships during long sea voyages was correctly traced to a nutritional deficiency (Lind, 1753) that could be prevented by a ration of limes. It is worth noting that effective prevention did not depend on a full understanding of the dietary lack; vitamin C was not isolated until 1928.

It is now generally accepted that epidemiologic study can be appropriately applied to all diseases, conditions, and health-related events. Further, since epidemiology aims for a comprehensive view of the dynamics of disease, it is concerned not only with epidemics but also with interepidemic periods and with sporadic and endemic occurrences of disease.

EPIDEMIC VERSUS ENDEMIC DISEASE

Endemic occurrence is defined as "the constant presence of a disease or infectious agent within a given geographic area . . . (or) the usual prevalence of a given disease within such area." The term is used in contrast with **epidemic**, "the occurrence in a community or region of a group of illnesses . . . of similar nature, clearly in excess of normal expectancy" (Benenson, 1980).

Examination of this definition of *epidemic* indicates that the term can have quite a broad meaning:

1.　It may include any kind of disease (or injury), including noninfectious conditions.

2.　There is no general rule about the number of cases that must exist for an outbreak to be considered an epidemic. Rather, an epidemic exists whenever the number of cases exceeds that expected on the basis of past experience for a given population. Clearly this level of expectation varies for different diseases and in different circumstances. Anywhere in the world today, even a single case of smallpox would exceed expectancy, whereas until recently 100 cases in a single year might have been within the expected number in Ethiopia or India.

3.　There is no specification of geographic extent; an epidemic may cover a few city blocks or an entire nation, or may even be worldwide in distribution, as is true of pandemics of influenza.

4.　An epidemic may encompass any time period; it may last a few hours (chemical intoxication or bacterial food poisoning), a few weeks (influenza or hepatitis), or several years (drug addiction). Many countries, including the United States, have been experiencing a lung cancer epidemic for the past 40 years.

A disease that remains epidemic over many years eventually may be considered endemic. Thus, in developed countries, most of the important chronic problems are endemic in nature. That is, they are widespread and do not exhibit great variability in frequency from year to year. For example, hypertension, one of the primary risk factors for cardiovascular, cerebrovascular, and renal disease, is one of the more prevalent conditions in the United States. Estimates as high as 60 million have been made for the prevalence of hypertension in the United States (Kopstein, 1980), and it is thought to contribute to at least 250,000 deaths annually. The strong relationship between diastolic blood pressure and risk of disease is apparent from Figures 1–4 and 1–5. Thus, endemic as well as epidemic conditions are of great public health concern.

CLASSIFICATION OF DISEASE

In studying disease as a phenomenon of populations, we define individuals as "well" or "ill." While acknowledging Selye's contribution that a common "adaptation syndrome" underlies all illness (Selye, 1956), we nevertheless find it fruitful to group ill persons together so that persons with the "same" disease are put into the same category.

The nature of the grouping and the assignment of causes of illness depends on the concepts of illness and health in a given culture. Anthropologic studies illustrate vividly the great range of interpretations put on illness by different groups. For example, years ago wasting disease might have been ascribed to malevolent spirits or to the work of sorcerers, while today we would look for physiologic causes.

In Europe, diseases used to be classified on the basis of symptomatology. There were poxes, fluxes, and fevers; in more modern terms, these conditions would be referred to as rash diseases, gastrointestinal disturbances, and febrile illnesses. As our understanding of pathology and physiology has increased, we have been able to move from pure description of symptoms to a classification of disease based on abnormal physiology or morbid anatomy. In other words, the level of classification beyond the merely descriptive is the categorization of disease by its manifestations. This level implies the need for understanding the mechanisms involved in the abnormality of structure or function. Over the centuries, astute clinicians have developed skills in identifying clinical features of different illnesses and in distinguishing diseases from each other.

An advance in classification arose from the advances in bacteriology in the late nineteenth century, when specific organisms were linked to such major disease entities as typhoid fever, cholera, plague, and tuberculosis. With the growing ability to associate particular microorganisms with specific disease states came the need to add *etiologic* classification to that based on the *manifestations* of disease.

To illustrate these different approaches, let us consider tuberculosis. In the nineteenth century, various clinical entities were known: Involvement of the cervical lymph glands was known as scrofula, and respiratory pulmonary tuberculosis as consumption, or the "white plague." Once the role of the tubercle bacillus in inducing disease was understood, these apparently discrete entities were then considered to be manifestations of the same disease. All of the manifestations are now seen to be related to each other by the presence of tubercle bacilli in the lesions.

The importance of etiologic classification is this: Whenever we are able to link an etiologic factor, or agent, to a disease, this gives us the insight necessary for developing rational preventive measures. Currently, the etiologic roots of many infectious, nutritional, and genetic diseases are known and have led to rational approaches to prevention and therapy.

Unfortunately, however, the origins of many of our major disease entities are still unclear. We still classify many conditions (i.e., cancer, musculoskeletal diseases, and joint conditions, as well as neurologic and psychiatric illness) by the manifestations of the disease rather than by its etiology.

The classification of psychiatric illness is a particularly vexing problem. In the United States, classification has been embodied in the Diagnostic and Statistical Manual of Mental Disorders. In the first two versions, DSM-I (1952) and DSM-II (1968), classification of disease was based on an impressionistic schema that implied an etiologic framework and labelled observable clinical entities. A major advance occurred with the publication of DSM-III in 1980 after several years of extensive field testing. DSM-III calls for the clinician to summarize a large number of observations on each patient along five axes:

Axis   I   Clinical syndromes
Axis   II   Personality disorders
Axis   III Physical disorders and conditions
Axis   IV   Severity of psychosocial stressors
Axis   V   Highest level of adaptive functioning during the past year

Table 2 – 1, the classification of affective disorders from DSM-III, gives the reader an idea of the wealth of detail that is called for by this classificatory schema. Of course, it is very important not to be led by the specificity of the association to regard any single factor as *the* agent of disease. The origins of disease are complex, and we need to invoke an

TABLE 2–1 Classification of Affective Disorders°

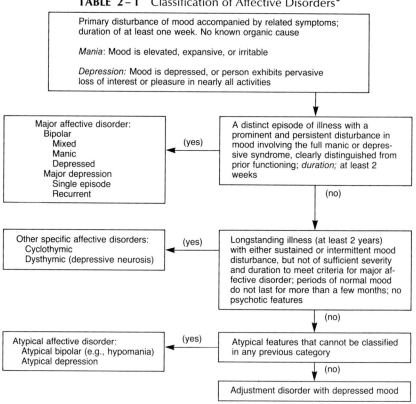

° Adapted from Diagnostic and Statistical Manual of Mental Disorders, 1980.

ecological model within which to develop ideas about causation and prevention.

MULTIPLE CAUSATION OF DISEASE

In medicine, we focus on the human and the forces within him and within the environment that influence his state of health. From this viewpoint, the human is the *host* organism; other organisms are considered only as they relate to human health. In veterinary medicine, the term "host" might refer to cats, dogs, or horses. However, many of the principles presented in this text apply equally to the study of health and disease in human and animal populations.

The egocentrism implicit in our view of the universe has been noted in the following poignant paragraph from Zinsser's *Rats, Lice and History* (1943). Epidemic typhus fever is a disease of humans likely to develop in cold climates when people are crowded together in unsanitary conditions. Zinsser points out that it may be equally reasonable to view typhus as a disease of lice or of humans.

Man is too prone to look upon all nature through egocentric eyes. To the louse, *we* are the dreaded emissaries of death. He leads a relatively harmless life — the results of centuries of adaptation; then, out of the blue, an epidemic occurs; his host sickens and the only world he has ever known becomes pestilential and deadly; and if, as a result of circumstances not under his control, his stricken body is transferred to another host, whom he, in turn, infects, he does so without guile, from the uncontrollable need for nourishment, with death already in his own entrails. If only for his fellowship with us in suffering he should command a degree of sympathetic consideration.

Humans and lice inhabit the same world. Although the term "ecology" has been overused in the popular press, it is still useful to think of humans and lice as parts of one ecological system. *Ecology* may be defined as the study of the relationship of organisms to each other as well as to all other aspects of the environment.

Since disease arises within an ecological system, a basic tenet of epidemiology is that an ecological approach is necessary to explain the occurrence of disease; disease cannot be attributed to the operation of any **one** factor. The requirement that more than one factor be present for disease to develop is referred to as *multiple causation* or *multifactorial etiology.*

At first glance it might seem that the introduction of an organism into a community would be enough to explain the development of an epidemic.

$$\text{Organism} \rightarrow \text{Human} \rightarrow \text{Disease}$$

However, the organism alone is not sufficient to account for the outbreak and cannot therefore be considered "*the* cause." The level of immunity of the population is also crucial. This can be seen from the sequence of events following introduction of measles or mumps into a *virgin population,* i.e., one in which an organism has not been present for many years, if ever. When this occurs, adults as well as children are affected. The upper age limit is determined by the number of years since the virus last circulated in the community. For example, Christensen and his colleagues (1953) found that when measles was introduced into Greenland for the first time in 1951, over 4200 cases developed in a total population of 4320. Those who escaped included abortive cases, patients who died without a definitive diagnosis, and some persons who either had had the disease previously in Denmark or had received prophylactic gamma globulin. Only five unprotected persons in the entire population appeared to have escaped infection entirely.

An additional set of factors, environmental conditions, also determines whether effective transmission of disease can occur in any given situation. These factors include degree of contact, level of hygienic practices, and presence of other organisms.

When a factor **must** be present (a sine qua non) for a disease to occur, it is called the *agent* of that disease. For example, influenza virus is the agent of influenza. Many, but not all, of the known agents of disease are located in the biologic environment. Examples of agents from the physical environment are lead, asbestos, beryllium, carbon monoxide in the inspired air, and ionizing radiation. A possible agent in the social environment is maternal deprivation. Numerous studies have demonstrated that the quality of parental care in the early years of life is intimately related to normal physical, emotional, and mental development (Bowlby, 1952). In keeping with the ecological view presented above, an agent is considered to be a **necessary but not sufficient cause** of disease because suitable conditions of the host and environment must also be present for disease to develop.

It is customary to divide factors affecting the development of disease into two groups, *host factors* (intrinsic) and *factors in the environment* (extrinsic). Host factors affect susceptibility to disease; factors in the environment influence exposure and sometimes indirectly affect susceptibility as well. The interactions of these two sets of factors determine whether or not disease develops.

Host Factors (Intrinsic)

The state of the host at any given time is a result of the interactions of genetic endowment with environment over the entire lifespan. For some conditions the relative contributions of genetic and environmental factors are quite clear; for others it is difficult to arrive at an assignment of weights.

An increasing number of genetically determined factors have been identified as related to either an increased or decreased susceptibility to certain diseases. A striking example is the risk of retinoblastoma among children born with the dominant retinoblastoma gene. Carriers of this gene have a 100,000-fold increase in risk of retinoblastoma compared to noncarriers. Similarly, the risk of cancer of the colon is more than 1000 times greater for persons with polyposis than for those without a predisposing gene (Knudson, 1977). ABO blood type is associated with several diseases. Persons with type A blood have an increased risk of gastric cancer (Aird et al., 1953), while those with type O are more likely to develop duodenal ulcer (Clarke et al., 1955). Sickle cell trait is associated with a decreased risk of malaria due to *Plasmodium falciparum* (Allison, 1954). Individuals who have xeroderma pigmentosum have a genetically determined inability to repair damage induced by ultraviolet light and are thus at unusually high risk of developing multiple neoplasms in areas of skin exposed to sunlight (Robbins et al., 1974).

Other attributes are primarily the result of past environmental exposures. Thus, one of the major components in resistance to infectious disease is *specific immunity*, a state of altered responsiveness to a specific substance acquired through immunization or natural infection. For certain diseases (e.g., measles, chickenpox), this protection generally lasts for the life of the individual. Other types of environmental exposure are chemical in nature and may come from an individual's personal environment, such as from cigarette smoking, from exposure at work (e.g., to asbestos), or from more generalized air or water pollution.

Personality is one host factor for which separation of intrinsic and extrinsic variables is difficult (Mischel, 1968). It is beyond our present scope to explore systematically the relation between personality and illness. However, we should note that personality variables do influence the course of illness, at least partly through their effect on tendency to seek medical care and to comply with medical advice.

One well-documented association between personality traits and disease concerns coronary heart disease (CHD). Since the late 1950s, Rosenman and Friedman, two California cardiologists, have been exploring with their co-workers the relevance of behavior to the development of CHD (1970). Over the years, they have produced evidence that a certain style of behavior is predictive of CHD. Their work, at first received with skepticism, is now widely accepted. The behavior they have identified, called type A, is characterized by aggressiveness, competitiveness, ambition, restlessness, and a sense of time urgency. Type B individuals, who do not exhibit these characteristics, have lower rates of CHD. By now numerous other investigators, some using different terminology (e.g., Jenkins' Activity Schedule [JAS]), have confirmed the association. Almost all of the work to date has used white upper- and middle-class employed males. Further work is in progress to investigate other populations and to determine which components of type A behavior are causally linked to CHD and whether the various manifestations of CHD (i.e., myocardial infarction, angina, sudden death) differ in their relationship to type A characteristics. One study, which compared individuals who actually developed CHD within the original cohort with controls who did not have CHD, found that two of the factors identified — competitive drive and impatience — were associated with the development of CHD (Matthews et al., 1977). A review panel has prepared a detailed evaluation of type A personality and has delineated the kinds of research efforts that are needed to clarify our understanding (Review Panel, 1981).

Social class membership is a host attribute that strongly reflects environmental influences. Because developmental experiences and lifestyle are intimately tied to social class, many diseases show a differential frequency among persons of different social classes. For example, the social class gradient in carcinoma of the cervix (i.e., rates inversely related to social class) is compatible with such class-related behavior as age at first intercourse and number of sexual partners (Doll and Peto, 1981).

There are many unanswered questions about the role of host factors in disease. We do not know, for example, why only some of the people exposed to large doses of x-rays develop leukemia, or why all heavy smokers do not develop lung cancer. Nevertheless, at least for certain diseases, our current state of knowledge does permit us to identify individuals with an increased probability of developing the disease and to concentrate preventive efforts on this group.

Environmental Factors (Extrinsic)

Extrinsic or environmental factors can be classified as biological, social, and physical.

Biological Environment. This sector of the environment includes (1) infectious agents of disease, (2) reservoirs of infection (other human beings, animals, and soil), (3) vectors that transmit disease (e.g., flies and mosquitoes), and (4) plants and animals (as sources of food, antibiotics, and other drug principles or as antigens). Most of these topics will be elaborated further in Chapter 11.

Social Environment. The social environment may be defined in terms of the overall economic and political organization of a society and of the institutions by which individuals are integrated into the society at various stages in their lives. All of these factors are relevant to health. Broadly speaking, overall socioeconomic and political organization affect the technical level of medical care, the systems by which that care is delivered, the extent of support for medical care and biomedical research, and the adequacy and level of enforcement of codes and laws controlling health-related environmental hazards (pollution, housing, occupational safety, and so on).

Particular social customs may affect health. The types of foods eaten and the thoroughness of cooking determine whether there will be exposure to parasites, such as fish tapeworm and trichinae. The practice of wearing shoes can prevent acquisition of hookworms in rural areas where these parasites are prevalent.

Another important aspect of social environment is the general level of receptivity to new ideas. When physicians and other health personnel try to encourage healthful practices, resistance may develop, at least in part, because these practices run counter to deeply held beliefs and values. This can apply equally to problems encountered in ensuring an adequate intake of milk in the diet of pregnant Zulu women (Cassel, 1955) and those found in persuading Americans to use seat belts. A number of other illustrations of similar phenomena are recorded and discussed in *Health, Culture and Community* (Paul, 1955).

The extent to which individuals are integrated into a society is vitally significant to health. In general, a high degree of integration is protective; social isolation and alienation are productive of disease. The pioneer work in this area was done by Durkheim (1897) in his studies of suicide. More recently, schizophrenia (Faris and Dunham, 1939; Hare, 1956) and depressed mental development in children (Spitz, 1945; Widdowson, 1951) have been found to be linked to circumstances of social isolation. Damaging effects from catastrophic losses in an individual's immediate social environment have also been demonstrated. Both suicide (MacMahon and Pugh, 1965) and entry into psychiatric care (Stein and Susser, 1969) tend to cluster in the period following bereavement. Recent work has indicated that being widowed, especially for men, is associated with higher mortality rates (Helsing and Szklo, 1981). Less dramatic life changes may also take a toll.

A phenomenon related to social loss is the upheaval associated with geographic mobility, particularly if it also involves a change in cultural milieu, such as a move from a rural to an urban area. Studies in North Dakota (Syme et al., 1964) and North Carolina (Tyroler and Cassel, 1964) indicate increased rates of coronary heart disease in persons exposed to cultural discontinuities.

Physical Environment. The physical aspects of the environment include heat, light, air, water, radiation, gravity, atmospheric pressure, and chemical agents of all kinds. In the technically developed areas of the world, humans have a great deal of control over the physical environment through provision of adequate shelter against extremes of weather, purification of drinking water, treatment of sewage, and year-round control of indoor temperature and humidity. Yet new environmental problems continue to arise as old ones are solved. Currently, the rapid growth of population, the increase in industrial wastes of all kinds, and the ever increasing number of motor vehicles interact to produce air, water, noise, and other types of pollution of the environment.

Air pollution, for example, has recently emerged as an urgent threat to health. When weather conditions are unfavorable, masses of polluted air can be trapped and hang over a city for several days at a time, exposing the inhabitants to a variety of noxious substances. A number of acute air pollution episodes have been documented. The largest, associated with a four-day fog in London in 1952, led to some 4000 deaths in excess of the usual number (as shown in Figure 11–8). Long-term exposure to pollution probably also produces damage. There are still many unanswered questions about the role of air pollution in certain chronic diseases, including lung cancer. However, air pollution probably contributes to the higher rates of chronic respiratory disease in urban than rural areas in several countries.

Pollution of air in indoor home environments is also of concern. Contamination of air may derive from such sources as building materials (formaldehyde) and cigarette smoke transmitted through passive smoking. Another source of indoor pollution may be heating systems and devices such as kerosene space heaters, which came into widespread use in the early 1980s for inexpensive heating. Excess emissions of nitrogen oxides, sulfur dioxide, and carbon monoxide have been reported from their use (Leaderer, 1982). The increasing costs of fuel have in some instances led to complete insulation of homes, with resultant decrease in ventilation and heightened exposure to indoor pollutants.

Although the physical environment is often regarded mainly as a source of stressors, its positive as well as negative aspects bear consideration. The range of environmental conditions (e.g., atmospheric pressure, oxygen supply, living space) compatible with human existence on earth is relatively narrow; in L. J. Henderson's words, there is a "fitness of the environment" (1913). Health-related environmental goals must be concerned with maintenance of this fitness as well as with elimination of identifiable stressors. A recently emerging science, known variously as environmental psychology or ekistics, is concerned with the design of living spaces. There is mounting interest in the effects of the arrangement of the physical environment on both physical and mental health (Proshansky et al., 1970).

Interrelations of Factors (Ecologic Models)

Although three discrete sectors of the environment (biological, social, and physical) have been identified, it should be emphasized that this separation is artificial; they are closely related to each other and to host factors. Several alternative models have been developed to depict the ways in which these interactions influence the occurrence of disease. Whichever model one uses, it is important to realize that the balance of forces that determines an individual's state of health at a given time is in a kind of dynamic equilibrium. A potentially harmful change in any of the components of the system may not lead to detectable disease if the other parts of the system have the capacity to compensate for the insult. If the existing balance is precarious, disease may develop after even a small insult. For example, flying at a high altitude, which would ordinarily not lead to illness, might precipitate a thrombotic crisis in a person with sickle cell hemoglobin. Exposure to organisms that usually cause no damage can be serious for a person with impaired immunologic defenses. This is a problem of increasing importance as persons are kept alive by drastic medical and surgical therapies (treatment of leukemia and other malignancies; organ transplantation) that require interference with immune mechanisms. With these considerations in mind, then, we will present three ecological models.

The Epidemiologic Triangle. This model was widely used for many years and still is referred to frequently in the epidemiologic literature. The epidemiologic triangle is considered to consist of three components — host, environment, and agent. The model implies that each must be analyzed and understood for comprehension and predictions of patterns of a disease. A change in any of the components will alter an existing equilibrium to increase or decrease the frequency of the disease.

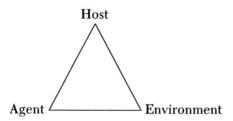

In the preceding pages, we identified host and environmental factors as determining, respectively, susceptibility and exposure to disease. The epidemiologic triangle highlights as a separate component the **agent** of disease, which is, of course, only one among many environmental factors.

When the focus of epidemiologic studies was limited to the infectious diseases, particularly the bacterial diseases, the infecting organisms were accorded a status separate from the other environmental factors and identified as *agents* of disease. However, with the recent application of epidemiologic concepts and methods to other categories of disease, we are dealing with conditions that have not been linked to specific agents, such as schizophrenia, coronary heart disease, and rheumatoid arthritis. Further, even for diseases with an identifiable agent, many epidemiologists prefer to regard the agent as an integral part of the total environment. Therefore, new models have been developed that deemphasize "agent" and, rather stress the multiplicity of interactions between host and environment. The two models to be presented next reflect this view.

The Web of Causation. The notion of a "web of causation" was put forth some years ago by MacMahon and his colleagues (1970). The essence of the concept is that effects never depend on single isolated causes, but rather develop as the result of chains of causation in which each link itself is the result of "a complex genealogy of antecedents." The large number of antecedents creates a condition that may appropriately be conceptualized as a "web, which in its complexity and origins lies quite beyond our understanding."

Figure 2–1 illustrates the web of causation underlying the occurrence of coronary heart disease. It is evident that multiple factors promote or inhibit the development of disease. Some of these factors are intrinsic to the host and thus immutable (e.g., genotypic LDL level). Others, such as components of the diet, smoking, physical inactivity, ingestion of hormones, and lifestyle (e.g., stress) are subject to manipulation. (See p. 18 for a discussion of the MRFIT trial as an attempt at primary prevention of coronary heart disease.)

The Wheel. A model that uses the wheel (Fig. 2–2) is another approach to depicting human-environment relations. The wheel consists of a hub (the host or human), which has genetic make-up as its core. Surrounding the host is the environment, schematically divided into the three sectors mentioned above—biological, social, and physical. The relative sizes of the different components of the wheel depend upon the specific disease problem under consideration. For hereditary diseases, the genetic core would be relatively large. For a condition like measles, the genetic core would be of lesser importance; the state of immunity of the host and the biological sector of the environment would contribute more heavily.

Like the web of causation, the model of the wheel implies a need to identify multiple etiologic factors of disease without emphasizing the **agent** of disease. For example, the wheel model lays no greater stress on rabies virus than on the animal reservoirs of the disease. However, in contrast to the web of causation, the wheel model does encourage separate delineation of host and environmental factors, a distinction useful for epidemiologic analyses.

Since the discussion of epidemiologic models has been rather abstract, we will illustrate the application of one model, the wheel, to two different health problems.

THE IRISH POTATO FAMINE. The interrelations of these various factors can be seen clearly in the great Irish potato famine of the late 1840s. In 1845, Ireland was an impoverished country with a dearth of natural resources, widespread unemployment, and a rapidly growing population largely dependent on agriculture, especially the potato, for subsistence. A wet spell in the summer of 1845 (change in the physical environment) was followed shortly by the appearance of a blight, a fungal disease, on the potato crop (biological change). The crop failure

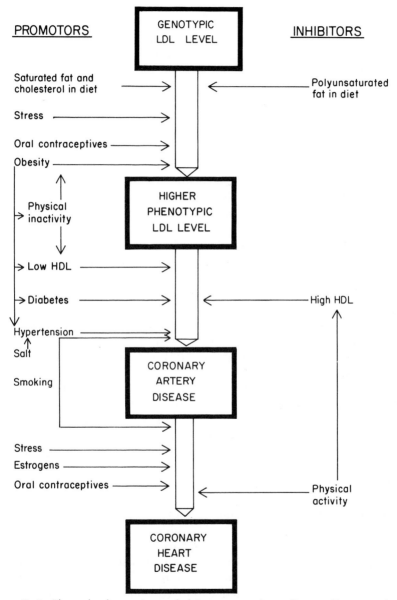

Figure 2-1 The web of causation underlying coronary heart disease. (Courtesy of Dr. Roger Sherwin, University of Maryland.)

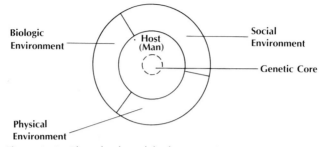

Figure 2-2 The wheel model of man-environment interactions.

was countered with successful relief measures (social and political organization) during the winter of 1845 – 46 in the form of purchase of food from the United States, provision of governmental loans, and relief measures. However, at this juncture there was a change of government in the United Kingdom. The new Whig government was strongly wedded to a laissez faire economic policy. Thus, when the crop failed again in 1846, they chose not to intervene. The famine that resulted was aggravated by a particularly severe winter. Starving mobs crowded into the towns in search of sustenance from soup kitchens and shelter in workhouses. Not surprisingly, epidemics of typhus and relapsing fever, both louse-borne diseases, broke out, adding to the miseries of dysentery, scurvy, and starvation edema. Over the five years from 1845 through 1850, Ireland lost about two million people, almost one-quarter of its population; half died, the rest emigrated.

Is it meaningful to ask about *the cause* of the starvation and of the diseases that developed during the famine, scurvy, and typhus fever? True, the agent of typhus fever (a Rickettsia) had to be present. But the lack of response in agricultural policy, even though potato blight had appeared in other countries before it hit Ireland, the blight itself, and the malnutrition, crowding, and lack of sanitary facilities, which favored the spread of louse-borne disease, all contributed to one of the greatest disasters in history.

LEAD POISONING. A contemporary example of an ecological problem is afforded by lead poisoning in children, a condition of insidious onset that is sufficiently widespread to have been referred to as a "silent epidemic." This man-made disease illustrates the concepts of natural history and levels of prevention presented in Chapter 1, as well as the interactions of factors in host and environment that lead to disease (Alpert, 1969).

Lead-based paints were commonly used for interior surfaces in this country until the 1940s when they were replaced by titanium-based paint because of the realization that lead in paint could be a source of danger for children. However, elimination of lead from interior paints did not eliminate the hazard of exposure from deteriorating houses built prior to the 1940s nor from improper use of exterior paint on interior surfaces.

In the decaying houses and apartments typical of urban slums, flaking and peeling paint may be ingested by young children with pica. *Pica* is defined as a tendency to eat nonedible materials. The concurrence of lead in the environment and a child with pica creates the conditions for lead poisoning (*stage of susceptibility*). If lead is in fact ingested and if the exposure is not overwhelming, there may be a period in which the child appears well despite accumulation of lead in his tissues (*stage of presymptomatic disease*). If this accumulation is not checked, symptoms eventually appear (*stage of clinical disease*). The effects of chronic lead poisoning are varied. Characteristic symptoms include hyperirritability, incoordination, loss of appetite, vomiting, and abdominal pain. Finally, lead encephalopathy with brain edema and outright convulsions may ensue. Untreated, the disease may progress to death or evolve into a chronic condition in which there is permanent residual damage in the form of depressed intellectual development and difficulty in learning (*stage of disability*).

Lead poisoning is preventable. The ideal approach, of course, is primary prevention so that the child does not become exposed to lead. If there is lead in the environment, it should be removed. Theoretically, at least, prevention of pica would also interrupt the chain of events leading to lead poisoning.

In the current state of affairs in which children are still being exposed to lead, preventive measures at a secondary level are needed. Screening efforts include testing the blood for lead and checking houses and apartments to detect lead in the environment. When elevated blood levels are found, treatment consists of deleading with chelating agents. If this is done early enough it can lessen permanent damage. It is not sufficient just to treat a child for accumulation of lead. The environment should be checked and corrected so that the child is not again subjected to an excessive exposure. Further, identification of a child with a high blood lead level or actual lead poisoning should be a signal for further case-finding efforts in that child's family and neighborhood.

Tertiary measures of prevention consist of rehabilitative efforts for all children seen after permanent damage has occurred, including special education classes and similar community facilities. It is to be hoped that tertiary and even secondary therapeutic measures will assume decreasing importance as communities move to combat the problem of lead poisoning.

To what extent does this problem exemplify the complexity of host-environment interactions extending beyond the harmful effects of a single agent, lead? As in the discussion of the Irish potato famine, we will use the wheel to examine this question.

The susceptible host is a child between one and five years of age in a stage of development when he needs oral gratification and has a real but limited degree of mobility, coupled with an unlimited desire to explore his environment. However, in the face of similar exposures to lead in the environment (flaking paint, peeling window ledges, and so on) not all children are equally likely to develop lead poisoning; only some children exhibit pica. If the tendency to pica is coupled with a substantial environmental exposure, the stage is set for lead poisoning to develop. The tendency to pica is only incompletely understood, but it seems to reflect the quality of parent-child interactions. In children with pica, there is often a background of inadequate mothering, supervision, and stimulation. Thus, the social environment contributes importantly to the problem.

In addition to the microlevel indicated above, i.e., the family, the social environment also determines the extent of the problem on a macrolevel through legislation governing availability of paints with lead, through economic patterns that encourage the continued use of substandard housing, and through local housing codes and their enforcement or lack of enforcement. Once excessive exposure has occurred, the availability of organized screening programs and skilled medical care are also important determinants of the outcome.

Finally, aspects of the physical environment other than the load of lead it imposes are also germane. There is a definite seasonal trend in lead poisoning, with a disproportionate number of cases becoming manifest during the summer months. The seasonality of onset is related to the fact that exposure to sunlight increases production of vitamin D, which in turn influences the metabolism of calcium and lead; there may be additional factors as well.

The Relationship Between Chronic and Infectious Disease Epidemiology

Traditionally, it has been believed that factors in the biological environment are linked solely with infectious diseases. Recent evidence suggests that certain infectious agents may be etiologically related to a number of chronic diseases, as illustrated by the following chart:

Agent	Disease
Hepatitis virus	Hepatoma
Herpes simplex virus	Cancer of the cervix
Epstein-Barr virus	Cancer of the nasopharynx
Epstein-Barr virus	Burkitt's lymphoma (Africa)

Likewise, demographic factors that are usually associated with chronic disease are also necessary to examine in studying infectious disease. One important element to consider is age at exposure. For example, the age at which a woman's breasts are irradiated influences her subsequent risk of breast cancer; radiation during puberty is associated with the highest risk (Tokunaga, 1979). Other examples of the effect of age on disease can be seen in the nature of the infections that develop following exposure to poliovirus and hepatitis virus: First exposure of young children to these agents leads to mild or inapparent infection, while first exposure at a later age results in a greater amount of apparent and even severe disease.

Etiologic Concepts and the Control of Disease

The multifactorial nature of disease has been emphasized because of its importance for prevention and control. Recognition of multifactorial causes has led to an awareness that studies of disease etiology must encompass multiple risk factors and their interactions. This also means that epidemiologic studies of most chronic diseases are necessarily complex in design, statistical analysis, and interpretation.

Although identification of risk factors for a disease is highly desirable, full knowledge of etiologic mechanisms is not necessary for effective control measures. We have already pointed out that this was true of scurvy in the eighteenth century. Goldberger (1914) quickly came to the conclusion that pellagra was related to nutritional deficiency; very shortly after he began his investigations, he suggested on an empiric basis that diet be supplemented by fresh meat, eggs, and milk in areas where pellagra was prevalent.

This principle is equally applicable today. Extensive epidemiologic evidence and experimental animal data support a direct causal relationship between cigarette smoking and cancer (Surgeon-General's report, 1979), although the precise mechanisms by which tobacco causes cancer are not fully understood. Despite these limitations in our knowledge, a reduction in tobacco use would have more of an impact on the number of deaths attributable to cancer than would manipulation of any other single agent (Doll and Peto, 1981).

Because of the multiplicity of ecological interactions, it is often possible to affect disease, even that with a known agent, by altering other aspects of human-environment interactions. In diseases in which an organism is carried by flies or mosquitoes, for example, successful control efforts have focussed on the insect, not the agent.

Since ecological relationships are complex, measures for disease control almost inevitably have far-reaching consequences. A striking example of this is the impact of malaria control through DDT spraying after World War II. The elimination of this disease from large areas of the world led to an unchecked growth of population and hence a new cycle of problems related to overpopulation and inadequate food supplies.

This principle actually pertains to any environmental manipulation. The effects of the substitution of detergents for soap on water quality are only now becoming fully apparent. We are now coming to appreciate the effects, shown in increased delinquency and other antisocial behavior, of the decisions made in the 1950s to build high-rise housing projects rather than units close to the ground. Thus, any proposed measure for control of disease should be evaluated in terms of the totality of effects it is likely to have on the ecosystem, at least as far as these can be estimated in advance. A forceful exposition of this thesis has been presented by Barry Commoner in *The Closing Circle* (1971).

SUMMARY

This chapter has delineated the broad scope of epidemiology as embracing both infectious and noninfectious diseases. Further, epidemiology was noted to be concerned with endemic and sporadic occurrence of diseases and conditions, as well as with the occurrence of epidemics.

We next discussed the classification of disease and the advance that is represented by the use of etiologic, rather than manifestational, classification. Several examples of classification were given, one of which was a new classification for psychiatric disorders.

The interrelation of host and environmental factors within an ecosystem and consequent implications for control of disease were presented in terms of three models—the epidemiologic triangle, the web of causation, and the wheel. The latter was applied to the analysis of two problems, the Irish potato famine and the modern problem of lead poisoning.

REFERENCES

Aird, I., Bentall, H. H., et al.: Relationship between cancer of stomach and ABO blood groups. Br. Med. J., *1*:799, 1953.

Allison, A. C.: Protection afforded by sickle-cell trait against subtertian malarial infection. Br. Med. J., *1*:290, 1954.

Alpert, J. J., Breault, H. J., et al.: Subcommittee on accidental poisoning, American Academy of Pediatrics. Prevention, diagnosis and treatment of lead poisoning in childhood. Pediatrics, *44*:291, 1969.

Baker, G.: An essay on the cause of the endemic colic of Devonshire, 1767. (Reprinted by Delta Omega Society, American Public Health Association, New York, 1958.)

Benenson, A. S. (Ed.): Control of Communicable Diseases in Man, 13th Ed. American Public Health Association, New York, 1980.

Bowlby, J.: Maternal Care and Mental Health, 2nd Ed. WHO, Geneva, 1952.

Cassel, J.: A comprehensive health program among South African Zulus. In Paul, B. D. (Ed.): Health, Culture and Community. Russell Sage Foundation, New York, 1955.

Christensen, P. E., Schmidt, H., et al.: An epidemic of measles in Southern Greenland, 1951. Measles in virgin soil. II. The epidemic proper. Acta Med. Scand., 144:430, 1953.

Clarke, C. A., Cowan, W. K., et al.: Relationship of ABO blood groups to duodenal and gastric ulceration. Br. Med. J., 2:643, 1955.

Commoner, B.: The Closing Circle. Alfred A. Knopf, Inc., New York, 1971.

Dembroski, T. M., Weiss, S. M., Shields, J. L., Haynes, S. G., and Feinleib, M.: Coronary-Prone Behavior. Springer-Verlag, New York, 1978.

Doll, R., and Peto, R.: The Causes of Cancer. Quantitative Estimates of Avoidable Risks of Cancer in the United States Today. Oxford University Press, 1981.

Durkheim, E.: Suicide: A study in sociology. 1897. (Reprinted by Free Press, Glencoe, Ill., 1951.)

Faris, R. E. L., and Dunham, H. W.: Mental disorders in urban areas: An ecological study of schizophrenia and other psychoses. University of Chicago Press, Chicago, 1939.

Goldberger, J.: The cause and prevention of pellagra. Public Health Rep., 29:2354, 1914. (Reprinted in Terris, M. (Ed.): Goldberger on Pellagra. Louisiana State University Press, Baton Rouge, 1964.)

Hare, E. H.: Mental illness and social conditions in Bristol. Br. J. Psychiatry, 102:349, 1956.

Helsing, K. J., and Szklo, M.: Mortality after bereavement. Am. J. Epidemiol., 114:1, 41, 1981.

Henderson, L. J.: Fitness of the Environment. Macmillan, New York, 1913. (Reprinted by Beacon Press, Boston, 1958.)

Jenkins, C. D.: Psychologic and social precursors of coronary disease. N. Engl. J. Med., 284:244, 307, 1971.

Knudson, A. G., Jr.: Mutation and cancer in man. Cancer, 39:1882, 1977.

Kopstein, A. N.: Hypertension-Related Mortality by Health Service Area. 1968–72. Statistical Notes for Health Planners, NCHS, No. 11, Sept., 1980.

Leaderer, B. P.: Air pollutant emissions from kerosene space heaters. Science, 218:1113, 1982.

Lind, J.: A Treatise of the Scurvy. Kincaird and Donaldson, Edinburgh, 1753. (Reprinted in Steward, C. P., and Guthrie, D. (Eds.): Lind's Treatise on Scurvy. University Press, Edinburgh, 1953.)

MacMahon, B., and Pugh, T. F.: Suicide in the widowed. Am. J. Epidemiol., 81:23, 1965.

MacMahon, B., and Pugh, T. F.: Epidemiologic Principles and Methods (Chap. 2). Little, Brown and Co., Boston, 1970.

Matthews, K. A., Glass, D. C., Rosenman, R. H., and Bortner, R. W.: Competitive drive, pattern A and CHD: A further analysis of some data from the Western Collaborative Group Study. J. Chronic Dis., 30:489, 1977.

Mischel, W.: Personality and assessment. John Wiley and Sons, Inc., New York, 1968.

Paul, B. D. (Ed.): Health, Culture and Community. Russell Sage Foundation, New York, 1955.

Proshansky, H. M., Ittelson, W. H., et al.: Environmental Psychology: Man and His Physical Setting. Holt, Rinehart and Winston, Inc., New York, 1970.

The Review Panel on Coronary-Prone Behavior and Coronary Heart Disease. Coronary-prone behavior and coronary heart disease: A critical review. Circulation, 63:1199, 1981.

Robbins, J. H., Kraemer, K. H., Lutzner, M. A., et al.: Xeroderma pigmentosum: An inherited disease with sun sensitivity, multiple cutaneous neoplasms and abnormal DNA repair. Ann. Int. Med., 80:221, 1974.

Rosenman, R. H., Friedman, M., et al.: Coronary heart disease in the Western Collaborative Group Study. J. Chronic Dis., 23:173, 1970.

Selye, H.: Stress of Life. McGraw-Hill, New York, 1956.

Spitz, R. A.: Hospitalism: An inquiry into genesis of psychiatric conditions in early childhood. The Psychoanalytic Study of the Child. I. International Universities Press, New York, 1945.

Stein, Z. A., and Susser, M. W.: Widowhood and mental illness. Br. J. Prev. Soc. Med., 23:106, 1969.

Syme, S. L., Hyman, M. M., et al.: Some social and cultural factors associated with the occurrence of coronary heart disease. J. Chronic Dis., 17:277, 1964.

Tokunaga, M., Norman, J. E., Jr., Asano, M., et al.: Malignant breast tumors among atomic bomb survivors, Hiroshima and Nagasaki, 1950–74. JNCI 62:1347, 1979.

Tyroler, H. A., and Cassel, J.: Health consequence of culture change. II. The effect of urbanization on coronary heart disease in rural residents. J. Chronic Dis., 17:167, 1964.

U.S. Public Health Service. Smoking and health. A report of the Surgeon General of the Public Health Service, U.S. Dept. of Health and Human Services, Office on Smoking and Health. Washington, D.C.: U.S. Govt. Print. Off. 1979.

Widdowson, E. M.: Mental contentment and physical growth. Lancet, 1:1316, 1951.

Zinsser, H.: Rats, Lice and History. Little, Brown and Company, Boston, 1943.

MEASUREMENT OF MORBIDITY AND MORTALITY

3 ▬▬▬▬▬▬▬▬▬▬▬▬▬▬▬▬▬▬▬

RATES, RATIOS, AND PROPORTIONS

In epidemiology, the most important tool for measuring disease is the rate, but we also use ratios and proportions.

A *ratio* expresses the relationship between two numbers in the form $x:y$ or $x/y \times k$. For example, the ratio of male to female births in the United States in 1979 was 1,791,000 : 1,703,000 or 1.052 to 1.

A *proportion* is a specific type of ratio in which the numerator is included in the denominator, and the resultant value is expressed as a percentage. For example, the male : female ratio is not a proportion but could readily be converted to one. The proportion of all births that were male is:

$$\frac{\text{Male Births}}{\text{Male + Female Births}} = \frac{179 \times 10^4}{(179 + 170) \times 10^4} = 51.3\%$$

A *rate* is a special form of proportion that includes specification of time. The rate is the basic measure of disease occurrence because it is the measure that most clearly expresses probability or risk of disease in a defined population over a specified period of time. Rates are defined as follows:

$$\frac{\text{Number of events in a specified period}}{\text{Population at risk of these events in a specified period}} \times k$$

In order to calculate a rate, we must be able to count accurately all events of interest that occur in a defined population during a specified period of time. For example, the death rate from cancer in the United States in 1980 was 186.3 per 100,000 population, which was calculated in accordance with the following formula:

$$\frac{\text{Deaths from cancer among U.S. residents in 1980}}{\text{U.S. population in 1980}} \times 100,000$$

INCIDENCE AND PREVALENCE RATES

A number of different rates of morbidity, or illness, are used in public health and epidemiology. All fall into two basic types, rates of incidence and rates of prevalence.

Incidence rates measure the probability that healthy people will develop a disease during a specified period of time; hence, it is the number of new cases of a disease in a population over a period of time. The *prevalence* rate measures the number of people in a population who have the disease at a given time. The formulas for incidence and prevalence rates are as follows:

$$\text{Incidence rate} = \frac{\text{Number of \textbf{new} cases of a disease}}{\text{Population at risk}} \text{ over a period of time}$$

$$\text{Prevalence rate} = \frac{\text{Number of \textbf{existing} cases of a disease}}{\text{Total population}} \text{ at a point in time}$$

Thus, incidence tells us the rate at which new disease occurs in a defined, previously disease-free group of people. Prevalence measures the probability of people having a disease at a given point in time (more specifically termed point prevalence). Prevalence depends on two factors: the number of people who have been ill in the past (i.e., previous incidence) and the duration of their illness. Even if only a few people in a group become ill each year, if the disease is chronic the number will mount and prevalence will be relatively large in relation to incidence. On the other hand, if the illness under consideration is of short duration (acute) because of either recovery or death, or if there is migration of diseased persons from the area, then prevalence will be relatively low.

The relation of prevalence (P) to both incidence (I) and duration (d) of disease is expressed in the formula $P \sim I \times d$, which states that prevalence varies directly with both incidence and duration. If the incidence and duration have both been stable over a long period of time, then this formula becomes $P = I \times d$. Under these circumstances, if two parts of this equation are known, it is possible to calculate the third.

Treatment that succeeds in prolonging life has a profound effect on disease prevalence. Outstanding examples are insulin treatment for diabetes and chemotherapy for childhood leukemia. In a thought-provoking article, "The Failures of Success," Gruenberg (1977) noted a paradox: a marked increase in prevalence of mental retardation and other handicaps, which resulted from the introduction of antibiotics and other agents that extend the life expectancy of children born with Down's syndrome and other congenital defects.

Incidence: Some Considerations

To determine incidence, it is necessary to follow prospectively a defined group of people and determine the rate at which new cases of disease appear. Certain basic requirements must be met if incidence rates are to be calculated.

1. Knowledge of the Health Status of the Study Population. There must be adequate grounds on which to assess the health of individuals in a population and to classify people as "diseased" or "not diseased." This information may be determined from health records, if these are accurate, or may require screening or more detailed examination of the population. If groups are to be compared, it is essential that an equivalent amount of information is available for all groups. It may be necessary to disregard certain information if it is available for only a single segment of the study group.

2. Time of Onset. Determination of date of onset is necessary for studies of incidence. For some events, this determination is relatively simple. The onsets of illnesses such as influenza, staphylococcal gastroenteritis, acute myocardial infarction, and cerebral hemorrhage can often be pinpointed to a specific hour. However, this is not true of certain other conditions, whose onsets may be indefinite. For these, the earliest definite, objectively verifiable event that can be identified must be taken as the time of onset. In cancer, the date of onset is defined by the date of definitive diagnosis, rather than by the date when symptoms were first noted or when a physician became suspicious that the person had cancer.

In epidemiologic studies of psychiatric outpatients, Bahn (1961) found it operationally useful to define "patient" in terms of date of first clinic visit rather than date of referral to the clinic or of commencement of treatment. On the basis of studies on the incidence of heroin use, de Alarcon (1969) and Hughes (1972) selected date of first heroin use as the standard time of onset. Apparently addicts are better able to recall this event than to specify a date on which they became addicted. Date of first heroin use also permits a fuller examination of the sequence of drug use over time.

3. Specification of Numerator: Number of Persons vs. Number of Conditions. In certain circumstances, more than one event can occur to the same person within a stated time period. This gives rise to two types of incidence rates from the same set of data. For example, since a person may have more than one cold in a year, the following two rates could be constructed:

$$\frac{\text{Number of people who developed a cold}}{\text{People at risk}} \text{ in one-year period}$$

$$\frac{\text{Number of colds}}{\text{People at risk}} \text{ in one-year period}$$

Each rate tells us something different. The first gives the probability that any person will develop a cold in one year. The second rate tells us the number of colds to be expected among the group of people in that year. When number of persons and number of events can differ, the numerator should be clearly specified. Without such specification, it is generally assumed that the numerator refers to persons and that an incidence rate represents a statement of probability or risk per person.

4. Specification of Denominator. The denominator in incidence rates must consist of a defined population, accurately enumerated. There are two points to be raised in relation to the denominator of incidence rates. First, since incidence covers a period of time, the numbers of persons at risk is likely to change. The simplest way to handle this problem is to let the population at the midpoint of the period represent the average population at risk. For annual rates, this would be the estimated midyear population.

Second, since incidence refers to new cases of disease, theoretically only those who are at risk of developing the disease under consideration, i.e., **population at risk,** should form the denominator. The denominator should not include those who have the disease or those who are not susceptible because they have already had it or have previously been immunized. Usually this correction to the denominator is not made because the disease is of low frequency and is being measured in a large population where this correction would make little statistical difference. However, if the condition is common or if precision is desired, or both, then the denominator should be corrected to include only those at risk.

For example, to test the effectiveness of measles vaccine in a group of six-year-old children, one should include only those who are still susceptible. Thus, in the trials of measles vaccines, children with antibodies at the beginning of a trial were either initially excluded from the study or eliminated from the analyses of results, since they were not at risk of developing measles. (In contrast, denominators in prevalence rates always include the general population, since the numerator contains "old" as well as "new" cases.)

5. Period of Observation. Incidence rates must always be stated in terms of a definite period of time. This is usually one year but can be any length of time. The time period for which a rate is calculated should be long enough to ensure stability of the numerator. For diseases of low frequency, incident cases may have to be accumulated over several years. In addition, one must be concerned about the accuracy of the denominator. When possible, the denominator should be drawn from a census year or from the years bracketing a census (i.e., 1979–1981).

For large populations, such as that of a city or state, an average annual rate is often calculated as follows:

$$\frac{\text{Number of new cases of a disease in an interval}}{\text{Midpoint population at risk during the interval}} \times \frac{1}{\substack{\text{Number of years} \\ \text{in the interval}}}$$

In large populations, it is not customary to correct the denominator by removing those not at risk. Thus, for example, tuberculosis case rates for a county or state are calculated by using census data for the denominator without correction for those who already have tuberculosis.

In a small population observed over a limited period of time, such as a family, school, or industrial group, the numerator of an incidence rate will be the exact number of new cases and the denominator will include only those who are disease-free at the start of the interval. When the study period spans the entire epidemic, a special term is used to describe infectious disease outbreaks; the incidence rate is then referred to as an *attack* rate. For example, in analyzing an outbreak of food-borne disease, the attack rate among those who ate a certain food is compared with the attack rate among those who abstained from that food (see Chapter 11).

UNEQUAL PERIODS OF OBSERVATION: PERSON-TIME DENOMINATORS. A different type of denominator, called a *person-time denominator,* must be used in the following situation. Let us say that a specific group of individuals is being followed for the incidence of peptic ulcer over the three-year time period of the study. There may be problems of attrition because individuals die, move away, or are otherwise lost to follow-up. Also, individuals may come under observation at different points after a study is initiated. Each of these possible events will result in unequal periods of observation of study subjects, which will cause subjects to contribute unequally to the calculation of population at risk. In order to utilize fully the period of observation for each individual, and to weigh properly each person's contribution to the study, a person-time unit, e.g., a person-year, is created for the denominator of any rates calculated. For example, in this hypothetical study of the incidence of peptic ulcer, 12 persons were observed for different periods of time, as shown in Table 3–1.

Altogether, the 12 people in the study were observed for a total of 66 person-years. That figure is the sum of the years of observation contributed by each person in the study. If, among the 12 people, 3 developed peptic ulcers, the incidence rate would be 3 in 66 person-years (i.e., ³⁄₆₆) or 4.5 per 100 person-years of observation.

The use of a person-time denominator is valid only under three conditions. The first is that the risk of disease or death is constant throughout the entire period of study; this assumption often does not hold true. For example, in a condition with a long latent period, the incidence rate may be relatively high in the latter part of the observation period. The opposite may also occur. The occurrence of contraceptive failures tends to decrease as the period of observation lengthens, since couples who are successful over long periods are likely to be conscientious users or low in fecundity or both (Potter, 1963). For these reasons, division of the observation period into several subperiods may be necessary.

Second, the rate of disease or death among those lost to follow-up should be the same as among individuals still under observation. This condition is particularly important; if the disease rate is higher among dropouts than within the group that continues under observation, then the true risk will be understated. For this reason, it is particularly desirable to ascertain the status of individuals even if they drop out of the study. If complete follow-up is impossible, one may calculate the two extremes of possibility, basing one rate on the assumption that the

TABLE 3–1 Person-Years Calculation in Incidence of Peptic Ulcer Study

Person	No. Years under Observation
1	3
2	8
3	10
4	9
5	6
6	4
7	1
8	2
9	8
10	7
11	5
12	3

dropouts had a favorable course and the other on the opposite assumption. The true value must lie between these two extremes.

Finally, if the disease under study is so rapidly fatal that certain individuals are observed for less than a full unit of time, then the rate will be artificially high. Each of these subjects will be counted as a new case, or as a "one" in the numerator, but as "less than one" person-time unit in the denominator.

Prevalence: Point vs. Period

There are two kinds of prevalence rates, *point* prevalence and *period* prevalence. When the term "prevalence" is used without further specification, it generally refers to "point prevalence."

$$\text{Point prevalence}^\circ = \frac{\text{Number of existing cases of a disease}}{\text{Total population}} \text{ at a point in time}$$

$$\text{Period prevalence} = \frac{\begin{array}{c}\text{Number of existing cases}\\\text{of a disease}\end{array}}{\text{Average population}} \text{ during a period or interval}$$

Requirements for the construction of a prevalence rate are similar to those enumerated in the prior section on incidence—i.e., one must know the health status of the study population, the numerator and denominator must be specified, the prevalence rate must be stated in terms of a definite period of time, and person-time denominators may be employed. A major difference between incidence and prevalence is that knowledge of time of onset is not required in a prevalence study. In addition, denominators in prevalence rates always include the entire related population, since the numerator contains "old" as well as "new" cases.

Point prevalence attempts to measure disease at one point in time. Despite this aim, the actual collection of data related to a specific day may take longer than that one day. For example, the census, which yields figures on prevalence, refers to the population as of April 1 of a given year, although the actual enumeration takes approximately three months.

Period prevalence is a compound measure and is constructed from prevalence at a point in time, plus new cases (incidence) and recurrences during a succeeding time period (e.g., one year). An example of period prevalence is found in the Hollingshead and Redlich study (page 130)

° Some epidemiologists refer to prevalence at a point in time as a "ratio," reserving the term "rate" for events or cases over a period of time. We will use the more general concept of rate to include any specification of time, instantaneous as well as interval.

of the relation between social class and mental illness in New Haven. In that study, a case was defined as a person in treatment with a private psychiatrist or under the care of a psychiatric clinic or mental hospital between May 31 and December 1, 1950. Thus, it included all people ill as of May 31 (point prevalence) plus those who became ill (incidence) or in whom illness recurred during the succeeding six months.

Period prevalence is frequently preferred to point prevalence or incidence for analyzing data on mental illness because of certain problems in the measurement of mental diseases. Exact date of onset needed for incidence is often difficult to determine, as is the presence or absence of mental illness on a given day (needed for point prevalence). Period prevalence, on the other hand, requires only a determination that the person was mentally ill at some time during a defined period.

For episodic diseases, such as some types of mental illness, the frequency of recurrence will affect prevalence. The same person will be counted as ill or not ill, depending on whether the disease is in remission at the time of the survey.

While a major use of period prevalence is in the study of mental illness, it may be used for other conditions as well. For example, for purposes of planning hospital beds, the medical administrator may be interested in the number of cardiac cases, both new and old, to be anticipated during a given year.

A variant of period prevalence is "lifetime prevalence," the proportion of a population that has a history of a given disorder at some point in time (Kramer et al., 1980). There are considerable problems with this term. The magnitude of lifetime prevalence depends not only on the incidence of disease but also on recollection of distant events, and it can be distorted by deaths from competing causes and losses due to migration. The fact that cases currently in remission are included in the numerator further reduces the usefulness of this measure for the planning of services. Nevertheless, investigators continue to use lifetime prevalence in epidemiologic studies of psychiatric illness to heighten awareness that psychiatric illness is a common occurrence.

Uses of Incidence and Prevalence

As mentioned earlier, incidence and prevalence rates serve different purposes. Prevalence is important, particularly in chronic disease, in determining workload, as it is a useful tool for the planning of facilities and manpower needs. Prevalence may also be used to express the burden of some attribute or condition in a population. Furthermore, for disease control, information is needed about factors that produce chronicity or recurrence once a disease has developed. Since prevalence reflects duration as well as incidence, it can be useful for monitoring control programs for chronic conditions such as mental illness. When data necessary for the calculation of incidence are not available, prevalence rates may be used to estimate the importance of a disease in a population, but with the realization that prevalence may not be a good estimator of incidence.

Periodic estimation of point prevalence is useful in tracking changes in disease patterns over time. Point prevalence can be determined by a series of cross-sectional surveys; this is easier and less expensive than longitudinal surveillance of one population over time. In addition, if the disease is chronic, a prevalence survey at one point in time will give an idea of the burden of the disease in the population. It is important to remember, however, that repeated cross-sectional surveys over time do not constitute a longitudinal study and, therefore, do not permit etiologic inference or estimates of changes in risk of disease over time.

Incidence rates are the fundamental tool for etiologic studies of both acute and chronic disease, since they are direct indicators of risk of disease. Incidence rates provide a direct measure of the rate at which individuals in a given population develop disease and thus provide a basis for statements about probability or risk of disease. By comparing incidence rates of a disease among population groups varying in one or more identified factors, we can test by analytic studies whether a factor affects the risk of acquiring a disease, and, if so, we can hypothesize about the magnitude of the effect.

As we have noted previously, incidence is a direct measure of risk. In contrast, high prevalence does not necessarily signify high risk; it may merely reflect an increase in survival, perhaps due to a change in virulence or in host factors in addition to improvements in medical care. Conversely, low prevalence may reflect a rapidly fatal process or rapid cure of disease as well as low incidence.

A limitation of prevalence is that it tends to produce a biased picture of disease: It favors inclusion of chronic over acute cases. Consider a hypothetical situation. Each month two cases of disease X arise in a population of 10,000. One case is chronic (i.e., lasting two months); the other is of shorter duration (i.e., lasting two weeks). The prevalence of disease is measured on the 15th of each month. Figure 3–1 makes it apparent that occurrence of an equal number of chronic and acute cases soon leads to a preponderance of prevalent chronic cases. (Note: Prevalence on May 15 shows $P_1 = 1$ chronic + 1 acute case; prevalence on July 15 or August 15 shows $P_2 = 2$ chronic cases + 1 acute case.)

The difference between prevalent and incident cases may be an important source of bias. This difference is crucial to an understanding of screening programs. The first screening of a population picks up

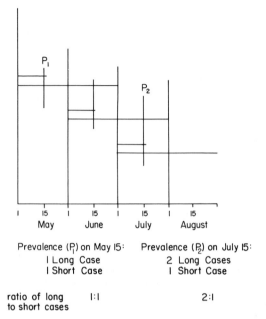

	Prevalence (P_1) on May 15:	Prevalence (P_2) on July 15:
	1 Long Case	2 Long Cases
	1 Short Case	1 Short Case
ratio of long to short cases	1:1	2:1

Figure 3–1 The effect of duration on prevalence.

prevalent as well as incident cases of disease. Rescreening detects only incident cases (i.e., those that developed between the first and subsequent screens).

A further limitation of prevalence data is seen in cross-sectional studies in which presence of an attribute and disease status are measured at the same time. In such studies, cause and effect are measured simultaneously, as in an instantaneous snapshot. In order to determine antecedents of disease, it is necessary to establish a time sequence and show that the presumed independent variable or variables antedated the dependent one. Such temporal relations cannot be established by cross-sectional data.

It is important to remember these limitations because it is often tempting to use prevalence data for causal inferences, since they are more readily obtained than incidence data. This is true because prevalence can be determined from one survey, while measurement of incidence requires at least two sets of observations of the same individuals: first a survey to determine whether each individual has the disease or has ever had it, then a resurvey of the nondiseased persons to see how many have become ill since the initial examination.

The different impressions that can be obtained from incidence and prevalence data will be demonstrated in material excerpted from the Framingham study of heart disease. This study started with a survey of

TABLE 3-2 Prevalence of Coronary Heart Disease (CHD) at Initial Examination among 4469 Persons 30-62 Years of Age, Framingham Study

Age (years)	Males Number Examined	Number with CHD	Rate per 1000	Females Number Examined	Number with CHD	Rate per 1000	Male/Female Ratio of Prevalence Rates
30–44	1083	5	5	1317	7	5	1.0
45–62	941	43	46	1128	21	19	2.4
Total	2024	48		2445	28		

the population to measure prevalence of coronary heart disease (CHD). Two years later, the population was resurveyed to ascertain incident cases that occurred over the lapsed two-year period. It should be noted that incidence, not prevalence, rates were used to calculate CHD rates in relation to specific risk factors (e.g., serum cholesterol, blood pressure, smoking status). In calculating incidence of heart disease, the prevalent cases identified on the first survey were subtracted from the denominator.

One can examine incidence and prevalence rates of CHD by sex, with quite different results (Tables 3–2 and 3–3). Looking at prevalence rates (Table 3–2), it appears that CHD exists with equal frequency in young males and young females (rate of 5 per 1000 in both sexes). However, the incidence figures (Table 3–3) indicate a risk more than 20 times higher in young males than young females. The explanation for this discrepancy lies in the different course of disease in young men and young women. In the men the disease manifests itself as myocardial infarction and sudden death. In women the disease is more likely to

TABLE 3-3 Incidence of Coronary Heart Disease (CHD) over an Eight-Year Period among 4995° Persons 30-59 Years of Age Free of Coronary Heart Disease at Initial Examination

Age (years)	Males Number Examined	Number with CHD	Rate per 1000	Females Number Examined	Number with CHD	Rate per 1000	Male/Female Ratio of Incidence Rates
30–39	825	20	24.2	1036	1	1.0	24.2
40–49	770	51	66.3	955	19	19.9	3.3
50–59	617	81	131.3	792	53	66.9	2.0
Total	2212	152		2783	73		

°It may be noted that there is a larger number of persons in Table 3–3 than in Table 3–2. Table 3–3 includes a volunteer group of 740 persons enrolled in the study before the formal sampling plan was fully developed and implemented. The addition of this group should not alter significantly the relationships being presented here.

present as anginal attacks, i.e., attacks of chest pain of brief duration that do not generally endanger life. With the longer duration of disease in women, prevalence can actually be equal in the two sexes despite the much greater incidence in males. One should also note that the sex differential in incidence rates declines with age. The male to female incidence ratio is 24.2 in persons 30 to 39, but only 3.3 and 2.0 for persons 40 to 49 and 50 to 59, respectively.

In spite of their limitations, prevalence figures are useful for determining the extent of a disease problem, and hence valuable for rational planning of facilities and services, e.g., number of hospital beds required, number of clinic visits anticipated, manpower needs, and so on.

CRUDE, SPECIFIC, AND ADJUSTED RATES

Any rate can be expressed for a total population (**crude** or **adjusted** rates) or for a population subgroup (**specific** rates).

Crude rates are summary rates based on the actual number of events (e.g., births, deaths, or diseases) in a total population over a given time period. Adjusted rates are summary rates that have undergone statistical transformation to permit fair comparison between groups differing in some characteristic that may affect risk of disease. For example, an age-adjusted rate is a summary rate that has been statistically transformed (adjusted) so that it is, in effect, independent of the age structure of the particular population being studied.

Crude Rates

Two factors contribute to the magnitude of a *crude* death rate: One is the probability of dying for individuals, and the other is the age distribution of the population. Since age is the major factor influencing risk of death, the higher the proportion of elderly people in the population, the higher the crude death rate for that population.

Two crude rates that are widely used in descriptions of populations are the crude birth rate and the crude death rate. They are defined as follows:

$$\text{Crude birth rate} = \frac{\text{Number of live births to residents in an area in a calendar year}}{\text{Average population}^\circ \text{ in the area in that year}} / 1000$$

° Usually midyear population (July 1). As a specific example, the 3,598,000 live births in the United States in 1980 occurring in the total resident population of 226,504,825 yielded a crude birth rate of 16.2 per 1000 persons. The 1,986,000 deaths in the same year were equivalent to a crude death rate of 8.9 per 1000.

$$\text{Crude death rate} = \frac{\begin{array}{c}\text{Number of deaths among residents} \\ \text{in an area in a calendar year}\end{array}}{\begin{array}{c}\text{Average population}^\circ \text{ in the area in} \\ \text{that year}\end{array}}/1000$$

Note that rates can be presented in any form that is convenient. That is, they may be expressed as a percentage (i.e., per 100), or per 1000, or per 100,000, depending on convention and the absolute magnitude of the numbers involved. In general, it is wise to avoid fractions: 4 per 100,000 is easier to interpret than 0.04 per 1000. Some rates are customarily presented in a specific format. For example, infant mortality is given as the rate per 1000 live births; crude birth and death rates are expressed per 1000 total population; and age-specific and cause-specific death rates are generally given per 100,000. Rates for rare diseases are sometimes given "per million" to avoid tiny fractions.

Crude rates, such as crude birth and death rates, which refer to the total population, may obscure the fact that subgroups of the population exhibit significant differences in risk. For example, the total population is really not an appropriate denominator for births, since these occur only in females of childbearing ages. Similarly, the total population is not an ideal denominator for a death rate since people in different age groups differ with respect to risk of death.

Suppose one wished to compare the crude death rates for two populations that differed in age distribution. Table 13–4 shows that, even though the two populations have identical age-specific death rates, the crude rates will differ if the two populations are dissimilar in age composition (see Chapter 13 for a discussion of adjustment of rates). Therefore, in evaluating crude rates, it is necessary to examine specific rates and age distributions to determine whether adjustment is necessary.

Despite their limitations, crude birth and death rates continue to be widely cited, in part because they are summary rates and in part because they can be constructed from a minimum of information. For example, crude birth rates require only knowledge of the number of births in a year and the total population of the area. A measure of births limited to females of childbearing age would require more refined information about the age and sex composition of the population. Therefore crude birth and death rates continue to be used for international and temporal comparisons of fertility and health.

Specific Rates

For understanding epidemiologic aspects of disease and population dynamics, detailed rates *specific* for age and other demographic components, such as sex or race, are needed. The J-shaped mortality curves presented in Figure 6 – 1 illustrate the great variation in death rates from all causes at different ages. The following is an example of an age-specific rate:

Age-specific death rate =
(ages 25 – 34)

$$\frac{\text{Number of deaths among residents aged } 25-34 \text{ in an area in a calendar year}}{\text{Average population aged } 25-34 \text{ in the area in that year}} \times \begin{matrix} 1000 \\ \text{(or } 100{,}000) \end{matrix}$$

Translated into actual numbers, the 44,973 deaths among the estimated population of 31,900,000 persons aged 25 to 34 years in the United States in 1977 yielded an age-specific death rate of 1.4 per 1000. In marked contrast, the age-specific death rate for those 65 to 74 years of age was 30.6 per 1000.

Adjusted Rates

While specific rates can provide valuable information for comparative purposes, there is a need for a summary type of rate free of the limitations of crude rates. Such a rate is the *adjusted* or *standardized* rate. Like the crude rate, the adjusted rate presents one summary figure for a total population, but statistical procedures are carried out to "remove the effect" of differences in composition of various populations. Age is the variable for which adjustment is most often required because of its marked effect on morbidity and mortality. Although the following discussion will refer to adjustment for age, one should remember that at times it may be necessary to adjust for variables other than age, such as sex, race, smoking status, and so on.

There are basically two methods for removing the effect of differences in composition of a population. In the *direct method*, age-specific rates observed in two or more study populations are applied to an arbitrarily chosen population of known age structure referred to as a "standard" population.

The *indirect method* is used to compare two populations, in one of which the age-specific rates are not known or, if known, are excessively variable because of small numbers. In this method, the more stable rates of the larger population are applied to the population of the smaller study group. Comparison of the number of expected deaths in the smaller population with the number actually observed yields a measure known as the *standardized mortality ratio*, or *SMR*.

$$SMR = \frac{\text{Observed deaths}}{\text{Expected deaths}}$$

Similarly, it is possible to use a standardized *morbidity* ratio if the event of interest is occurrence of disease rather than death.

A detailed discussion of the direct and indirect methods of adjustment, and their computational requirements, is presented in Chapter 13.

Many of the tables and figures in this book show standardized mortality or morbidity ratios. For example, in Table 7–4 the age-specific death rates of nonsmokers are applied to the age distribution of various smoking categories to derive expected deaths for each group. The observed deaths divided by the expected deaths yields the standardized mortality ratio for that group. In the Framingham data (see Fig. 7–5), the age-specific incidence rate of stroke or CHD for the total study cohort is applied to the age distribution of each subgroup (e.g., hypertension absent, hypertension present) to first obtain expected cases and then a standardized morbidity ratio.

Sometimes the direction or magnitude of differences in rates is not consistent across all age groups. Under such circumstances, an overall summary rate will mask some of the details of the comparison. For example, Figure 6–1 shows higher age-specific death rates for non-whites than whites in the United States at all ages except past 80 years of

TABLE 3–4 Advantages and Disadvantages of Crude, Specific, and Adjusted Rates

	Advantages	Disadvantages
Crude Rates	Actual summary rates Readily calculable for international comparisons (widely used despite limitations)	Since populations vary in composition (e.g., age), differences in crude rates difficult to interpret
Specific Rates	Homogeneous subgroups Detailed rates useful for epidemiologic and public health purposes	Cumbersome to compare many subgroups of two or more populations
Adjusted Rates	Summary statements Differences in composition of groups "removed," permitting unbiased comparison	Fictional rates Absolute magnitude dependent on standard population chosen Opposing trends in subgroups masked

age. After that, the picture reverses and whites have higher death rates. Because trends may differ for different age groups, one should always compare age-specific rates before doing any age adjustment.

Table 3–4 summarizes the advantages and disadvantages of the three kinds of rates we have been discussing—crude, specific, and adjusted.

MAJOR SOURCES OF ERROR IN MEASUREMENT OF DISEASE

In all scientific endeavors one must be concerned with the possibility of error in the measurements being made. There are two basic kinds of error, random (chance) and systematic (bias).

Random error refers to fluctuations around a true value because of sampling variability. The magnitude of this error can be estimated from statistical theory (Armitage, 1974). *Systematic error,* also known as *bias,*° may be formally defined as any difference between the true value and that actually obtained that is the result of all causes other than sampling variability. Of the two sources of error, systematic error is generally the more important, the more insidious, and the more difficult to measure.

For a simple example of systematic error, consider the effects of an inadequate measuring instrument. If a sphygmomanometer is incorrectly calibrated, there will always be an error in the measurement and it will always be in the same direction. The only way to detect such an error is to compare the results with those obtained by an independent standard (i.e., a correctly calibrated instrument). Several sources of bias are particularly likely to enter epidemiologic studies, and some of these particularly affecting descriptive studies will be discussed briefly. Some errors of measurement may predominantly affect the numerator of a rate; others affect the denominator. These will be discussed in turn.

Use of Nonrandom Samples of the Target Population

In order to make correct inferences about a population, one must first define the group of interest and study either the total group or a representative sample of it. Whether the group selected for study is the

---

° In statistics and epidemiology the term "bias" carries no imputation of prejudice or other subjective factor, such as the experimenter's desire for a particular outcome. This differs from conversational usage in which bias refers to a particular, partisan point of view.

total population or a sample, every person in the target group must have an opportunity to be selected. For example, to describe the total prevalence of disability in a population, one must include in the sampling frame not only those people living independently in the community, but also those living in institutions.

A classic example of bias due to nonrandom sampling of the population is provided by the Literary Digest poll that attempted to forecast the outcome of the Presidential election of 1936. The poll-takers predicted a victory for the Republican candidate, Alfred Landon; Franklin Roosevelt actually won the election by a landslide. How could the prediction have been so wrong? The sample of people queried was obtained from telephone listings. People who had telephones in those days were typically prosperous citizens likely to vote for Republican candidates. This example is not intended to imply that telephone surveys cannot be used effectively today, as long as appropriate methods are used to account for persons who have unlisted telephones or no telephones at all.

Much of our epidemiologic information comes from nonrandom samples of the population—from findings based on hospitalized patients and autopsy series, from the data of insurance companies and the employed population. The biases inherent in autopsy data are discussed in Chapter 4; the effects on disease rates of self-selection into occupational groups will be mentioned in Chapter 12. A major advance toward reducing certain of these biases is achieved by the use of population-based samples to replace or supplement more readily obtained data from nonrandom samples of the population.

Nonparticipation of Members of the Target Group

Another problem in making inferences about a population stems from the fact that some of the people designated as the target group decline to participate or are not available for the study. If the participants are either more or less healthy, on the average, than the nonparticipants, or more or less likely to have had some specific exposure related to the purposes of the study, then a serious source of bias is introduced.

This is a problem that bedevils all kinds of studies. In household surveys, for example, if no one is home in a previously designated household, then it might seem convenient and harmless to substitute the family next door. This may make the sample unrepresentative since the fact of being home may be related to illness, employment status, lifestyle, and so on. It is therefore necessary to make as many revisits as practicable to complete the study.

Nonparticipation or nonresponse is particularly troublesome in mailed surveys. Unless the survey is of particular interest to the respondents, or is sponsored by an organization viewed as prestigious, substantial nonresponse is the rule.

Differences between participants and nonparticipants have been demonstrated repeatedly in surveys based on clinical examination. For example, in the Framingham study of arteriosclerotic heart disease mentioned previously, the initial nonresponse rate was a little over 30 per cent. On follow-up, both male and female nonrespondents were found to have a higher death rate than respondents.

There are several approaches to the reduction of bias from nonparticipation. First, diligent efforts should be made to keep nonparticipation at a minimum. Participation should be as convenient and painless as possible. Flexible schedules and use of mobile examination vans have been found helpful. However, even under the most favorable circumstances problems of nonresponse should be anticipated. The number of call-backs planned for a household interview survey, for instance, should be specified and provided for in the budget of the study. Second, the final group of nonrespondents should be evaluated if possible to see whether they differ in demographic characteristics and health status from the respondents. This might be done by search of death certificates or hospital records or by extraordinary efforts (e.g., repeated telephone calls or home visits) to gain some basic information about a subsample of the nonparticipants. Finally, analyses can be carried out based on extreme assumptions, i.e., that *all* or *none* of the nonrespondents would have a disease or factor. The maximum and minimum possible values for the item obtained in this way establish the outer limits of variation around the true value.

Observer Variation

Epidemiologic studies generally require observations of large numbers of persons. This makes it necessary to pool data from multiple observers, often working in different institutions or different countries and under differing organizational, technical, and climatic constraints. Other sources of variation are differences in diagnostic practices among the physicians participating in the study and variations in the correctness of diagnostic labels assigned for the coding of data. Additional problems can arise if there are variations in the degree of completeness with which cases are reported to a registry (e.g., by institution or area of residence). Efforts should be made to identify sources of incomplete reports and strategies developed to circumvent the problem. For example, one might survey periodically the pathologic and radiation treatment records of an institution that had been deficient in reporting. The main approaches to reducing this kind of variation lie in a common protocol, standardization of methods and training of personnel to carry out procedures and record observations, and in the use of duplicate or multiple observers.

Variability in findings due to variation among observers (*observer variation*) has been of concern for several decades. A major impetus to awareness of the phenomenon was a study in the late 1940s by Yerushalmy to compare the value of different types of chest x-rays for mass screening purposes. Several kinds of miniature films had recently been developed and it was hoped that they would provide a cheaper way to x-ray larger numbers of persons than the standard (14 × 17) chest films. However, it was not known whether the results would be as dependable. To test this, some 1200 persons were each x-rayed, using four different techniques. The resulting films were read independently by five experts. Yerushalmy concluded that the four techniques were essentially equivalent for tuberculosis case-finding in mass survey work (1947). Surprisingly, the variations in reading for each technique were so great that in effect they exceeded the variation among techniques. One conclusion from the study was the recommendation that survey films be read independently by at least two observers and that all persons whose films were read as positive or suggestive for tuberculosis by either reader be recalled for further study.

In the years since this study the phenomenon of variability among observers, as well as inconsistency for the same observer, has been documented for many kinds of medical data—history-taking, physical examination, and laboratory tests of various kinds.

Different Response Patterns

Much of the information required for carrying out epidemiologic studies must be obtained by interview (e.g., dietary history, history of drug ingestion, and so on). The interview may be carried out in person or by telephone. This process may seem simple to design and carry out, but detailed studies indicate that a variety of factors can influence the amount and validity of information obtained (Cannell, 1977). For example, the Survey Research Center of the University of Michigan and the National Center for Health Statistics have collaborated over the years in investigations of response problems. They have done a number of tests on the validity of data from household interviews. The concern has been about underreporting, which is more of a problem than overreporting.

The questionnaire used in the study is essentially the same as that used in the Health Interview Survey (Chap. 4). Records of visits to physicians and to clinics and of hospital discharges were compared with information obtained by interview to determine the extent of underreporting on the interview and the factors related to this tendency to underreport. They found that reporting of hospitalization varied with the time since discharge. From a low of 3 per cent omissions at one to 10 weeks, the percentage of discharges not reported increased to 42 per cent at one year. With respect to visits to physicians, people were asked to report the number of visits they had made to physicians within the last two weeks. The rate of underreporting for the second week preceding the interview was double that for the week immediately preceding the interview (30 per cent vs. 15 per cent). In addition to time elapsed, events that are threatening or cause embarrassment tended to be under-reported.

Demographic factors were not found to be strongly related to completeness of reporting. Men and women were similar in their extent of reporting; educational level and income had little effect on reporting. Positive findings were that whites reported more completely than non-whites, young people (under 35 years of age) were more likely to report than older people (especially those over 55 years of age), and self-reports were better than proxy reports. (The latter is relevant to choice of persons to be accepted as respondents in a household visit). The overall conclusion of the study was that the characteristics of the respondent were not nearly as consistent, nor as strong an influence on the completeness of the report, as was the nature of the event being reported on. Knowledge of these factors in reporting is clearly important to the design of studies and evaluation of findings.

Variation in Perceptions of Illness (Illness Behavior)

One factor contributing to biased morbidity statistics is *illness behavior*. This has been defined (Mechanic, 1962) as "the ways in which given symptoms may be differentially perceived, evaluated, and acted (or not acted) upon by different kinds of persons." Differences in the perception of disease and consequent action will affect all kinds of morbidity statistics.

Severe, life-threatening symptoms almost always lead to specific action. As one moves along the spectrum to less severe symptoms, the likelihood that medical aid will be sought decreases. Conversely, personal and environmental factors assume increasing importance in determining what, if any, action is taken. Thus, a moderately severe respiratory infection might have different outcomes in different individuals. One person might carry on his daily activities and seek no medical advice; another might continue to work but visit a doctor; a third might not only seek medical consultation but take one or more days off from work. In the first example, the illness would be known only to the person himself; in the second and third examples, the person would contribute to morbidity statistics; but only in the third example would the person's actions be reflected in statistics on days lost from work, a measure of disability. Among the reasons for the differences in illness behavior are (1) the past history of the person; (2) the cultural, ethnic, and family background, as well as situational factors, such as whether the person is a civilian or a member of the military; and (3) the nature of his arrangements for medical care (i.e., whether he must pay for care, whether he receives paid sick leave, whether reporting of minor illnesses is encouraged by his employer, whether care is accessible, and so on).

Measures of utilization of medical care have importance in their own right. However, they have serious weaknesses as tools for etiologic studies of disease, for the reasons just discussed. When etiologic hypotheses are being tested, it is important to be aware of the potential contribution of illness behavior to the statistics.

Variation in Availability of Treatment Resources

Differences in the availability of treatment facilities between areas can lead to misleading statistics on disease rates. For example, the rate of hospitalization may reflect availability of hospital beds as well as frequency of illness. This is shown clearly in Figure 3–2, which compares rates of first hospitalization in two time periods for certain psychoses for Hagerstown, Maryland, and for the remainder of the county in which Hagerstown is located. The striking increase in first admissions for psychosis for Hagerstown in the second time period as compared with the rest of Washington County reflects primarily the building of a new hospital in Hagerstown in 1959 (Silverman, 1968).

In concluding this section on sources of error one should note that

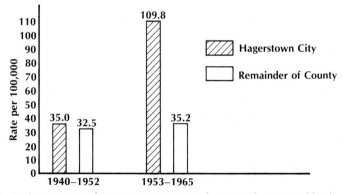

Figure 3–2 Average annual rates per 100,000 population aged 15 to 64 of first hospitalization for specified psychoses, Washington County, Maryland, 1940–1952 and 1953–1965. (Based on data from Silverman, C.: The Epidemiology of Depression. Johns Hopkins University Press, Baltimore, 1968.)

inaccuracies in the denominator, as well as problems with the numerator, can be serious sources of bias. The denominators are derived from census data that contain errors of omission and commission, especially the former. In Chapter 4 we point out some of the inaccuracies of the census and their impact on calculations of disease occurrence.

SUMMARY

This chapter has discussed the principal methodologic tools developed to ensure unbiased measurement and analysis of disease. Incidence and prevalence are the fundamental measures of morbidity. The differences between the two measures were stressed, as were the advantages of using incidence rather than prevalence data whenever possible.

These morbidity rates, as well as mortality rates, may be expressed as total (crude or adjusted) rates or as specific rates. The need for adjustment to prevent biased comparisons of populations differing in composition is emphasized; age is the most common factor for which adjustment is necessary.

A variety of sources of error in measurement were enumerated. These included selection of biased (i.e., nonrandom) samples of the target population; nonparticipation of members of the target group; variation among observers; different patterns of response; differences in perception of illness (i.e., illness behavior); and difference in availability of treatment resources.

REFERENCES

Armitage, P.: Statistical Methods in Medical Research. John Wiley and Sons, New York. 1974.

Bahn, A. K.: Methodologic Study of Population of Outpatient Psychiatric Clinics, Maryland 1958–1959. USPHS Pub. No. 821 (Public Health Monograph No. 65), U.S. Govt. Printing Office, Washington, D.C., 1961.

Cannell, C. F.: A summary of research studies of interviewing methodology, 1959–1970. Vital and health statistics: Series 2, Data evaluation and methods research; No. 69. DHEW Pub. No. (HRA) 77–1343.

Dawber, T. R., Kannel, W. B., and Lyell, L. P.: An approach to longitudinal studies in a community: The Framingham study. Ann. N.Y. Acad. Sci., 107:593, 1963.

Dawber, T. R., Meadors, G. F., and Moore, F. E., Jr.: Epidemiological approaches to heart disease: The Framingham study. Am. J. Public Health, 41:279, 1951.

de Alarcon, R.: The spread of heroin abuse in a community. Bull. Narc., 31:17, 1969.

Gruenberg, E. M.: The failures of success. Milbank Mem. Fund Q., 55:3, 1977.

Hollingshead, A. B., and Redlich, F. C.: Social Class and Mental Illness: A Community Study. John Wiley & Sons, Inc., New York, 1958.

Hughes, P. H., Barker, N. W., et al: The natural history of a heroin epidemic. Am. J. Public Health, 62:995, 1972.

Kramer, M., von Korff, M., Kessler, L.: The lifetime prevalence of mental disorders: Estimation, uses, and limitations. Psychol. Med., *10*:429, 1980.

Mechanic, D.: The concept of illness behavior. J. Chronic Dis., *15*:189, 1962.

Potter, R. G., Jr.: Additional measures of use-effectiveness of contraception. Milbank Mem. Fund Q., *41*:400, 1963.

Silverman, C.: The Epidemiology of Depression. Johns Hopkins University Press, Baltimore, 1968.

Yerushalmy, J.: Statistical problems in assessing methods of medical diagnosis, with special reference to x-ray techniques. Public Health Rep., *62*:1432, 1947.

SOURCES OF DATA ON COMMUNITY HEALTH

4

There are numerous sources of data on morbidity and mortality in the community. Each source has advantages and limitations. Complete and unbiased ascertainment is carried out by special surveillance systems, such as population-based registers, and must be balanced against costs. Existing data sources, such as data from health insurance companies, are relatively inexpensive for the investigator but are based on segments instead of the whole population. We will outline some of the major data sources and the health indices that may be derived from them.

THE CENSUS

Health planning and programming depend on knowledge of the size and composition of a population, the forces that determine these variables, and the trends anticipated in the future. The importance of accurate population data is recognized by governments everywhere. The United States Congress allocates large monetary sums for periodic enumerations of the population. Census data are necessary for accurate description of the health status of the population, since they are the principal source of denominator data for rates of disease and death.

The term *census*, which comes from the Latin word meaning "to estimate or assess," means periodic counts or enumerations of a population. Records of population enumerations go back over 5000 years to the Babylonians, Chinese, and Egyptians. Following the disintegration of the Roman Empire, there were relatively few attempts to maintain accurate population records in Europe until the late eighteenth century, when a number of Western European countries instituted a formal census.

In this country, the Census of Population has been taken every 10 years since 1790. In addition, other censuses are regularly carried out, including censuses of agriculture, of business, and of housing. The original purpose of the Census of Population was to count heads in order to apportion the number of legislators each state would send to the House of Representatives. Since its beginnings, the census has gradually been expanded to encompass data on many characteristics of the population. Name, address, age, sex, race, marital status, and relationship to the head of the household, as well as some characteristics of housing, are obtained from all persons. Information on nativity, migration, education, parity, employment status, income, and so on are obtained from a sample. Information from the census is vitally important to each jurisdiction because it forms the basis for the allocation of federal and state funds under a variety of programs. This has recently become particularly important owing to the decentralization of federal activities and the introduction of revenue-sharing.

There are two principal methods for enumeration of a population: *de facto*, which allocates persons according to their location at the time of enumeration, and *de jure*, which assigns them according to their usual place of residence. For example, a salesman living in Cincinnati but working in Boston on the day of the census would be assigned to Boston on a de facto census, to Cincinnati if the de jure method were employed. The United States Census uses de jure enumeration because it provides a better indication of the permanent population and household composition of an area.

The Bureau of the Census has attempted to compensate for the cost and complexity of enumerating an ever-increasing population by utilizing technological advances, such as punched cards (1890) and optical scanning of forms (1960). Through 1950, the census was taken primarily by trained enumerators who visited each household to collect data. The 1960 census introduced self-enumeration by households, and in 1970 the census relied on the mails for distribution and return of census forms. In the latter year, enumerators were used in urban areas only to obtain missing information and to verify questionable items.

In 1980, reliance on mailing of forms continued. The entire population received a "short form" that included information about age, sex, education, family type, marital status, relationship to head of family, and presence of children. In addition, 20 per cent of households received a longer questionnaire that included information about place of birth, place of residence in 1975, labor force participation, and family income.

Census information is analyzed and presented for the country as a whole and for progressively smaller subdivisions — four regions (Northeast, North Central, South, and West), nine divisions (e.g., New England, Middle Atlantic), states, counties, cities or municipalities, census tracts, blocks, and, whenever requirements for anonymity permit, block faces. Areas are also classified as urban or rural. The definitions of urban and rural have changed from time to time. The term "urban" is now normally used for places with at least 2500 inhabitants, but the complete definition specifies a number of exceptions.

Since 1950, emphasis has been placed on classification of areas as metropolitan or nonmetropolitan as well as rural or urban. The political boundaries of cities in the United States no longer describe meaningful units. The proliferation of a network of highways in and around cities has been followed by the establishment of not only dormitory suburbs and shopping centers but also industrial parks and commercial complexes. Because of the extensive interactions between a city and its surrounding areas, a unit encompassing both is needed as a base for statistical description.

The concept of a *Standard Metropolitan Statistical Area* (or *SMSA*) was introduced in 1949 to furnish such a unit. To qualify as an SMSA, an area has to meet certain criteria. It must have (1) a large population nucleus (e.g., usually one city with at least 50,000 residents), (2) a total population of at least 100,000 (75,000 in New England), and (3) adjacent communities that are well-integrated socially and economically with the major population nucleus. In the 1980 census, there were 318 SMSAs in the United States. Three-quarters of the population (75 per cent) lived within an SMSA. Of this segment, 43 per cent lived outside and 30 per cent lived inside the central city of the SMSA. The actual level of integration among the political entities within an SMSA varies greatly. The degree to which the metropolitan area functions as a unit has profound import for the planning and delivery of health services.

Within cities there is often a need for statistical analysis of smaller geographic areas. To meet this need, units called "census tracts" were established. These are relatively permanent subdivisions of large cities and adjacent areas. The boundaries of tracts were originally set so that each tract would contain 3000 to 6000 persons and would be relatively homogeneous in ethnic and socioeconomic composition. However, with the passage of time many tracts have become quite heterogeneous, and population growth has necessitated subdivision of some tracts.

Between 1970 and 1980, the Bureau of the Census further developed a fine geographic grid code that is linked to latitude and longitude cross-points. These grids can be agglomerated into geographic areas such as political entities, tracts, or SMSAs, but they can also be agglomerated into previously unidentified geographic areas—e.g., health service areas that may cross political boundaries.

The Bureau of the Census makes detailed studies to check on the completeness and accuracy of the census. The 1980 census has been estimated to err by a net undercount of about 2.2 per cent, but the percentage is much higher for certain groups—young children (especially infants), young males, and blacks. In 1970, the underenumeration of blacks was estimated to be 7.6 per cent. The preliminary figures from 1980 reveal some improvement in accuracy. There is an overcount of 0.4 per cent for the total country, and an undercount of 4.8 per cent for blacks. However, the estimated population does not account for illegal immigration; every million illegal aliens adds about 0.4 to 0.5 per cent to the undercount.

The accuracy of censuses may vary from one census to the next. Marked changes in the completeness of population coverage must be considered in assessing time trends in disease rates. Undercounting by the Bureau of the Census has recently become a political issue, as minority groups become concerned lest undercounting deprive them of a fair allotment of resources.

A serious current limitation of the census is that a decennial count cannot provide the accurate and up-to-date information needed by a growing, highly mobile population. This limitation is partially overcome by a monthly sample survey called the Current Population Survey (CPS), which investigates about 70,000 households. However, this survey cannot provide information in sufficient detail to meet all intercensal needs. There is continued interest in reducing the interval between total population censuses to five years.

The information furnished by individuals to the census is confidential and is not available to private or other government agencies except in the form of summary statistical compilations. Tabulations for small areas are suppressed if they would permit identification of individuals. Despite this, in the past there have been complaints about invasion of privacy. Indignation has been expressed at such questions as whether the toilet and bathroom in a house are shared with another household. The consensus of reactions among public health workers to these objections was well expressed in an editorial in the American Journal of Public Health (1969).

[While] this controversy may appear to have its humorous aspects, it is potentially serious in its implications. . . . Valuable statistical information is provided by the census and it is necessary, in fact essential, to have it so as to know where we are and to plan for the future.

VITAL STATISTICS

Probably the major source of information about the health of a population is its vital statistics. By *vital statistics* we mean the data collected from ongoing recording, or registration, of all "vital events"—births and adoptions; deaths and fetal deaths; marriages, divorces, legal separations, and annulments. We will discuss only those aspects of registration with which physicians are mainly concerned—certification of death, birth, and fetal death.

Although certificates are filed locally, legal responsibility for registration of vital events is centralized in the governments of individual states and territories and several large cities. Figure 4–1 outlines the flow of information through the Vital Statistics Registration System in the United States. Although each state determines the format and content of its own certificates, the federal government, through its National Center for Health Statistics (NCHS) and its Cooperative Health Statistics System (CHSS), recommends standard forms that the states tend to adopt. The standard certificates were last revised in 1978.

Historically, registration of vital events goes back a variable length of time for the different states. In Virginia and Massachusetts, the pioneer states, registration of births, marriages, and deaths had been instituted by the middle of the seventeenth century. The federal government began to compile national statistics on deaths in 1880 and on births in 1915 on the basis of copies of certificates submitted by the states. Over the years, the minimum standards for reporting established by the federal government have been met by an increasing number of states. By 1933, all states were included in what is known as the Birth and Death Registration Area. Since then, registration of births and deaths has continued to improve, partly because an increased proportion of these events take place in hospitals and partly because registration is advantageous to each individual and family. Proof of birth is required for obtaining a passport and for school entrance. Death certificates are needed for establishing insurance claims, for receipt of veterans' or Social Security benefits, and so on. Advances in computer technology have greatly facilitated the collection and analysis of vital statistics data.

Epidemiologic studies are often based on mortality data. In the United States, it used to be very difficult to trace people who had died because each state maintained a separate system for the recording of vital events. In response to this problem, the NCHS established the National Death Index (NDI) in 1979. This is a central, computerized index of information about deaths compiled by the NCHS from tapes provided by the various state offices of vital statistics. Use of the NDI is restricted to approved research projects.

RESPONSIBLE PERSON OR AGENCY	BIRTH CERTIFICATE	DEATH CERTIFICATE	FETAL DEATH REPORT (Stillbirth)
Hospital Authority	1. Completes entire certificate in consultation with parent(s) 2. Files certificate with local office or State office, per State law.	When death occurs in hospital, may initiate preparation of certificate: Completes name, date of death, and place of death information; obtains certification of cause of death from physician; and gives certificate to funeral director.	1. Completes entire report in consultation with parents(s) 2. Obtains cause of death from physician. 3. Obtains authorization for disposition of fetus. 4. Files report with local office or State office, per State law.
Funeral Director		1. Obtains personal facts about decedent and completes certificate. 2. Obtains certification of cause of death from physician or medical examiner or coroner. 3. Obtains authorization for disposition, per State law. 4. Files certificate with local office or State office, per State law.	If fetus is to be buried, the funeral director is responsible for obtaining the authorization for disposition. NOTE: In some States the funeral director, or person acting as such, is responsible for all duties shown above under hospital authority.
Physician or Other Professional Attendant	Verifies accuracy of medical information and signs certificate.	Completes certification of cause of death and signs certificate.	Provides cause of fetal death information.
Local Office* (may be Local Registrar or City or County Health Department)	1. Verifies completeness and accuracy of certificate and queries incomplete or inconsistent certificates. 2. If authorized, makes copy or index for local use. 3. Sends certificates to State registrar.	1. Verifies completeness and accuracy of certificate and queries incomplete or inconsistent certificates. 2. If authorized, makes copy or index for local use. 3. If authorized by State law, issues authorization for disposition upon receipt of completed certificate. 4. Sends certificates to State registrar.	If State law requires routing of fetal death reports through local office, the local office will perform the same functions as shown for the death certificate.

City and county health departments use data derived from these records in allocating medical and nursing services, followups on infectious diseases, planning programs, measuring effectiveness of services, and conducting research studies.

State Registrar, Office of Vital Statistics	1. Queries incomplete or inconsistent information. 2. Maintains files for permanent reference and as the source of certified copies. 3. Develops vital statistics for use in planning, evaluating, and administering State and local health activities and for research studies. 4. Compiles health-related statistics for State and civil divisions of State for use of the health department and other agencies and groups interested in the fields of medical science, public health, demography, and social welfare. 5. Sends copies of records or data derived from records to the National Center for Health Statistics.
Public Health Service—National Center for Health Statistics	1. Prepares and publishes national statistics of births, deaths, and fetal deaths; and constructs the official U.S. life tables and related actuarial tables. 2. Conducts health and social-research studies based on vital records and on sampling surveys linked to records. 3. Conducts research and methodological studies in vital statistics methods including the technical, administrative, and legal aspects of vital records registration and administration. 4. Maintains a continuing technical assistance program to improve the quality and usefulness of vital statistics.

*Some States do not have local vital registration offices. In these States the certificates or reports are transmitted directly to the State office of vital statistics.

Figure 4–1 The Vital Statistics Registration System in the United States. (From Medical Examiners' and Coroners' Handbook on Death Registration and Fetal Death Reporting.) DHEW Pub. No. (PHS) 78-1110, National Center for Health Statistics, August 1978.

Death Certificate

The death certificate is so important for epidemiologic study that it deserves further comment. Death certificates provide information not only on the number of deaths and the decendent's characteristics (e.g., age, sex, race, usual occupation) but also on the conditions that led to death. (Figure 4–2 shows the recommended standard form.)

It is important to be aware of some problems inherent in obtaining and interpreting information on cause of death. The amount of information available about decendents varies; it depends on the extent to which the person had been studied medically before death, on the familiarity of the certifying physician with the deceased, and on whether or not an autopsy was done. Problems of particular importance for comparative purposes are variation from one area to another in medical practices and diagnostic labelling.

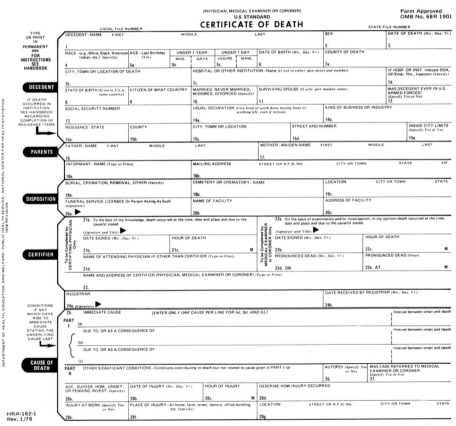

Figure 4–2 U.S. Standard Certificate of Death. National Center for Health Statistics, 1978 Revision.

In this connection we might consider the value of autopsy data. The pathologic information obtained from the autopsy is often the basis for a final judgment about the individual patient and is, therefore, of great value in the continuing education of physicians. Autopsy data have contributed significantly to an understanding of the natural history of disease and knowledge of trends in frequency. For example, an important piece of information about atherosclerotic heart disease was the finding of a high prevalence (77 per cent) of atherosclerotic lesions in the coronary arteries of young soldiers killed in action in the Korean War (Enos et al., 1951). Among the earliest indications of a rise in the incidence of lung cancer were reports that this condition was being found in autopsies with increasing frequency.

However, autopsy results can be misleading for epidemiologic purposes, because autopsies are done on a nonrandom sample of all deaths. Failure to obtain permission for some autopsies because of religious or other reasons adds yet another selective process to those already involved in gaining admission to a hospital. These selective processes make autopsy series quite unrepresentative of all deaths.

It is probably unfortunate that the proportion of autopsies has been going down over the past decades. Currently, only 15 per cent of deaths come to autopsy.

Medical Examiners' and Coroners' Cases. If death is due to an accident, if there is any suspicion of either homocide or suicide, or if a physician has not been in attendance, then the private physician cannot complete the death certificate. Instead, the physician must notify a local authority, i.e., a medical examiner or coroner. The **medical examiner** is a public official who must be a physician and who is usually trained in forensic pathology. It is the function of the medical examiner to investigate the cause of death, under the circumstances just described. A **coroner** is also a public official but need not be a pathologist or even a physician. In fact, the coroner's qualifications are often more political than scientific.

Not surprisingly, more and better information is available from autopsies performed by medical examiners than from those done by coroners. Unfortunately, however, most jurisdictions still have a coroner's system. For example, in Pennsylvania, which has 67 counties, only Philadelphia and Delaware counties have medical examiners' offices. Even using the medical examiner's system does not guarantee adequate information in all cases of sudden death. Investigation of an unexplained death is not mandatory; rather, the medical examiner decides on the need for an autopsy on the basis of a preliminary investigation. For persons previously under medical care but not attended by a physician immediately prior to death, the medical examiner may defer to the judgment of the decedent's physician.

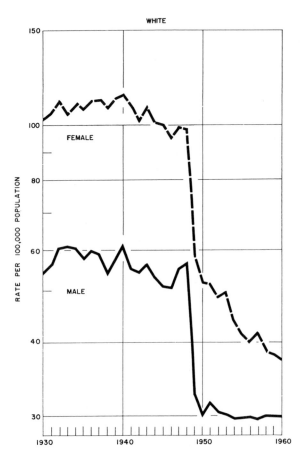

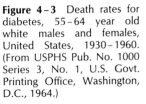

Figure 4-3 Death rates for diabetes, 55-64 year old white males and females, United States, 1930-1960. (From USPHS Pub. No. 1000 Series 3, No. 1, U.S. Govt. Printing Office, Washington, D.C., 1964.)

Assignment of Cause of Death. The physician's major contribution to the death certificate is certification of the cause of death (Fig. 4-2). For each death, one condition must be assigned on the death certificate as the "underlying cause of death" (part I, item 25c). There is also provision for reporting the immediate cause or causes of death (items 25a and 25b), as well as other significant conditions that contributed to the death (part II).

The diagnostic terms on the certificate must conform to an internationally accepted classification, the International Statistical Classification of Diseases, Injuries and Causes of Death (ICD), which is revised every 10 years to reflect medical advances and to be responsive to the changing profile of health problems (i.e., the increasing importance of chronic diseases in industrialized nations). With each revision of the ICD, the National Center for Health Statistics of the United States calculates comparability ratios for major classifications of disease. These ratios summarize the effect of changes in ICD classification on rates of disease by coding a large number of death certificates according to both the current and preceding ICD classifications. When marked changes occur, they must be taken into account in assessing time trends in death rates.

In 1949, a major change was introduced in the method of assigning cause of death. Before that date, if more than one cause was recorded on a certificate, the official cause of death was assigned by a statistical clerk according to a system of fixed priorities that tended to favor diagnoses of infectious disease. Since 1949, the cause of death that is incorporated into all statistics is the one recorded on the death certificate as the underlying cause by the individual physician. In this way, practicing physicians contribute directly to the official vital statistics system.

This change in the system had a pronounced effect on the recording of some diseases. Figure 4–3 shows an apparently abrupt drop in mortality from diabetes in 1949, when deaths attributed to diabetes decreased by almost 50 per cent. About half of this deficit was accounted for by attributing deaths to arteriosclerotic heart disease, and the other half to several other conditions. In contrast, at the same time rates for malignant neoplasms showed an abrupt upward shift.

In earlier times, when the major causes of death were infectious diseases, it was relatively easy to assign deaths to cholera, typhoid fever, tuberculosis, or a similar cause. Today, with increased life expectancy, people are more likely to die with multiple afflictions (e.g., diabetes and a malignant neoplasm) or conditions that affect multiple organ systems (cardiovascular-renal disease). As a result, assignment of one cause of death is increasingly difficult and unsatisfactory as an indication of the major disease processes present in an individual.

The impact on mortality statistics of coding only one cause of death was studied by Dorn and Moriyama (1964). Their analysis of United States death certificates for 1955 revealed that, overall, limiting the tabulations to a single cause resulted in the loss of about half of the diagnostic information on the death certificate. This was more of a problem for some diseases than for others. For cancer, the loss of information was relatively small, since about 95 per cent of the certificates that mentioned cancer cited it as the underlying cause of death. On the other hand, generalized arteriosclerosis and hypertension without indication of heart disease were listed as contributing to death about eight times as often as they were cited as the underlying cause of death. Statistics based on one cause of death would miss such information. To extend the amount of medical information available from the death certificate, the National Center for Health Statistics has since 1968 used a computer-based system called Automated Classification of Medical Entities (or ACME), which not only records the underlying cause of death but also prepares tabulations reflecting multiple causes of death.

The death certificate is also used as a source of demographic and occupational information about the decedent. This information is usually obtained by the funeral director from the available next of kin. The completeness and accuracy of such data are therefore questionable for certain population groups. For example, women who have worked outside the home for many years tend to be described as housewives. This obscures the effects of occupational exposures.

Certificate of Live Birth

As noted before, registration of live births is one of the cornerstones in the system of vital statistics. In addition, it provides identification essential to individuals as citizens.

The standard certificate of live birth is shown in Figure 4–4. Note that the certificate contains two parts. The first, which is an open public record, primarily identifies the child and his parents. A separate section, marked "information for medical and health use only," contains information useful for epidemiologic study. This section calls for information on the race and education of the parents, the mother's previous pregnancies, month of pregnancy in which prenatal care began, total number of prenatal visits, date of last live birth, date of last fetal death, birth weight, complications of pregnancy and delivery, and congenital abnormalities. Most of this information, although gathered previously by some states, was added to the standard certificate only recently.

There has been some controversy over whether sensitive items, such as race and legitimacy status, should be included in the certificate. As a partial answer to such concerns, race, which has always been on the standard certificate, was moved to the confidential portion, where illegitimacy is also recorded. Inclusion of both these items is recommended because they help in the evaluation of social and health problems. Not all states require, or even permit, reporting on illegitimacy. Since there is undoubtedly underreporting even in the states where the information is requested, estimates of the extent of illegitimacy from birth certificates are certainly below the actual level.

The data on birthweight, birth injuries, and congenital malformations are potentially useful for identifying children likely to need special health, educational, and social services. In addition, they provide information for epidemiologic studies of prematurity and congenital defects. However, there are limitations to the use of birth certificates for such purposes. Whether a given birth defect is entered on the certificate depends on its severity and manifestation at birth, the thoroughness with

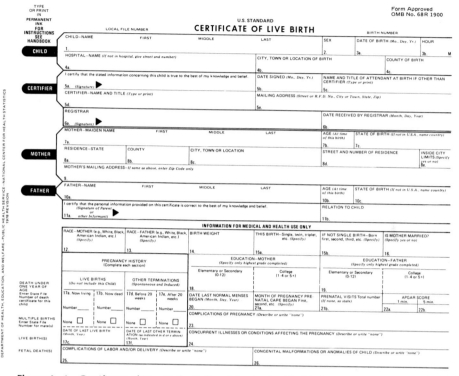

Figure 4-4 Certificate of Live Birth, National Center for Health Statistics, 1978 Revision.

which the child is examined, and the care with which the certificate is completed. Milham (1963) found, for example, that in a series of 143 cases of cleft lip and palate, one-fourth were not noted on the birth certificates. Hospital records may also yield an underestimate. One-fifth of these defects were not noted on the hospital records of these infants.

Certificate of Fetal Death

Statistics on fetal death provide some information on fetal wastage. These data are undoubtedly inferior to those on births and deaths in completeness and in comparability of different areas. There are minor differences from one jurisdiction to another in the criteria specified for determining the presence or absence of life at birth (live birth versus fetal death), but the major problems result from incomplete registration and from differences among states in the stage of gestation at which registration is required. The definition of fetal death adopted by the World Health Assembly includes all fetal deaths, regardless of age of gestation. Although this definition has been recommended for use in the

United States, in practice most states require registration only after 20 completed weeks of gestation.

MORBIDITY DATA

The earliest attempts by government authorities to investigate disease occurrence were related to the urgent need to contain serious infectious diseases, such as smallpox, diphtheria, yellow fever, typhoid fever, and cholera. To this pragmatic goal was added that of studying the distribution of these diseases.

More recently, attempts have been made to extend systematic collection of data to a range of conditions broader than the group of catastrophic infectious diseases. Through the Centers for Disease Control (CDC), records are kept on abortions, congenital anomalies, rubella, nosocomial infections, tuberculosis, and other conditions that may have a preventable component. In addition, the federal government and many states have established cancer reporting networks because of the seriousness and frequency of this disease. This section of the chapter will contain an outline of major sources of morbidity data and some comments on the utility and limitation of these sources.

Reports of Notifiable Disease

In their focus on patients as individuals, practicing physicians are likely to be relatively unconcerned with their role in contributing to a community-wide network of information about disease. We will try to give a picture of that network, and also, if possible, to stimulate awareness of the important role physicians can and should play in transmitting information about cases of *reportable disease.*

Effective control of communicable disease requires that responsible officials know the nature and extent of the health problems in their jurisdiction so that they can take appropriate action. The reporting of disease that originates with physicians and laboratories forms the basis for action by public health officials. For example, when a case of typhoid fever or an outbreak in a newborn nursery is reported, an investigative team must be dispatched to determine the source of the infection so that control measures can be instituted. Prompt reports on food-borne illness are of importance in preventing future common-vehicle epidemics.

Today, with the possibility of eradication of measles, health departments are most anxious to learn about its occurrence. They can then search out unimmunized segments of the population and set up immunization campaigns. Cases of venereal disease provide an entry into a chain of infection that includes the source on the one hand and persons possibly infected by the reported case on the other. Thus, control activities not only serve the immediate need for containment of a disease but also generate additional information about its distribution and transmission.

As with the collection and recording of vital statistics, the responsibility and authority for control of disease is legally vested in the individual states. The list of diseases that must be reported varies somewhat from state to state. Diseases reportable in all states are shown in Table 4–1. Note that four — cholera, plague, smallpox, and yellow fever — are covered by international regulations. Some states also require reporting for epidemics of any kind and for occupationally acquired disease; in a few areas, cancer is reportable.

Unfortunately, the reporting of disease is often neglected. The more serious and rare infectious diseases, such as plague and rabies, are probably reported quite consistently, because physicians can see the need for notifications of such illnesses. The value of reporting the more common diseases is less obvious. In addition, physicians are often reluctant to report diseases that carry a social stigma, such as syphilis and gonorrhea. Nonetheless, the dangers to the community as a whole from uncontrolled communicable diseases are such that legally and ethically a physician is bound to report the occurrence of these diseases to the proper authorities.

Recognition of the incompleteness of reporting has led health departments to streamline and simplify the reporting process, to establish multiple sources for reporting (i.e., physicians, hospitals, and laboratories), and, at times, to solicit reports from a sample of interested physicians rather than the total group. For example, in a three-year trial in Rhode Island (1966 to 1969), 40 physicians, mostly general practitioners and pediatricians, were paid a token honorarium to report each week the communicable illnesses in their own practices. During this trial period the 40 consultants reported more cases of three common conditions — chickenpox, mumps, and streptococcal infections — than did the 400 general practitioners and pediatricians in the entire state in the period prior to the trial (Schaffner et al., 1971).

The exact procedures for reporting vary in the different states. In general, the attending physician is responsible for reporting cases to the local health authority. Hospital and laboratory directors may also be required to report. The information is channelled to the state health department, from there to the CDC in Atlanta, and eventually to the World Health Organization for inclusion in international statistics. The CDC prepares a weekly report (the Morbidity and Mortality Weekly Report, or MMWR) that summarizes the current incidence of certain notifiable diseases, as well as the week's deaths in 121 large cities throughout the country. Other items in the MMWR consist of reports of

TABLE 4-1 Summary of Reported Cases of
Notifiable Disease, United States, 1981, with the
Total Number of Cases[*]

Disease	Total
Amebiasis	6,632
Anthrax	—
Aseptic, Meningitis	9,547
Botulism, total	103
Food-borne	22
Infant	76
Brucellosis (undulant fever)	185
Chickenpox	200,766
Cholera	19
Diphtheria	5
Encephalitis, primary	322
Indeterminate	1,156
Post childhood infections	38
Gonorrhea[1]	990,864
Hepatitis A	25,802
Hepatitis B	21,152
Hepatitis, unspecified	10,975
Legionellosis[2]	408
Leprosy	256
Leptospirosis	82
Malaria	1,388
Measles (rubeola)	3,124
Meningococcal infections, total	3,525
Civilian	3,514
Military	11
Mumps	4,941
Pertussis (whooping cough)	1,248
Plague	12
Poliomyelitis, total	6
Paralytic	6
Psittacosis	124
Rabies, human	2
Rheumatic fever	264
Rubella (German measles)	2,077
Rubella congenital syndrome	19
Salmonellosis	39,990
Shigellosis	19,859
Syphilis, primary & secondary[1]	31,266
Tetanus	72
Trichinosis	206
Tularemia	288
Typhoid fever	584
Typhus fever	
Flea-borne (endemic, murine)	61
Tick-borne (Rocky Mountain spotted)	1,192

[1] Civilian cases only.
[2] Sporadic cases only.

[*] From Centers For Disease Control. Annual Summary, 1981:
Reported Morbidity and Mortality in the United States. Morbidity
and Mortality Weekly Report 30:54, 1982.

current epidemiologic investigations, recommendations from official committees on immunization policy, and reviews of disease surveillance. Because of a system of weekly telegraphic reports from state and territorial health officers to the CDC, only a few days elapse between transmittal of information to Atlanta and its publication and dissemination. The CDC also publishes yearly summaries of morbidity and mortality from notifiable diseases. Additional information about certain infectious diseases is derived from a series of national surveillance programs (see Chap. 11).

The fact that most infectious diseases are underreported does not mean that data from official notifications have no epidemiologic value. It is possible, at least for some diseases, to estimate the level of underreporting; data on reported illness can be used to study trends over time and place. Such data, albeit incomplete, can lead to hypotheses about the etiology and mode of transmission of disease.

Other Statistics on Morbidity

Information about illness is available from a number of sources other than compulsory notifications, as a byproduct of the ongoing activities of various organizations. Among these sources are hospital records, records of private physicians, data from insurance programs, industrial health plans, school records, and federal agencies, such as the armed forces and Veterans Administration.

Hospital Records. On first thought it might seem that records from general hospitals would be a good source of morbidity data. Unfortunately, this is not true in the United States for most types of illness. Data based on hospital admissions or discharges provide a biased picture of the illnesses in a community. Acute minor illnesses treated in a physician's office and cases that do not come to medical attention would be missed. In addition, serious chronic diseases, such as cancer and rheumatoid arthritis, followed on an outpatient basis would not appear in prevalence data based on hospital inpatients. Further, admission to a given hospital results from many selective factors, such as access to the hospital, availability of beds, desire for care by a specific physician, and insurance policies that promote inpatient care. Thus, there is usually no defined population base associated with any one hospital or even, in many instances, with all the hospitals in an area; therefore, rates of disease cannot be generated. However, if a disease is so serious that almost all patients affected are hospitalized, and if medical care tends to be sought in a defined geographic area, then hospital data may be used to estimate incidence rates of disease for the area, with the census data providing the appropriate denominators. An example of this is the Greater Delaware Valley Pediatric Tumor Registry which covers southern New Jersey, eastern Pennsylvania, the state of Delaware, and north-eastern Maryland. This population-based registry relies on reporting of cases of pediatric cancer from 150 hospitals in a 31-county area with a pediatric population base of two million (Kramer, 1983).

Further, hospital statistics even on primary diagnosis are generally difficult to collect, at least in part because of the lack of automated systems. In the United States, at the present time there is no centralized and uniform mechanism for collecting epidemiologic and utilization data from general hospitals. However, a nonprofit system, the Professional Activity Study (PAS) system, was formed in 1953 in response to the need for such information. This organization, which is sponsored by several professional groups, currently collects and compiles reports on discharges from almost 2000 short-stay hospitals. The information, which is collected on a standard abstract form, includes demographic characteristics, length of stay, diagnosis, treatment, complications, status at discharge, and details of diagnostic work-up and management.

Additional impetus to the reporting of hospital data now comes from the statistical requirements of various government programs. Examples are the utilization review mandated by Medicare and the data required by the Children's Bureau for those cared for under the Children and Youth Programs. These should serve to increase the value of hospital records for the study of morbidity.

Despite their many deficiencies, data on morbidity from hospitals lend themselves to surveillance of certain conditions. The defined populations of inpatients provide denominators for rates of events occurring during hospitalization. Two problems that have been studied in this manner are adverse drug reactions and hospital-acquired (nosocomial) infections.

When the problem of adverse drug reactions was first investigated, it was estimated (National Academy of Sciences, 1971) that as many as 15 per cent of patients suffer an adverse drug reaction during their hospital stay. More recently, attempts have been made to classify adverse reactions more clearly and to focus only on those that cause a severe or life-threatening condition. With this newer approach, it became apparent that the risk of serious complications is actually smaller than previously thought. One large-scale study from the Boston Collaborative Drug Surveillance Program (Jick, 1974) indicated that life-threatening reactions occur at a rate of about 3 per cent and that the drug-related fatality rate is approximately 2.4 per 1000 patients admitted to the medical services of hospitals.

Nosocomial infections, infections that occur in an institutional setting such as a hospital, convalescent home, or skilled nursing facility, are also of concern, so much so that two nationwide conferences were called in 1970 and 1980 to deal with this problem. The incidence of nosocomial infections has been relatively constant over the years; about 5 per cent to 6 per cent of hospitalized patients eventually develop a nosocomial infection. Considering the extensive efforts of hospitals toward infection control, the efficacy of such procedures is of great importance. Several recent carefully designed projects have provided definitive data that indicated lack of value of several previously widely used control procedures (e.g., lack of effectiveness of irrigation and daily meatal care for catheterized patients, and lack of effectiveness of reverse isolation). In the late 1970s, the Centers for Disease Control developed an ambitious nationwide project known as the Study on the Efficacy of Nosocomial Infection Control, or SENIC. The results of the SENIC study are to be released shortly and should provide further grounds for rational decisions about expenditures for control of infection.

Data on mental illness and retardation form one of the more useful categories of sources of health data. Most public and private mental hospitals and psychiatric outpatient clinics routinely report uniform data on characteristics and diagnoses of patients to the state mental health agency and the National Institute of Mental Health. In chronic or remitting disease such as mental illness, there is a great likelihood that individuals will have multiple admissions to one or more facilities during a time period. The use of case registers obviates the problem of multiple counts of the same individual. Of course, one must be aware that treated mental illness represents only a small and atypical fraction of the illness in the general population.

Prepaid Group Practice Insurance Programs. Increasing use is being made of illness data available from large prepaid group practice services, such as the Health Insurance Plan (HIP) of Greater New York and the Kaiser-Permanente Group that started on the West Coast. Although the membership of these groups does not form a "representative" sample of the population, their large size and excellent computerized records of illnesses and services rendered have made it possible to obtain morbidity data not available from other sources. An example of the usefulness of such records can be found in a study of outcome of pregnancy initiated by HIP in 1958 (Shapiro and Abramowicz, 1969). Using primarily routinely recorded information, they were able to study the outcome of approximately 12,000 pregnancies and to identify factors related to an unfavorable result. They found that about one-quarter of the pregnancies ended unfavorably (i.e., in fetal or neonatal death, a low-birth-weight infant, or a significant congenital anomaly) and that the history of the outcome of previous pregnancies was a useful predictor of risk for subsequent pregnancies.

Private Physicians. The records of private physicians have been little used in this country. In contrast, in England approximately 95 per cent of the population is covered by the National Health Service, and each individual is on the list of one general practitioner who is paid on a per capita basis. This defined relationship has made it possible to use general practitioners' records for morbidity studies that could not be duplicated in this country.

However, in 1973 the National Center for Health Statistics embarked on a sample survey of office-based physicians, the National Ambulatory Care Survey (NAMCS). In this ongoing survey, randomly selected physicians are asked to report on the demographic characteristics and medical problems of a limited number of patients seen in office visits during one week of practice. It is estimated that participation in the survey should take approximately 15 minutes a day during the week the physician participates. Participation rates have been good (over 80 per cent). This survey, which provides the first national statistics on the use of ambulatory services in this country, is a part of the National Health Survey (page 85).

Disease Registers. A limited application of the concept of record linkage (see p. 87) is found in the disease register. A disease register is a mechanism for identifying and recording information on the salient characteristics of all the people who have been diagnosed as having a given condition in the area covered by the registry. Cancer, tuberculosis, rheumatic fever, and mental illness are some of the major conditions for which registers have been established. In a register, all newly diagnosed cases meeting specified criteria are identified through routine reporting to a central repository (e.g., state or local health department). Incoming case reports are matched against the current roster to eliminate duplication of reports, and new cases are added to those already enrolled. The roster is kept current through periodic follow-up.

For diseases such as tuberculosis and cancer, a register helps in the care of patients by facilitating regular follow-up. A well-designed and conducted case register can also provide information not readily available from any other source on the natural history of a disease. In addition, if the register is population-based, it can yield information on incidence and prevalence as well as survival. Some notable population-based registers have been the Psychiatric Case Registers in Maryland and in Monroe County, New York, and the Connecticut Cancer Registry. The latter has been in operation continuously since 1935.

In the years between 1940 and 1973, information on treatment and survival rates in cancer was collected by an agency composed of three state and 10 hospital registers, known as the End Results Group. This was replaced by a cancer research program of Surveillance, Epidemiology and End Results Reporting (SEER), which gathered data from population-based registers and provided information on incidence as well as treatment and survival.

In view of the substantial work and expense entailed in establishing and maintaining a population-based register, the decision to set up a new register should not be made without careful consideration. A register should be attempted only in situations in which there are good prospects for exploiting the information to be collected for research in etiology or survival. The existence of a register necessitates cooperation from the local medical community and stable financial support for a competent professional staff.

Morbidity Surveys. Unfortunately, routinely collected data on illness from physicians, hospitals, and other sources of medical care do not yield a complete picture of the illness and disability experience of the total population of a defined region. To provide more comprehensive data for monitoring the health status of a population, sample surveys, known as *morbidity surveys*, have been undertaken.

Large-scale surveys of illness in selected geographic areas of the country were first carried out in the early years of this century. Some were single-visit surveys (e.g., the National Health Survey conducted by the United States Public Health Service in 1935 and 1936). In others, the same households were revisited periodically over months or years (e.g., Hagerstown, Maryland, 1921 to 1924). The most extensive and ambitious survey undertaken to date is the current National Health Survey, which has been in operation for over two decades.

The National Health Survey. The National Health Survey was established by an Act of Congress in 1956 to provide a continuing source of information about the health status and needs of the entire country. Conducted by the National Center for Health Statistics, it includes several major survey programs.

HEALTH INTERVIEW SURVEY. Throughout the year, interviews are conducted with a probability sample of about 40,000 households across the country, providing a cross section of the civilian, noninstitution- alized population. Included are queries about any limitation of activity associated with an acute or chronic condition, about visits to a doctor or dentist, and about hospitalization. Most of the questions cover the two-week period preceding the interview.°

Responses in a household survey must be interpreted cautiously. Among the limiting factors is that the respondent knows only about diagnoses the doctor has transmitted. Also, one person reports for the entire household; reports about others are likely to be even less com- plete and accurate than self-reports. The National Center for Health Statistics has carried out studies to validate the self-reports of illness and

---

° Examples of questions from the National Health Survey: During the past two weeks, did anyone in the family go to a dentist? Has anyone in the family been a patient in a hospital during the past two weeks? (During the past two weeks) has anyone in the family been to a doctor's office or clinic for shots, x-rays, tests, or examinations?

hospitalization obtained from household interviews. It has been found that certain chronic illnesses (e.g., mental illness and cancer) are greatly underreported in interviews.

HEALTH EXAMINATION SURVEY (HES). To augment the information that may be obtained appropriately by household interviews, additional population samples have been studied through physical examinations, conducted in specially designed mobile units and supplemented by laboratory tests (e.g., serum cholesterol and blood glucose). These examinations have been carried out in cycles, each requiring approximately three years for completion. The first cycle was designed to study the prevalence of certain chronic conditions in adults 18 to 79 years of age; this was done between November 1959 and December 1962. The second cycle included children 6 to 11 years of age and was conducted between July 1963 and December 1965. In the third cycle, adolescents aged 12 to 17 years were examined between March 1966 and early 1970.

In 1971, the HES was renamed the Health and Nutrition Examination Survey (HANES). In this continuing survey, persons aged 1 to 74 years are examined, with particular attention to the detection of nutritional deficiency. It is planned that nationwide surveys will be held every 10 years, with subsamples of the population to be examined between cycles.

Two additional surveys are maintained by the National Center for Health Statistics. These are the National Hospital Discharge Survey and the National Nursing Home Survey. Both of these surveys were initiated in 1973 and were designed to collect data about these facilities and the people they serve.

NATIONAL FAMILY GROWTH SURVEY. This survey, in operation since 1973, provides information on fertility patterns and trends and family planning practices. Originally a biennial survey, in the future it will be carried out every five years through personal interviews.

SURVEYS LINKED TO VITAL RECORDS. In these "follow-back surveys," information supplementary to death or birth certificates is obtained from the family, physician, or hospital. For deaths, this includes data on morbidity and hospitalization in the last year of life; for births, information is sought on prenatal care and fertility history.

Quality Control in the National Health Survey. To improve the quality of the data from these surveys, the National Center for Health Statistics carries out many pilot tests of procedures and conducts various types of checks to detect sources of error and bias. For example, hospital records have been reviewed to validate self-reports of hospitalization obtained through household interviews. As noted previously, such studies have shown that certain chronic illnesses (e.g., mental illness and cancer) are greatly underreported on interview. Among the probable reasons are the social stigma associated with certain diseases and people's lack of knowledge of the specific diagnoses made by physicians.

Other limitations to the National Health Survey are that it represents primarily prevalence rather than incidence data, and that sample sizes are such that analyses can be presented only for major geographic regions and for relatively common conditions. Nevertheless, despite these limitations, the National Health Survey is the only source of nationwide data on minor illnesses, disabilities, functional deficits, physiologic measurements, and patterns of utilization of medical care. To provide data of greater value to state and local areas, the National Center for Health Statistics is developing cooperative arrangements among the various levels of government (the Cooperative Health Statistics System).

Surveys for Specific Diseases. The National Health Survey attempts to collect comprehensive data on illness. In contrast are surveys that focus on a specific disease or group of diseases, e.g., cancer, mental illness, and diabetes. Examples of this approach are the cancer surveys conducted by the National Cancer Institute (1937, 1947, and 1969 to 1971) for selected urban and rural areas. These surveys have yielded basic data on the incidence of cancer by primary site, histologic type, and stage of disease at diagnosis.

LINKED HEALTH RECORDS

The various sources of data cited so far lead to fragmented records for many individuals. A person's birth certificate may be on file in one jurisdiction, his marriage certificate in another, his children's birth certificates in a third. In addition, he may be entered in the records of a number of hospitals and individual physicians. There are some exceptions. Many states link birth certificates and death records for infants who die within the first few years of life. In addition, in some states cancer registries link the death certificates to hospital records for patients who have died from cancer. The possibility of integrating all of this information into one record system is attractive. The term *record linkage* was first used by Dunn in 1946 to denote a comprehensive approach to linking events of significance for health. In the words of a speech by Dunn:

Each person in the world creates a book of life. This book starts with birth and ends with death. Its pages are made up of the records of the principal events in life. Record linkage is the name given to the process of assembling the pages of this book into a volume.

Two aspects of contemporary life in particular make such linkage highly desirable: the increase in life expectancy, with its concomitant burden of chronic disease; and widespread population mobility. With the advent of computer technology it became reasonable to consider the feasibility of linking records on vital statistics and health events for entire populations or subpopulations. The initial concept of linkage of events for individuals (personal record linkage) has since been broadened to encompass family record linkage; as the name implies, this means that the records of individuals are assembled in family units.

In the past quarter-century, several projects have been developed to evaluate the feasibility of record linkage and to demonstrate its usefulness. The Oxford Record Linkage Project was established in 1962 (Acheson, 1967). In that project, files are built up through entries on all births and deaths within the defined area, all episodes of in-hospital treatment, and all deliveries in hospital and at home. The files have provided material useful for planning and administration of health services, as well as findings of epidemiologic significance. Newcombe's work in British Columbia with family linkage has yielded knowledge about such matters as familial aggregation of disease and maternal fertility following stillbirth and birth of children with various diseases (Newcombe, 1966; Newcombe and Tavendale, 1965). To search for causal factors in cancer, Sweden linked data from its national cancer registry for the years 1961 to 1973 with occupational information from the 1960 census. This made it possible, through a case-control study, to determine that there was no excess risk of leukemia among telephone workers , as had been suggested previously (Wiklund, 1981).

Data banks of computer-linked vital and health records theoretically have great potential for studies in demography, fertility, genetics, and natural history of disease. However, the high cost of initiating and maintaining such files and the need for sophisticated technical and analytical skills to exploit the data, as well as questions of confidentiality, suggest that linked records will find limited application in the near future.

There would be many advantages to having an individual's health and other records united through a unique identifying number; the Social Security number has been proposed to serve this purpose. However, many people have expressed fear that, despite official safeguards, the information on file might improperly become available to potential employers, to sources of credit, and to a variety of government agencies. No really satisfactory solution to this problem has yet been devised.

In this chapter we have presented a variety of sources of data for determination of the frequency of disease. It is important to realize that a number of factors determine the choice of source and methods for the study of a given disease problem.

Of primary importance is the nature of the disease, i.e., whether it is common or rare, acute or chronic, typically mild or severe, and whether it regularly serves to bring people to medical attention. For example, we might contrast lung cancer with arthritis and rheumatism. Death certificates would be a good source of information about the former, the National Health Survey about the latter.

We should also point out that in rapidly fatal conditions (e.g., acute myelogenous leukemia) mortality data are practically equivalent to data on incidence. However, in most instances, mortality and morbidity are not synonymous, and the problems of collecting information about these two aspects of a disease must be considered separately.

Other factors relevant to choice of study method include current state of knowledge about the condition, the relative costs of different methods of study, and the specific purposes of the investigation.

Definitive answers about the etiology of disease often cannot be reached through any of the sources of data discussed so far. Instead, a special study may have to be initiated to test a specific hypothesis. A number of illustrations of such studies have been cited. The Framingham study, the various studies of the effects of cigarette smoking, and the fluoridation trials are but a few examples of research in which new data had to be generated to answer specific questions.

SUMMARY

This chapter has outlined the major sources of data about the population for monitoring health status and for epidemiologic investigation. The decennial census provides the basic information on the numbers of persons and their demographic, socioeconomic, and household characteristics. It thus provides the denominator of morbidity and mortality rates.

The numerators of these rates are derived from a variety of other sources. Chief among them is the reporting of vital events, principally births and deaths. The accurate information furnished on documents by the physician, particularly with respect to the cause of death, was highlighted as our main source of intelligence about the causes of death and trends in these causes.

Especially for nonfatal diseases and conditions, mortality data must be supplemented by data on illness. The uses and limitations of various types of morbidity data were enumerated. The reporting of notifiable diseases, principally communicable diseases and cancer, although incomplete, provides useful information on trends in disease.

Other routinely collected morbidity statistics are derived (or potentially derived) from the ongoing records of hospitals, private practitioners, and large prepaid group practices. A more modern source of information is the morbidity survey. This rubric includes not only surveys of specific diseases but also the more comprehensive ongoing National Health Survey, in which random samples of the population are studied through such means as household interviews, physical examinations, and analysis of vital records and utilization of health care facilities. Finally, the concept, potentialities, and problems of linking records of vital and health events were outlined.

REFERENCES

Acheson, E. D.: Medical Record Linkage. Oxford University Press, London, 1967.
Dorn, H. F., and Moriyama, I. M.: Uses and significance of multiple cause tabulations for mortality statistics. Am. J. Public Health, 54:400, 1964.
Editorial: Support the 1970 census now. Am. J. Public Health, 59:897, 1969.
Enos, W. F., Holmes, R. H., et al.: Coronary disease among United States soldiers killed in action in Korea. J.A.M.A., 152:1090, 1951.
Jick, H.: Drugs—Remarkably nontoxic. N. Engl. J. Med., 291:824, 1974.
Kramer, S., Meadows, A. T., Jarrett, P., and Evans, A. E.: Incidence of childhood cancer: Experience of a decade in a population-based registry. J.N.C.I., 70:49, 1983.
Milham, S., Jr.: Underreporting of incidence of cleft lip and palate. Am. J. Dis. Child., 106:185, 1963.
National Academy of Sciences: Report of the International Conference on Adverse Reactions Reporting Systems. Washington, D.C., 1971.
Newcombe, H. B.: Familial tendencies in diseases in children. Br. J. Prev. Soc. Med., 20:49, 1966.
Newcombe, H. B., and Tavendale, O. G.: Effects of father's age on the risk of child handicap and death. Am. J. Hum. Genet., 17:163, 1965.
Schaffner, W., Scott, H. D., et al.: Innovative communicable disease reporting. HSMHA Health Rep., 86:431, 1971.
SENIC Project. Special Issue: The SENIC Project. Am. J. Epidemiol., 111:465, 1980.
Shapiro, S., and Abramowicz, M.: Pregnancy outcome correlates identified through medical record-based information. Am. J. Public Health, 59:1629, 1969.
Wiklund, K., Einhorn, J., and Eklund, G.: An application of the Swedish cancer-environment registry. Leukemia among telephone operators at the telecommunications administration in Sweden. Int. J. Epidemiol., 10:373, 1981.

SELECTED INDICES OF HEALTH

5

We will now focus on a number of commonly used indices of health. These are summarized in Table 5–1, along with the values for the United States for the year 1980. Note that the rates have been grouped according to the base to which they refer: total population, live births, and live births plus fetal deaths. As you consider each rate, try to identify the source of information for the numerator and the denominator (census, vital registration, and so on). For example, in the crude birth rate, the numerator is derived from vital registration and the denominator from census data.

The Crude Death Rate

Many of the health indices reviewed in this chapter focus on rates of death, because mortality data are routinely collected and are widely available. Incidence rates may be preferable as measures of risk of disease, but morbidity statistics are not maintained for most conditions and, where they do exist, are generally underreported. The crude death rate is defined and discussed on p. 54 and in Table 5–1.

Figure 5–1 shows annual crude and age-adjusted death rates for the United States from 1930 to 1981. You will observe that the age-adjusted rate shows a much greater decline than the crude death rate. Again, this is a reflection of the changes in age composition over the time period. Note also that the two lines cross each other at 1940, because the rates were standardized to the 1940 population. This means that the crude and standardized death rates were the same at that point in time.

Crude death rates (CDRs) from many countries are presented in Table 5–2. Note that the variation in range is smaller for crude death rates (4.1 to 26.5) than for infant mortality rates (IMRs) (7.3 to 142.1).

TABLE 5–1 Major Public Health Rates°

Rates	Usual Factor	Rate for United States, 1980
Rates Whose Denominators Are the Total Population		
Crude birth rate = $\dfrac{\text{number of live births during the year}}{\text{average (midyear) population}}$	per 1000 population	15.9
Crude death rate = $\dfrac{\text{number of deaths during the year}}{\text{average (midyear) population}}$	per 1000 population	8.8
Age-specific death rate = $\dfrac{\text{number of deaths among persons of a given age group in a year}}{\text{average (midyear) population in specified age group}}$	per 1000 population	5–14 years — 0.3 65–74 years — 29.9
Cause-specific death rate = $\dfrac{\text{number of deaths from a stated cause in a year}}{\text{average (midyear) population}}$	per 100,000 population	Diseases of the heart — 336.0 Malignant neoplasms — 183.9
Rates and Ratios Whose Denominators Are Live Births		
Infant mortality rate = $\dfrac{\text{number of deaths in a year of children less than 1 year of age}}{\text{number of live births in same year}}$	per 1000 live births	12.6

$$\text{Neonatal mortality rate} = \frac{\text{number of deaths in a year of children}}{\text{number of live births in same year}} \quad \text{per 1000 live births} \quad 8.5$$

$$\text{Fetal death } \textit{ratio} = \frac{\text{number of fetal deaths** during year}}{\text{number of live births in same year}} \quad \text{per 1000 live births} \quad 9.1$$

$$\text{Maternal (puerperal) mortality rate} = \frac{\text{number of deaths from puerperal}}{\text{number of live births in same year}} \quad \substack{\text{per 100,000 (or 10,000)} \\ \text{live births}} \quad \substack{\text{9.2 per 100,000} \\ \text{live births}}$$

Rates Whose Denominators Are Live Births and Fetal Deaths

$$\text{Fetal death rate} = \frac{\text{number of fetal deaths during year}}{\text{number of live births and fetal deaths during same year}} \quad \substack{\text{per 1000 live births} \\ \text{and fetal deaths}} \quad 9.0$$

$$\text{Perinatal mortality rate†} = \frac{\substack{\text{number of fetal deaths 28 weeks or more and} \\ \text{infant deaths under 7 days of age} \\ \text{plus fetal deaths 28 weeks or more gestation}}}{\substack{\text{number of live births and fetal deaths 28} \\ \text{weeks or more during the same year}}} \quad \substack{\text{per 1000 live births} \\ \text{and fetal deaths}} \quad 12.8$$

*From Monthly Vital Statistics Report, Vol. 32, No. 4 Supplement, August 1983; and from National Center For Health Statistics, unpublished data.
**Includes only fetal deaths with stated or presumed period of gestation of 20 weeks or more.
†This rate is for Perinatal Definition I.

TABLE 5–2 Crude Birth, Crude Death, and Infant Mortality Rates for Selected Countries (1978 or 1979 unless otherwise specified)[a]

Continent and Country	Crude Birth Rate per 1000 Population		Crude Death Rate per 1000 Population	Infant Mortality Rate per 1000 Live Births	Expectation of Life (yrs) M	F
Africa						
Botswana	50.7	(1970–75)	19.4	—	44.3	47.5
Gambia	46.7	(1970–75)	23.1	—	39.4	42.5
Kenya	50.5	(1970–75)	14.0	51.4	46.9	51.2
Malawi	50.5	(1970–71)	26.5	142.1	40.9	44.2
Sierra Leone	45.6	(1970–75)	21.1	—	41.8	45.0
North America						
Canada	15.3	(1978)	7.2	12.0	69.3	76.4
Costa Rica	31.8	(1978)	4.1	22.3	66.3	70.5
Guatemala	42.9	(1978)	7.1	69.2	48.3	49.7
Mexico	42.0	(1970–75)	8.6	60.2	62.8	66.6
United States	15.8	(1979)	8.7	13.0	68.7	76.5
South America						
Argentina	25.2	(1978)	8.9	40.8	65.2	71.4
Bolivia	46.6	(1975)	18.0	77.3	46.5	51.1
Chile	21.2	(1978)	6.7	40.1	60.5	66.0
Uruguay	20.4	(1977)	9.8	48.5	65.5	71.6

Asia					
India	34.4	(1976)	15.0	12.2	46.4	44.7
Indonesia	41.5	(1970–75)	16.7	12.5	47.5	47.5
Israel	24.7	(1979)	6.9	16.0	71.5	75.0
Japan	14.3	(1979)	5.9	8.0	72.1	77.4
Philippines	41.0	(1970–75)	10.3	47.6	56.9	60.0
Yemen	48.7	(1970–75)	26.3	—	37.3	38.7
Europe					
Albania	33.3	(1971)	8.1	86.8	64.9	67.0
Belguim	12.6	(1979)	11.4	11.2	67.8	74.2
Denmark	11.6	(1979)	10.7	9.1	71.5	77.5
England and Wales	13.0	(1979)	12.1	12.6	69.6	75.8
Finland	13.5	(1978)	9.2	7.6	68.5	77.1
France	14.1	(1979)	10.2	9.8	69.7	77.8
Italy	11.8	(1979)	9.5	15.3	69.0	74.9
Sweden	11.6	(1979)	11.0	7.3	72.2	78.1
Oceania					
Australia	15.5	(1979)	6.9	12.5	67.6	74.1
New Zealand	16.9	(1979)	8.2	13.8	68.6	74.6
Union of Soviet Socialist Republics (USSR)	18.2	(1978)	9.7	27.7	64.0	74.0

* From Demographic Yearbook, 1979, United Nations, New York, 1980.

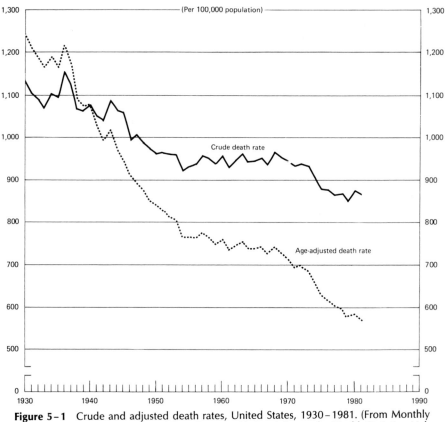

Figure 5-1 Crude and adjusted death rates, United States, 1930-1981. (From Monthly Vital Statistics Report, Provisional Data from the National Center for Health Statistics, Vol. 3Q, No. 3, December 20, 1982.)

This occurs because CDRs reflect the age composition of the population as well as the age-specific death rates for the component segments of the population.

CAUSE-SPECIFIC INDICES

The *cause-specific death rate*, which approximates the risk of death from a specific condition, is probably the most important epidemiologic index available. As pointed out earlier, differences in the magnitude of this measure in subgroups and by time and place suggest etiologic hypotheses and document the need for control measures. Cause-specific death rates are, of course, subject to the various errors and limitations previously discussed, such as difficulties in assigning cause of death (inaccurate numerator) and underenumeration of certain segments of the population (inaccurate denominator).

As we have noted, mortality rates are inadequate for study of the dynamics of diseases that either are not fatal or produce death only after a protracted course. For such conditions, data on morbidity are required. In examining morbidity data, it is always necessary to consider whether a specific index represents incidence or prevalence. Infectious diseases are generally reported as annual incidence rates (i.e., new cases of hepatitis per 100,000). Reports on chronic disease may represent incidence (e.g., new cases of cancer in the population of Connecticut each year) or prevalence (chronic conditions such as diabetes reported in the National Health Survey).

In the next section, trends in cause-specific deaths are presented. Figure 5–2 shows the 10 leading causes of death in 1900 and 1981. Note the marked shift from infectious diseases in the earlier year to primarily chronic, noninfectious disease and trauma as major sources of mortality in 1981. This obviously creates new challenges for health care providers.

Figure 5–3 shows trends in death rates for a number of the leading

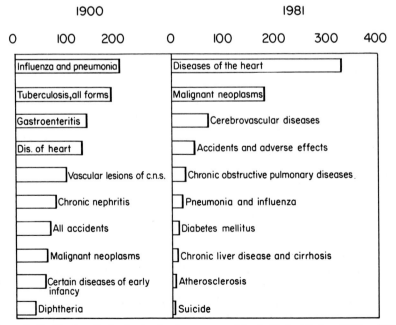

Figure 5–2 Death ratio for the ten leading causes of death, United States, 1900 and 1981.

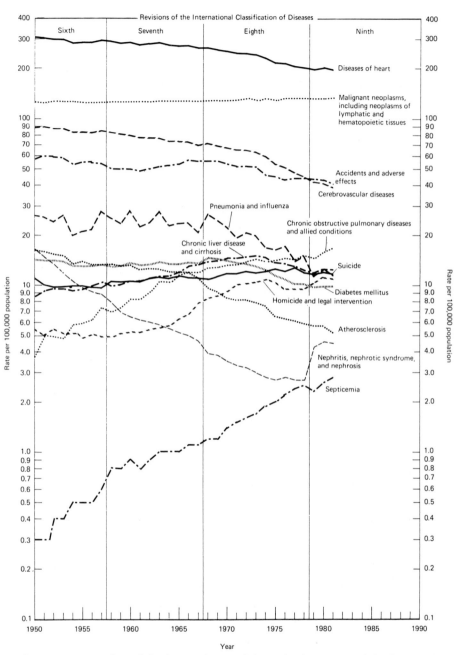

Figure 5–3 Age-adjusted death rates for 13 of the 15 leading causes of death, United States, 1950–1981.

causes of death and indicates the independence of trends for different diseases. Note, for example, the decreasing rates of death from heart disease and cerebrovascular diseases, in contrast with the slight increase in malignant neoplasms and the sharp increases in chronic obstructive pulmonary disease, homicide, and septicemia. (Also note that the vertical axis of the graph is drawn on a log scale. This permits visual comparison of the rate of change over time.)

Proportionate Mortality Ratio

A measure that is often confused with the cause-specific death rate is the *proportionate mortality ratio*, or PMR. This measure tells us the relative importance of a specific cause of death in relation to all deaths in a population group.

$$\text{Proportionate mortality ratio (PMR)} = \frac{\text{Number of deaths from a given cause in a specified time period}}{\text{Total deaths in the same time period}} \text{ per 100 (i.e., percentage)}$$

The PMR is defined somewhat differently in occupational epidemiologic studies, and its formulation in that context is described in Chapter 11. Note that the proportionate mortality ratio is not a rate, since the denominator is derived from deaths and not from the population at risk. This measure answers the question, "What proportion of deaths is attributable to disease X?" In contrast, a cause-specific death rate answers the question, "What is the risk of death from disease X for members of a population?"

From the viewpoint of public health, the proportionate mortality ratio is useful because it permits estimation of the proportion of lives to be saved by eradication or reduction of a given cause of death. On the other hand, proportionate mortality ratios can be misleading. Because

TABLE 5–3 Death Rates per 100,000 Population, All Causes and Accidents, and Proportionate Mortality Ratio for Persons aged 1–4 and 65–74 Years, United States, 1975°

Age	Death Rate per 100,000 All Causes	Accidents	Proportionate Mortality Ratio for Accidents (%)
1–4	70	28.2	40.0
65–74	3190	65.5	2.1

° From National Center for Health Statistics: Vital Statistics of the United States, 1975, Vol. IIA. U.S. Govt. Printing Office, Washington, D.C., 1979.

the denominator refers to total deaths, its magnitude depends on the number of deaths from other causes besides the condition under consideration. For example, Table 5 – 3 shows that, although the *proportion* of deaths due to accidents is greater for young children than for elderly persons, death *rates* from accidents are actually higher among the elderly. The explanation of this seeming paradox is, of course, that the total number of deaths from all other causes is also considerably higher in the elderly.

INFANT AND NEONATAL MORTALITY

Losses early in life (i.e., fetal wastage and deaths shortly after birth) present important challenges to those concerned with community health. Several measures (see Table 5 – 1) are used to indicate the stages of development at which these losses occur. These terms are clarified in Figure 5 – 4, which presents schematically the relationships of the various time periods.

The infant mortality rate traditionally has been considered of great significance in public health. A high rate has been taken to indicate unmet health needs and unfavorable environmental factors — economic conditions, nutrition, education, sanitation, and medical care. Figure 5 – 5 shows the trend in infant mortality rates in the United States over the years from 1930 to 1981. A sharp drop in rates from 1930 to 1950 was followed by more than a decade of little change. In the late 1960s, however, considerable improvement was once again apparent. The percentage decline in infant mortality rate was greater for the five-year period from 1965 to 1970 than for the preceding fifteen years, from 1950 to 1965.

Figure 5 – 5 also shows the trend in *neonatal mortality* (deaths under 28 days of age) and, by subtraction, *postneonatal mortality* (deaths between 28 days and one year). It can be seen that in 1930 the neonatal mortality was slightly higher than the postneonatal. Although both rates declined over the next 50 years, the improvement in the postneonatal mortality rate has been considerably greater, largely because of the control of infectious diseases and better nutrition. The mortality rate for neonates, on the other hand, which reflects such factors as prematurity and congenital defects, shows less dramatic improvement. By 1980, the neonatal mortality rate was more than twice the post-neonatal rate.

A further breakdown of deaths within the first year is shown in Figure 5 – 6. It is clear that the deaths are concentrated in the first week of life, and within that time period, in the first day. Accordingly, there has been an increasing focus on the hazards of the early days of life.

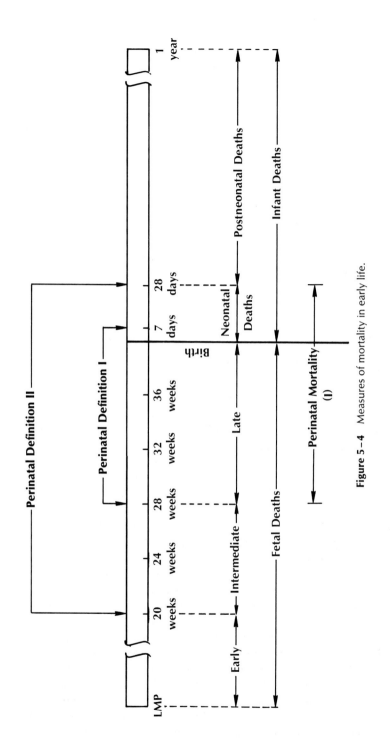

Figure 5-4 Measures of mortality in early life.

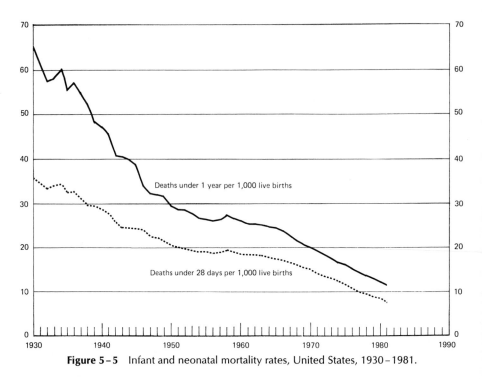

Figure 5–5 Infant and neonatal mortality rates, United States, 1930–1981.

Evidence of this can be found in the emergence of neonatology as a major subspecialty within pediatrics.

International Comparisons

The variations in infant mortality rates, along with crude birth and death rates, are shown for selected countries in Table 5–2. In general, the infant mortality rate is highly correlated with the crude birth rate and, to a lesser extent, with the crude death rate. The extraordinarily high infant mortality rates (per 1000 live births) in Malawi (142), Albania (87), Bolivia (77), and Guatemala (69) are in striking contrast to the rate of 7 in Sweden and of 8 in Japan.

Like the crude death rate, the infant mortality rate is a composite figure that reflects both the distribution of birth weights and mortality rates specific for birth weight. In the United States between 1970 and 1982, the infant mortality rate fell from 20 to 11.2 per 1000 live births. The distribution of birth weights did not change substantially over this period. The improvement was due almost entirely to improvement in birth weight–specific survival rates. The United States leads all other countries in birth weight–specific survival rates but its overall figures

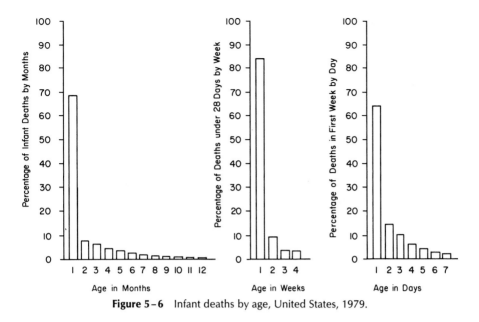

Figure 5 – 6   Infant deaths by age, United States, 1979.

on infant mortality are nevertheless unimpressive. For example, in 1980 the United States was eighteenth in infant mortality rate because of a high proportion of low-birth-weight infants (7.1 per cent of U.S. births, as compared with 4.3 per cent of all births in Sweden). Within the United States, the proportion of low-birth-weight infants is about twice as high for blacks as whites.

Since our birth weight – specific survival rates are so good, the approach to prevention of low-birth-weight infants must focus on shifting the distribution of birth weights to the right. Approaches should include the detection of preterm labor and prevention of preterm delivery (Guyer et al., 1982; Herron et al., 1982). In addition, the public and the medical profession must be made aware of the factors that could improve the situation — i.e., the need for good nutrition, good care of infections, and avoidance of smoking, alcohol, and drugs. And, finally, early antenatal care should be available to all, especially to minority groups and those at high risk.

There are also significant economic considerations in the care of preterm infants. A factor that may encourage the development of preventive services is awareness that intensive neonatal care is exceedingly expensive and that prevention of preterm births would result in great savings. For example, the average stay in a neonatal care unit is estimated at costing $8000 (range, $1000 to $40,000). If the preterm birth rate could be halved, the savings might be as great as $550 million per year in the United States.

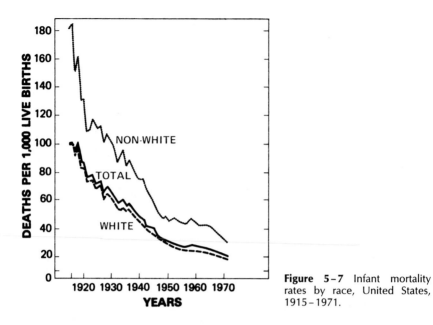

Figure 5-7 Infant mortality rates by race, United States, 1915-1971.

Much concern has centered on the extent of black-white differences in infant mortality in the United States (Fig. 5-7). Note that there is a persistent difference in rate for whites and nonwhites, even though black rates have declined impressively. The differences are undoubtedly due to numerous factors, including the socioeconomic conditions of life (e.g., nutrition, general health status) and the quality and availability of medical care.

FETAL AND PERINATAL MORTALITY

Emphasis has shifted from earlier concern over maternal mortality to concern about fetal and perinatal mortality. For intrauterine deaths, the term "fetal death" is now used in place of the older terms "abortion" and "stillbirth." While in most instances the product of gestation can readily be classified as a "live birth" or a "fetal death," there are instances in which it is difficult to make this distinction. For these reasons the following definitions have been adopted by the World Health Assembly and recommended for use in the United States by the Surgeon General of the United States:

Live Birth—Live birth is the complete expulsion or extraction from its mother of a product of conception, irrespective of the duration of pregnancy, which, after such separation, breathes or shows any other evidence of life, such as beating of the heart, pulsation of the umbilical cord, or definite movement of voluntary muscles, whether or not the umbilical cord has been cut or the placenta is attached;_each product of such a birth is considered liveborn.

Important: If a child breathes or shows any other evidence of life after complete birth, even though it be only momentary, the birth should be registered as a live birth and a death certificate should be filed also.

Fetal Death—Fetal death is death prior to the complete expulsion or extraction from its mother of a product of conception, irrespective of the duration of pregnancy; the death is indicated by the fact that after such separation the fetus does not breathe or show any other evidence of life, such as beating of the heart, pulsation of the umbilical cord, or definite movement of voluntary muscles.°

The definition of fetal death just given includes all fetal deaths "irrespective of the duration of pregnancy." However, in the United States, most of the states require registration only at or after 20 weeks of gestation. National statistics for the United States are based on all deaths in gestations 20 weeks or longer plus those for which length of gestation is unspecified.

The perinatal mortality rate combines losses of late fetal life and early infancy. Thus it spans both intrauterine and extrauterine life. Its utility derives from the fact that it reflects the collaborative efforts of obstetricians and neonatologists in the care of these tiny infants. In contrast to fetal deaths, statistics on perinatal mortality are usually based on fetal deaths occurring 28 weeks or later rather than 20 weeks or later in gestation (i.e., Perinatal Definition I rather than II).

MATERNAL MORTALITY

Maternal mortality rate is a measure that reflects not only the adequacy of obstetric care but also the general level of socioeconomic development. Maternal deaths represent particularly tragic losses because they affect young adults, often at the peak period of family responsibility.

The definition of maternal mortality rate is given in Table 5–1. It can be seen that this rate is approximately 1 per cent of the infant mortality rate. Note that the denominator consists only of live births. If this were a true rate, the denominator should include all pregnancies, since each pregnancy puts the woman at risk regardless of the outcome for the fetus. However, since registration is more complete for live births than for fetal deaths, it has been customary to express this rate in terms of live births only.

° From Physicians' Handbook on Medical Certification: Death, Birth, Fetal Death. DHHS Publication No. (PHS) 81-1198, National Center for Health Statistics, June, 1978.

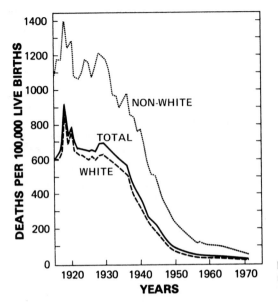

Figure 5–8 Maternal mortality rates by race, United States 1915–1971.

The decreases in maternal mortality rates in many parts of the world in recent decades have been dramatic. Figure 5–8 shows the decline in the rates for white and nonwhite women in the United States between 1915 and 1971. As with infant mortality, rates of maternal mortality have been consistently higher for blacks than for whites. Although the rates have declined for both groups, the ratio of the rates for nonwhite women compared with those for white women has increased, from 2.2 in 1940 to 3.9 in 1979. The larger number of maternal deaths among nonwhites reflects a variety of social and economic handicaps, and a lack of family planning and antenatal and delivery services.

Although the maternal mortality rate has been dropping over the years, one component of maternal deaths, deaths from ectopic pregnancy, has been increasing in a number of countries, at least since 1970. In 1979, 45 of the 336 maternal deaths in the United States (13.4 per cent) were due to ectopic pregnancy.

The causes for the increase are not clear. Several large studies give conflicting results. IUDs were suggested by several workers as related to the increase (Beral, 1975), but a large-scale case-control study in the United States (Ory, 1981) examined the role of IUDs and concluded that IUD use did not explain the increased incidence of ectopic pregnancies. Other factors that have been suggested as related to the occurrence of ectopic pregnancies are age of the woman (the rate is three times higher for ages 30 to 39 than for teenagers) and salpingitis (causing a sevenfold increase in rates [Weström et al., 1981]). Additional factors, such as

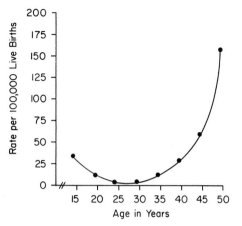

Figure 5-9 Maternal mortality rate per 100,000 live births, by maternal age. United States, 1978.

tubal surgery, progestogen-only oral contraceptives, and induced abortion are also being studied as possibly relevant.

Age appears to be a key factor in risk of death for the mother. Figure 5-9 shows a J-shaped curve for maternal mortality, with high rates at both extremes of age. Specific medical problems associated with these high rates are toxemia in very young mothers, and a greater tendency to hypertension and uterine hemorrhage in older women. However, it is difficult to say how much of the risk can be attributed to maternal age per se. For one thing, maternal age and parity are inevitably intertwined. Further, a woman's social class position influences the likelihood that she will bear children at the extremes of her reproductive period.

Until recently in this country effective methods of contraception have been utilized largely by those favored in educational opportunity and social position. More widespread availability and use of effective contraception will decrease maternal mortality, since it will probably increase the proportion of births among mothers in the relatively favorable third decade of life and would decrease parity (Hellman, 1973).

It is known that, over the years, a significant portion of the maternal mortality in this country was related to the indeterminate but large number of illegal abortions performed yearly. Indirect evidence of this can be found in the sharp drop in maternal mortality (from 53 to 29 per 100,000 live births) in New York City between 1969 and 1971 after the laws of that state were changed to permit abortion on demand.

We have referred to the beneficial effects of contraception and induced abortion on maternal mortality. However, we should also note that even the best available methods of contraception are not without some risk. The increased risk of thromboembolism among users of oral

TABLE 5–4 Mortality Associated with Pregnancy and Childbirth, Legal Abortion, Oral Contraceptives (by smoking status), and IUDs, by Age[*]

Age (years)	Pregnancy and Childbirth[a]	Legal Abortion[b]	Oral Contraceptives[c]		IUDs[c]
			Nonsmokers	Smokers	
15–19	10.4	1.0	0.6	2.1	0.8
20–24	9.5	1.4	1.1	4.2	0.8
25–29	12.1	1.8	1.6	6.1	1.0
30–34	22.8	1.8	3.0	11.8	1.0
35–39	43.7	2.7	9.1	31.3	1.4
40–44	68.2	2.7	17.7	60.9	1.4

[*] From Tietze, C., Lewit, S.: Life risks associated with reversible methods of fertility regulation. Int. J. Gynaecol. Obstet., 16:456, 1979.
[a] Per 100,000 live births (excluding abortion).
[b] Per 100,000 first trimester abortions.
[c] Per 100,000 users per year.

contraceptives is well established (Sartwell et al., 1969; Vessey and Doll, 1968), but the risk is related to age and cigarette smoking as well as to oral contraceptive use (Table 5–4). There is concern that oral contraceptives may have a carcinogenic potential as well, but there is no evidence that this is so. They have been found to be actually protective against ovarian cancer (Relative Risk = 0.6) (CDC, 1983c) and endometrial cancer (R.R. = 0.5) (CDC, 1983a) and to have no effect on risk of breast cancer (R.R. = 0.9) (CDC, 1983b) or carcinoma of the cervix (Thomas, 1972).

A different set of hazards exists with the use of intrauterine devices (Mishell, 1979). While there are no adverse systemic effects from these devices, their risks include increases in local pathology—increased menstrual blood loss, pelvic infections, complications related to pregnancy, increase in ectopic pregnancies, and, rarely, perforation of the uterus.

In Table 5–4, from Tietze and Lewit (1979), calculations from a computer model are summarized. This model attempts to measure the risks of pregnancy and childbearing in relation to the risks of various contraceptive methods. The risks of pregnancy and childbirth exceed by a considerable margin those of the contraceptive methods. Note also the effect of smoking in potentiating the risk from use of oral contraceptives.

Tietze and Lewit noted that "at all ages, the lowest level of mortality by far is achieved by a combined regimen, i.e., use of barrier contraceptives with recourse to early abortion in case of failure." Of course, the hope is that effective contraception will largely eliminate the need for abortion.

Abortion

Abortion has been a controversial issue for many decades. In 1973, a ruling by the Supreme Court (Roe versus Wade) legalized abortion. Even before the Supreme Court decision, the Centers for Disease Control (CDC) had started to collect data from a number of sources on induced abortions. After the Supreme Court decision, the CDC expanded its surveillance of abortion. In addition, through the Alan Guttmacher Institute (AGI) the availability of abortion services has been monitored periodically. There is now almost a decade of nationwide data collection that provides information about the number of abortions performed, the demographic characteristics of the women who have abortions, the stage of pregnancy at which the abortion is performed, the type of procedure used, the site of performance, and the availability of services. Mortality associated with abortion has also been analyzed in relation to these factors. We will present some of the highlights of this information.

There has been a consistent increase in the number of abortions since 1972, when the number of abortions was approximately 750,000,

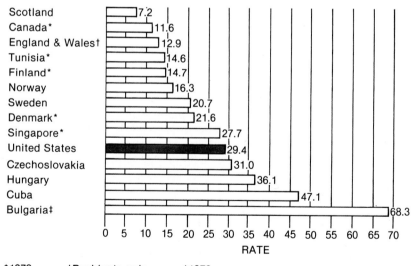

*1979   †Residents only   ‡1978

Figure 5–10 Rates of legal abortion per 1,000 women aged 15–44, various countries, 1980. (Sources: C. Tietze, *Induced Abortion: A World Review,* The Population Council, New York, 1981; and data collected by C. Tietze from various sources.) (From Henshaw, S. K., Forrest, J. P., Sullivan, E., and Tietze, C.: Abortion services in the United States, 1979 and 1980. *Family Planning Perspectives 14:*6, 1982.)

or 16.5 per 1000 women aged 15 to 44 years. The increase slowed during the late 1970s, and in 1980 (a year in which there were 3.6 million births and 1.5 million abortions) the abortion rate stabilized at about 30 abortions per 1000 women aged 15 to 44 years. In 1980, 30 per cent of all pregnancies ended in induced abortion, and this represented about half of all the unintended pregnancies. Put another way, one of every two unintended pregnancies went to term.

Figure 5–10 shows the position of the United States in relation to other countries in rate of abortion. It is plain that the rate of the United States is higher than those of the United Kingdom and Scandinavian countries but substantially lower than the rates of Cuba and Bulgaria. The overall rate for the United States masks an ethnic differential, with abortion rates about three times as high for blacks as for whites. Another typical characteristic of women who receive abortions is that they are young—almost one third are under 19 years of age and another third are between 20 and 24. Also, most of them (70 per cent) are unmarried.

Over the past decade, there has been an increase in early abortions, and by 1978 half of all abortions were done before nine weeks of gestation. It is fortunate that abortions are being performed at this early stage of gestation, because the death-to-case rate for legal abortions is lowest at or before eight weeks of gestation. The overall death rate at eight weeks' gestation is 0.6 deaths per 100,000 abortions, and it then climbs steadily according to increasing duration of pregnancy (MMWR, 1979).

There has also been a trend to do fewer abortions in hospitals. In 1973, half of all abortions were performed in hospitals; in 1980, less than a quarter of all abortions were done in hospitals, the remainder being performed in free-standing health centers. A 1980 AGI survey indicated that despite recent advances many women still lack the availability of abortion services (Henshaw et al., 1982).

Interest has also centered on the comparative mortality from childbirth and abortion. The data for making this comparison have to be adjusted because of differences in demographic and medical characteristics between women whose pregnancies go to full-term and those who seek abortions. When this was done (LeBolt et al., 1982), it was found that between 1972 and 1978 the relative risk of death from childbirth was seven times greater than the risk from abortion, and the gap widened during the second half of the decade. The MMWR has confirmed the low risk of death from legal abortion. In 1979, it reported an overall risk of two deaths per 100,000 procedures, in contrast to the 10.6 deaths per 100,000 women from pregnancy- and childbirth-related causes.

Obviously there are many religious, ethical, legal, and political factors involved in abortion, all of which affect the allocation of public resources to abortion services. The complexity of such issues places them outside the scope of this text.

LIFE EXPECTANCY

Life expectancy, the average number of years an individual is expected to live, is a very important summary measure for comparing death rates within and between countries and over time. One practical application of this measure is its use for life insurance purposes.

The term "life expectancy" is generally used to refer to expectation of life at birth, the average number of years of life that a newborn infant is expected to live. However, expectation of life can be calculated for any age. Expectation at age 20, for example, indicates the average number of remaining years of life for those who have attained the age of 20.

There has been an impressive change in life expectancy in the United States since the turn of the century. On the average, white males born in 1900 could expect to live only 48 years. By 1981, life expectancy for this group had increased to 71 years. While similar increases have occurred for all race-sex groups, life expectancy has consistently been highest for white females and lowest for nonwhite males. For 1981, these rates were 78.5 and 66.1 years, respectively.

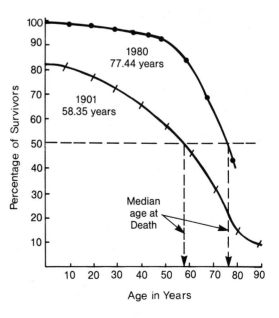

Figure 5–11 Percentage of survivors at specified ages from the life tables of 1900 and 1980. (Median age at death, 1901, 58.35 years; 1980, 77.44 years.)

The biggest advance has come from the salvage of life in infancy and early childhood. Both the expectation of life and the percentage of survivors at different ages (Fig. 5–11) for children born in 1980 are higher than for those born in 1901. This advance is reflected also in the change over time in the median length of life, the age at which half of a cohort remains alive and half have died. This measure of survival increased from 58.4 years in the 1901 life table to 77.4 years in 1980.

There has been proportionately less change in the expectation of life for those who survive to middle age. Figure 5–11 suggests that there has been relatively little progress in extending the lifespan, a reflection primarily of the toll of cardiovascular disease and cancer.

As might be expected, the populations of different countries vary greatly in life expectancy. Table 5–5 shows the extent of international variation in life expectancy for a few selected countries during approximately the same time period. The range of values for expectation of life at birth varies from approximately 35 to more than 75 years of life for females. Note also that expectation of life is appreciably greater for females than for males in demographically advanced countries. In contrast, in India the expectation of life is slightly less for women than for men, which probably reflects the hazards associated with pregnancy and childbirth.

Life expectancy is calculated from tables known as *demographic life tables*. These tables are constructed from current age-specific death rates as if these rates would remain unchanged throughout the lifetime of the cohort, about 85 or more years. That is, life expectancy for infants born in 1980 is calculated from 1980 age-specific death rates even though the 1980 birth cohort will, as it ages, be subjected to the

TABLE 5–5 Expectation of Life at Specified Ages by Sex for Selected Countries

Area and Period	Sex	Expectation of Life in Years at Age				
		0	1	5	30	60
Ghana						
African population	M	37.08	47.95	45.46	29.83	11.6
196	F	—	—	—	—	—
Guatemala	M	48.29	52.49	54.4	35.53	14.77
1963–65	F	49.74	53.37	55.8	36.9	14.67
India	M	41.89	48.42	48.72	29.03	11.77
1951–60	F	40.55	46.02	47.01	27.86	12.98
Netherlands	M	71.2	71.1	67.4	43.4	17.0
1971–75	F	77.2	77.0	73.1	48.7	21.0
Canada	M	69.34	69.76	66.02	42.5	16.95
1970–72	F	76.36	76.56	72.79	48.51	21.39
United States	M	68.7	68.9	65.1	41.7	16.8
1975	F	76.5	76.6	72.8	48.5	21.8

age-specific rates prevailing in 1990, 2000, and so on. This limits the accuracy with which demographic life tables can predict life expectancy over the lifetime of the cohort.

MEASUREMENT OF DISABILITY

Most of this chapter has focussed on measures of mortality. While these measures tell us much about a society, they convey little information about the quality of life. Information that life expectancy is high in a given population does not tell us whether the population is predominantly well or is heavily burdened with chronically ill or disabled individuals.

It is only recently that life expectancy has increased to the point where concern has become focussed on functional measures of ill-health. For many years, statistics have been available from public agencies on persons with severe impairments (e.g., blindness, severe physical disability). More recently, information is becoming available on more subtle deviations from optimal function, and on the extent and causes of such problems.

Disability can be defined in a variety of ways. For insurance purposes, disability is usually defined as inability to engage in gainful employment. The National Health Interview Survey defines *disability* more broadly as "any temporary or long-term reduction of a person's activity as a result of an acute or chronic condition." It specifies three measures of disability. The most general is the "restricted-activity day," defined as follows:

Restricted-activity day — one on which a person cuts down on his usual activity for the whole of that day on account of an illness or injury.

Within this general definition, more severe restrictions of activity are specified by the work-loss day and the bed-disability day:

Work-loss day — one on which a person would have worked but instead lost an entire work day because of an illness or injury.

Bed-disability day — one on which a person stays in bed for all or most of the day (i.e., more than half the daylight hours). Hospital days are classed as bed-disability days even if the person is ambulatory within the hospital.

The National Health Interview Survey has produced much information on extent of disability for the population as a whole and for subgroups according to age, sex, geographic region, race, and family income. In 1981, for example, the overall yearly average per person was 19.1 days of restricted activity; of these, 4.9 were work-loss days, 5.3 were school-loss days, and 6.9 were bed-disability days. Disability rates are higher for nonwhites than for whites, and within racial groups, for

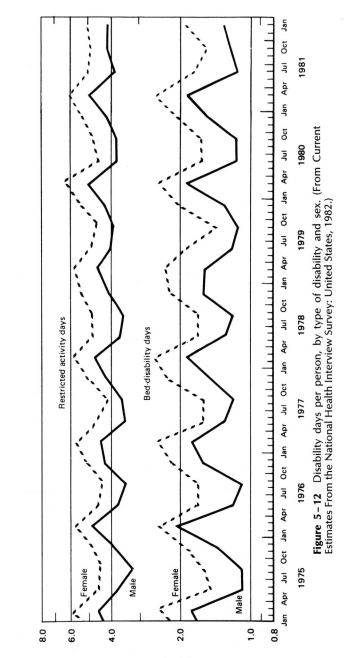

Figure 5–12 Disability days per person, by type of disability and sex. (From Current Estimates From the National Health Interview Survey: United States, 1982.)

low-income compared to high-income families (National Health Interview Survey, 1981).

The average number of restricted-activity and bed-disability days per person per quarter-year over a six-year period is shown in Figure 5-12. The marked seasonality can be attributed mainly to seasonal fluctuations in acute diseases, especially respiratory conditions.

OTHER HEALTH-RELATED INFORMATION

Additional types of information relevant to the general mental, physical, and socioeconomic health of a community are available from a variety of sources—vital statistics, the United States census, data routinely collected by health and mental health departments and law enforcement agencies, and surveys of the labor force. These indices may be categorized according to the age-group and stage of life-cycle that they reflect (Table 5-6). While many of these are not direct measures of health and the supporting data are often incomplete, they are important indices of the quality of life in a community and may indicate deviations from "complete physical, mental and social well-being" (WHO, 1948).

Of particular concern is the "nesting" of health and social problems in certain areas, both urban and rural, and in certain "hard core" families. This was demonstrated in a classic study that showed that 6 per cent of the families in St. Paul, Minnesota, absorbed 25 per cent of the total social and health service efforts (Buell et al., 1952). An ecological analysis of Baltimore by Klee et al. (1967) combined data from the Maryland Psychiatric Case Register and the 1960 census with information supplied by a variety of agencies. This analysis showed that census tracts that ranked high on various indices of poverty, social disorganization, and public health problems tended also to have high total psychiatric admission rates. In one tract (1960 population of 1400, mainly white) there were 48 arrests per 100 adults yearly, a three-year tuberculosis morbidity rate of 1 per 100, and a three-year psychiatric admission rate of 11 per 100.

The difficulties of elucidating the etiologic relationships in such a complex of medical and social pathology are noted in relation to schizophrenia on page 129. To what extent does living in this tract cause a high arrest, tuberculosis, or psychiatric admission rate? To what extent do the high rates represent the drift or migration to this area of persons already incapacitated mentally and physically? Whatever the contribution of each factor, the findings certainly underscore the need for comprehensive approaches to the measurement of health.

TABLE 5-6 Health Indices in Relation to Stage of Life-Cycle

Stage of Life-Cycle	Community Health Index
Conception to Birth	Infertility rate
	Rate of fetal loss
	Rate of perinatal loss
	Proportion of mothers with no or inadequate pre- natal care
Infancy to Childhood	Perinatal mortality
	Infant mortality
	Rate of congenital malformations
	Rate of low birth weight
	Illegitimacy Rate
	Immunization status and injuries
Childhood to Adolescence	Immunization and injuries
	Growth and development
	Learning disabilities
	Nutrition
	Smoking/alcohol/drug use
	Rates of crime and juvenile delinquency
	Sexual activity and rates of sexually transmitted disease
Adults	Marriage and divorce rates
	Rate of unemployment
	Adult crime
	Drug and alcohol use
	Smoking status
	Utilization of psychiatric facilities
	Proportion of population in substandard housing
	Proportion of population living below poverty level
Older Adults (Senior Citizens)	Economic status
	Activities of daily living (functional level)
	Proportion living alone
	Proportion living in institutions

SUMMARY

In this chapter, we focussed on the major measures of morbidity and mortality needed for epidemiologic study and for monitoring the health status of a community. Death rates from all causes were noted, as were trends in cause-specific death rates. Cause-specific death rates are fundamental to epidemiologic knowledge and control programs. Proportionate mortality ratio (i.e., proportion of all deaths due to a disease) was contrasted with the death rate from a disease; only the latter indicates risk of death.

We next reviewed indices related to early life. The infant mortality rate is an indicator not only of the adequacy of medical care but also of general conditions of health, nutrition, and education. It is to this early period that preventive measures should be directed. Reproductive care should be viewed as a continuum, extending from preparation for pregnancy, through childrearing and child spacing.

There has been a marked decline in the maternal mortality rate, particularly for nonwhites. Factors related to maternal risk include age of the mother and parity, as well as adequacy of medical care. The widespread use of contraceptives and liberalization of the restrictions against abortion have had a significant impact on decreasing this rate.

Finally, life expectancy, a measure that summarizes current levels of mortality, was described. While life expectancy has changed markedly largely owing to reduction of death in infancy and early life, it is apparent that there has been no significant extension of the lifespan of man during this century. The international ranking of the United States on several measures indicates that advances being achieved elsewhere are yet to be made here.

The chapter concluded with a discussion of measures of the quality of life, such as disability rates and indices of other health-related problems. The nesting of problems in certain families and areas was also noted.

REFERENCES

Beral, V.: An epidemiological study of recent trends in ectopic pregnancy. Br. J. Obstet. Gynecol., *82*:775, 1975.

Buell, B., et al.: Community Planning for Human Services. Columbia University Press, New York, 1952.

The Centers for Disease Control: Morbidity and Mortality Weekly Report. Annual Summary 1979. U.S. Dept HHS. Vol. 28, No. 54, Sept. 1980.

The Centers for Disease Control Cancer and Steroid Hormone Study: Oral contraceptive use and the risk of ovarian cancer. JAMA, *249*:1956, 1983a.

The Centers for Disease Control Cancer and Steroid Hormone Study: Oral contraceptive use and the risk of endometrial cancer. JAMA, *249*:1600, 1983b.

The Centers for Disease Control Cancer and Steroid Hormone Study: Long term oral contraceptive use and the risk of breast cancer. JAMA, *249*:1591, 1983c.

Constitution of the World Health Organization, 1948. *In* Basic Documents, 15th Ed., WHO, Geneva, 1964.

Guyer, B., Wallach, L. A., and Rosen, S. L.: Birth-weight–standardized neonatal mortality rates and the prevention of low birth weight: How does Massachusetts compare with Sweden? N. Engl. J. Med., *306*:1230, 1982.

Hellman, L. M.: Conception control as a health practice: An emerging concept in government and medicine. Perspec. Biol. Med., *16*:357, 1973.

Henshaw, S. K., Forrest, J. D., Sullivan, E., and Tietze, C.; Abortion services in the United States, 1979 and 1980. Family Planning Perspectives, *14*:6, 1982.

Herron, M. A., Katz, M., and Creasy, R. K.: Evaluation of a preterm birth prevention program: Preliminary report. Obstet. Gynecol., *59*:452, 1982.

Klee, G. D., Spiro, E., et al.: An Ecological Analysis of Diagnosed Mental Illness in Baltimore in Psychiatric Epidemiology and Mental Health Planning. *In* Monroe, R. R., Klee, G. D., et al. (Eds.): American Psychiatric Association (Psychiatric Research Report No. 22), 1967.

LeBolt, S. A., Grimes, D. A., and Cates, W.: Mortality from abortion and childbirth. Are the populations comparable? JAMA, *248*:188, 1982.

Mishell, D. R., Jr.: Intrauterine devices: Medicated and nonmedicated. Int. J. Gynaecol. Obstet., *16*:482, 1979.

National Health Survey: Health Household—Interview Survey. USPHS Pub. No. 584–A3, U.S. Govt. Printing Office, Washington, D.C., 1972.

National Health Interview Survey 1981, The National Center for Health Statistics. Unpublished data.

Ory, H. W., and the Women's Health Study. Ectopic pregnancy and intrauterine contraceptive devices: New perspectives. J. Am. Coll. Obstet. Gynecol., *57*:137, 1981.

Sartwell, P. E., Masi, A. T., et al.: Thromboembolism and oral contraceptives: An epidemiologic case-control study. Am. J. Epidemiol., *90*:365, 1969.

Sullivan, D. F.: A single index of mortality and morbidity. HSHMA Health Rep., *86*:347, 1971.

Thomas, D. B.: Relationship of oral contraceptives to cervical carcinogenesis. Obstet. Gynecol., *40*:508, 1972.

Tietze, C., and Lewit, S.: Life risks associated with reversible methods of fertility regulation. Int. J. Gynaecol. Obstet., *16*:456, 1979.

Vessey, M. P., and Doll, R.: Investigation of relation between use of oral contraceptives and thromboembolic disease. Br. Med. J., 2:199, 1968.

Weström, L., Bengtsson, L. P. H., and Mardh, P. A.: Incidence, trends, and risks of ectopic pregnancy in a population of women. Br. Med. J., *282*:15, 1981.

DESCRIPTIVE EPIDEMIOLOGY: PERSON, PLACE, AND TIME

6

It is customary to consider epidemiologic studies as falling into two broad categories: study of the *amount* and *distribution* of disease within a population by person, place, and time (called **descriptive** epidemiology) and more focussed study of the *determinants* of disease or *reasons* for relatively high or low frequency in specific groups (called **analytic** epidemiology). This chapter will focus on descriptive epidemiology. Descriptive epidemiology identifies nonrandom variations in the distribution of disease to enable an investigator to generate testable hypotheses regarding etiology.

To describe the occurrence of a disease fully, some broad questions must be answered: **Who** is affected? **Where** and **when** do the cases occur? In other words, it is necessary to specify **person, place,** and **time.**

PERSON

Although people may be characterized with respect to an almost infinite number of variables, in practice the number must be limited according to the purposes and resources of the specific study and the information available. In epidemiologic study it is almost routine to specify three characteristics of a person — age, sex, and ethnic group or race. These demographic variables will be discussed first.

Age

Overall, age is the most important determinant among the personal variables. Mortality and morbidity rates of almost all conditions show some relation to this variable. We will first consider relation of age to mortality. Figure 6–1 shows death rates from all causes in the United States by age, sex, and race. Compare the relative impact of these three variables on death rate.

The four curves portraying age-specific death rates for each race-sex group are quite similar; all are J-shaped. In all four groups the death rate is fairly high in infancy, then decreases markedly, reaching its lowest point between ages 5 and 14. The rate then climbs gradually until age 40, after which it increases almost exponentially, virtually doubling with each decade. These sharp differences in death rate by age make it necessary to correct ("adjust") for any differences in age composition of population groups if their death rates are to be compared (see p. 339).

We turn now to a consideration of the relationship of age to patterns of morbidity. In general, chronic conditions tend to increase with age whereas the relation of age to acute infectious diseases is less consistent.

Young children readily acquire acute respiratory infections. Maternal antibodies transmitted during fetal life protect the infant for approximately the first half-year after birth. Thereafter, protection wanes and the number of respiratory infections increases, tending to peak in the period when the child starts to attend school.

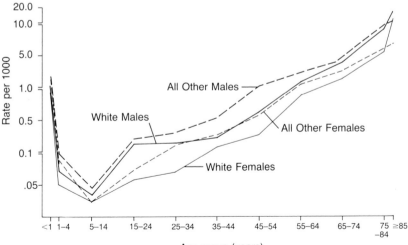

Figure 6–1 Death rates per 1000 by age, color and sex, United States, 1980. (Note: graph is on a semilogarithmic scale.) (Data from National Center for Health Statistics: Vital Statistics of the United States. Vols. I and II. U.S. Govt. Printing Office, Washington, D.C., 1980.)

Before immunization against infectious disease was available, the infections that conferred lifelong immunity (e.g., measles, chickenpox, mumps) occurred mainly in young children. As immunization programs were developed and patterns of immunity in the population changed, there were changes in modal age of infection. For example, measles used to be primarily a disease of preschool children. In more recent years the peak has occurred later, between 5 and 15 years of age. Figure 6–2 depicts schematized age curves for several diseases, to demonstrate the marked differences in age that are possible. Note, for example, the peak incidence of California encephalitis in preschoolers, of measles and mumps in older children, of rubella in adolescents, and of legionnaires' disease in older people (primarily males).

The age and sex distribution of certain infections reflects occupational exposure; an example would be brucellosis or anthrax in adult males who are exposed to the agents of these diseases in the course of their work. The striking age-sex distribution of cases of brucellosis in a Midwestern agricultural state in the late 1940s is shown in Figure 6–3.

Age is related not only to the *frequency* of infectious disease but also to *severity*. Certain organisms, e.g., Pneumococcus and Salmonella, tend to produce particularly severe disease in the very young, the very old, and the debilitated. Newborns and the aged are particularly sensitive to

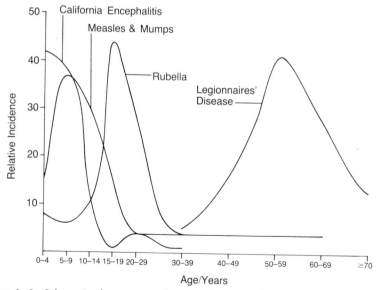

Figure 6–2 Schematized age curves for several acute infectious diseases. (Data from Centers for Disease Control. Morbidity and Mortality Weekly Report Annual Summary, 1981. Vol. 30, October, 1982.) Centers For Disease Control. Morbidity and Mortality Weekly Report. 27:439, 1978.)

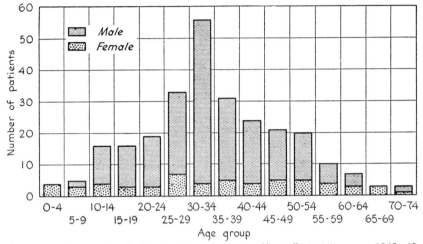

Figure 6–3 Age-sex distribution of 268 proven cases of brucellosis, Minnesota, 1945–48. (From Magoffin, R. L., Kohler, P. et al.: An epidemiologic study of brucellosis in Minnesota. Public Health Rep., 64:1021, 1949.)

bacteria, such as coliform organisms and *Staphylococcus aureus*, which are usually nonpathogenic in other age groups.

Age is related to deaths from noninfectious as well as infectious causes. The finding of a high rate of injury in a specific age group can identify a particular health hazard. For example, Karwacki and Baker (1979) noted that children under the age of 1 year were overrepresented among all motor vehicle deaths of children under age 15 (Fig. 6–4). The figure shows death and injury rates by year of age. Overall injury rate did not vary much by age, but the death rate for infants under

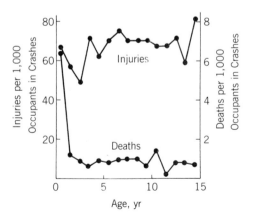

Figure 6–4 Deaths and injuries in Maryland automobile crashes. (From Karwack; J. J., and Baker, S. P.: Children in motor vehicles. Never too young to die. J.A.M.A., 242:2848, 1979.)

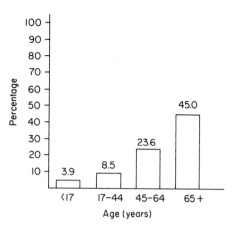

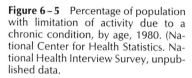
Figure 6–5 Percentage of population with limitation of activity due to a chronic condition, by age, 1980. (National Center for Health Statistics. National Health Interview Survey, unpublished data.

age 1 was much higher than for children between ages 1 and 14. Further, it was found that head injuries predominated in the group under age 1. This finding became the basis for a widespread crusade to restrain infants in specially designed carriers. Some examples of public enthusiasm in this campaign are the practice of sending infants home from the hospital in carriers, instead of in the mother's lap, and the slogan "Let the first ride be a safe ride."

The tendency for chronic diseases to increase with age is shown in Figure 6–5, which depicts the proportion of the general population in different age groups who, on home interviews, reported having a limitation of activity due to one or more chronic conditions. The effect of age on frequency of certain diseases is especially marked. For example, "arthritis" is ten times more common among persons 45 to 64 than among those under 45 and the rate doubles again for those 65 and over. Other ills that befall people as they age are dental problems — edentia and periodontal disease. One-third of persons 65 and over have no teeth, and less than 10 per cent are free of periodontal disease.

Sex

The most striking aspect of analysis of disease rates by sex is the contrast between mortality and morbidity rates. Death rates are higher for males than females, but morbidity rates are generally higher in females.

Figure 6–1 shows that death rates from all causes are higher for males than for females at every age; this is true of both whites and nonwhites. In utero and neonatal death rates are also higher for males. The higher death rates for males throughout life may be due to sex-linked inheritance or to differences in hormonal balance, environment,

TABLE 6–1 Ratio of Age-Adjusted Death Rates for 15 Leading Causes of Death, by Sex*

Cause of Death	Ratio of Male Rate to Female Rate
All causes	1.80
Homicide and legal intervention	3.88
Chronic obstructive pulmonary disease	3.13
Suicide	3.05
Accidents and adverse effects	2.96
Chronic liver disease and cirrhosis	2.19
Diseases of the heart	2.01
Pneumonia and influenza	1.86
Nephritis, nephrotic syndrome, and nephrosis	1.58
Malignant neoplasms	1.51
Septicemia	1.40
Atherosclerosis	1.29
Certain conditions originating in the perinatal period	1.26
Cerebrovascular diseases	1.19
Congenital anomalies	1.15
Diabetes mellitus	1.04

* From National Center for Health Statistics. Advance Report, Final Mortality Statistics, 1979. U.S. Govt. Printing Office, Washington, D.C., September 1982.

or habit patterns. The sex-differential varies greatly for specific disease entities, as shown in Table 6–1, ranging from a male-to-female ratio of almost four for homicides and three for chronic respiratory disease to near-equality for diabetes mellitus. The sex difference is not as large for ischemic heart disease as for certain other conditions. However, because this condition accounts for such a high proportion of deaths, the excess mortality in males from this cause alone is tremendous.

As we indicated earlier, the higher mortality rates for men are not paralleled by higher rates of illness. Data from several sources indicate that, in almost all age groups and for a number of different conditions, women have more episodes of illness and more physician contacts than men have (i.e., 5.2 physician visits per woman per year compared with 4.0 for men in 1981). This is true for women over 45 as well as those in the reproductive years of life (National Center for Health Statistics). Possible explanations for the relatively high morbidity and low mortality in women are (1) that women seek medical care more freely and perhaps at an earlier stage of disease and (2) that the same disease will tend to have a less lethal course in women than in men.

A good example of male-female differences in pattern of disease and death is depression. Rates of depression were found to be almost twice as high in women as in men (Eaton and Kessler, 1981), and the rate of attempted suicide is also higher in women. However, completed sui-

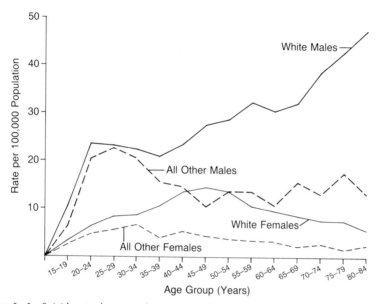

Figure 6 – 6   Suicide rates by age, color, and sex, 1974. (From the National Center for Health Statistics, Vol. IIA, U.S. Govt. Printing Office, Washington, D.C., 1978.)

cides are more common in men, particularly among the elderly (Fig. 6 – 6).

An example of extreme sex differences in incidence of disease is seen in the occurrence of toxic shock syndrome, a recently identified syndrome of great severity. A study carried out in Wisconsin from 1975 to 1980 (Davis et al., 1980) revealed that 37 of the 38 cases occurred in women; there was only one male patient.

Ethnic Group and Race

The classification and recording of data by ethnic group or race present conceptual and practical difficulties. Nevertheless, even though it is controversial, such classification has been traditional in health statistics, since (1) many diseases differ markedly in frequency, severity, or both in different racial groups, and (2) statistics by race are helpful for identifying health problems. The fact that many of the observed differences are related to differences in socioeconomic status does not detract from the usefulness of race as an indicator of groups with particular deficiencies in health care.

In 1980, 83.1 per cent of the United States population was classified as white, 11.7 per cent as black, and 5.2 per cent as "other" (i.e., American Indian, Japanese, Chinese, Filipino). The nonwhite popula-

TABLE 6-2 Vital Statistics of the United States, 1980*

	Total Population	White	Black & Other
Mortality Rates			
Infant	12.6	11.0	21.4
Neonatal (<28 days)	8.5	7.5	14.1
Fetal death ratio	9.1	8.1	14.5
Maternal (per 100,000 live births)	9.2	6.7	21.5
Life Expectancy at Birth (yrs)	73.7		
Male		70.0	63.7
Female		78.1	72.3

* From National Center for Health Statistics. Advanced Report, Final Mortality Statistics, 1980. U.S. Govt. Printing Office, Washington, D.C., August, 1983.

tion in the United States is at a marked disadvantage with respect to mortality, as shown in Table 6-2; every major index shows higher rates for nonwhites. Figure 6-1 shows that nonwhites had higher death rates than whites for each age-sex group until the age of 80, after which whites had higher rates. The gap between blacks and whites has been narrowing in past years but clearly is far from obliterated.

Certain racial differences in morbidity and mortality are noteworthy. Blacks have substantially higher rates (adjusted for differences in age composition) of deaths caused by hypertensive heart disease, cerebrovascular accidents, tuberculosis, syphilis, homicide, and accidental death. Whites have higher rates of death from arteriosclerotic heart disease, suicide (see Fig. 6-6), and leukemia. On the other hand, cancer of the cervix is markedly higher in blacks, so much so that it is a leading cause of cancer deaths in black females. In contrast, cancer of the breast is appreciably higher in whites. As previously noted, some racial differences, such as the virtual restriction of sickle cell anemia to blacks, are genetically determined. Conversely, Ewing's sarcoma is almost absent from black populations throughout the world. However, many differences in rates of disease and death reflect at least in part differences in various environmental exposures, in lifestyle, and in the extent and quality of medical care.

Like race, ethnic stock is a variable whose effect must be separated from the effects of environment. Studies of international migrants have been particularly valuable for this purpose. Any differences in rates of disease between migrants and those who remained at home must be interpreted cautiously, since migrants are usually self-selected. When the differences are marked, the importance of environment in development of disease is suggested. For example, the rate of cancer of the stomach is very high in Japan. The appreciably higher rate for native Japanese than for Japanese descendants in the United States suggests that an environmental factor is important in the etiology of this disease (Haenszel and Kurihara, 1968; Buell and Dunn, 1965).

While the "melting pot" effect in the United States has tended to reduce differences in lifestyle among the many ethnic groups in the population, there is still variation in patterns of disease, part of which may be attributed to cultural differences. For example, alcoholism is markedly less common among Jews than among many other ethnic groups, although increasing remoteness from old world religious patterns among Jews born in this country is reducing the difference in patterns of alcohol use (Snyder, 1958).

Social Class

Social class is a widely used concept for ranking or stratifying a total population into subgroups that differ from each other in prestige, wealth, and power. These three dimensions are usually related; a person high in one tends to be high in the others, and vice versa. Despite some discrepancies among the dimensions of social class (e.g., in the United States university professors and skilled blue collar workers differ more in prestige than in income), the concept of "class" is a useful summarizing variable linking occupation, education, area of residence, income, and, in fact, total lifestyle. In view of the pervasiveness of social class in so many aspects of life, it is not surprising that a marked gradient by class in morbidity and mortality is the rule rather than the exception in

TABLE 6-3 Mortality Rates by Social Class 1970-1972: Men Aged 15-64 and Infant Mortality by Sex*

Social Class	Crude Death[1] Rate	Age-Standardized Death Rates	Standardized Mortality Ratios (SMRs)	Infant Mortality Rate[2] Male	Female
I Professional	399	462	77	14	10
II Intermediate	554	486	81	15	12
III Nonmanual, skilled	580	591	99	17	12
III Manual, skilled	608	633	106	19	15
IV Partly skilled	797	681	114	22	17
V Unskilled	989	832	137	35	27
All men[3] aged 15-64, all infants	597	597	100	20	15

[1] Deaths per 100,000 men per year.
[2] Deaths per 1000 live births.
[3] Includes those not assigned to a social class.
* From Great Britain Office of Population Censuses and Surveys: Occupational Mortality: The Registrar General's Decennial Supplement for England and Wales, 1970-72. H. M. Stationery Off., London, 1978.

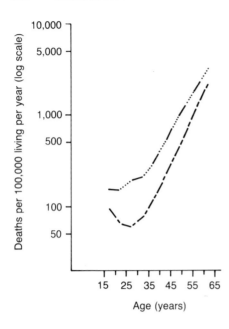

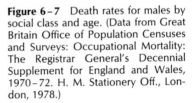

Figure 6–7 Death rates for males by social class and age. (Data from Great Britain Office of Population Censuses and Surveys: Occupational Mortality: The Registrar General's Decennial Supplement for England and Wales, 1970–72. H. M. Stationery Off., London, 1978.)

epidemiologic studies. For a comprehensive survey of the historical literature on life expectancy and mortality by social class, Antonovsky (1972) may be consulted.

Because of practical considerations, occupation alone is often used in epidemiologic studies as a measure of overall socioeconomic status. In Great Britain for over a hundred years it has been customary to present social and health data in terms of five well-defined occupational ("social") classes. A very large body of information has thus been developed. Table 6–3 shows the classification scheme, along with deaths from all causes for males and infant mortality rates. Both the infant mortality rates and the mortality of adult males show a distinct class gradient. Further analysis of social class differences by age (Fig. 6–7) shows that the differential for deaths from all causes according to social class is greater for younger than for older males.

In the United States, the relatively poor health status of blacks is probably due largely to the fact that a disproportionate number of blacks live in conditions of poverty. The median family income of blacks in 1980 was $12,670 as compared to $21,900 for white families. In that year, one-third of the black population and only one-tenth of the white was living below the poverty level. A marked gradient in mortality rate among nonwhites by occupational level (Guralnick, 1962) confirms that socioeconomic status contributes importantly to differentials by race. Of

course, nutritional status, crowding, and personal hygiene also contribute to the differential.

Poverty affects utilization of medical care services for a variety of reasons. In addition to having limited financial resources and restricted access to medical care, the poor tend to underutilize available preventive services. Motivation to seek such care entails a concern about present health, and about future health problems. Surveys of perceived needs among the urban poor show that problems such as unemployment and inadequate housing are so overwhelming that health needs tend to have relatively low priority.

The relationship between economic status and health care can be clearly identified in Figure 6–8, which shows opposing trends for number of teeth filled and number of teeth decayed in American children 6 to 11 years of age, grouped according to family income.

With respect to mental illness, a heavy concentration of schizophrenia in the lowest social classes of urban communities has been found in a number of studies. Two conflicting hypotheses have been developed to account for this phenomenon. According to the *breeder* hypothesis, the conditions of life in lower class society contribute to the development of schizophrenia (Faris and Dunham, 1939). The other explanation, the *drift* hypothesis, states that the inverse relationship between rate of schizophrenia and social class exists not because low socioeconomic status predisposes to schizophrenia, but because the illness itself leads to a downward drift in potential for employment and hence in socioeconomic position. Strong evidence has been developed in support of the

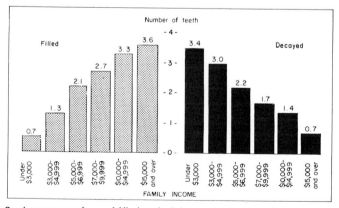

Figure 6–8 Average numbers of filled and of decayed primary and permanent teeth per child aged 6–11, by family income, United States, 1963–65. (From the Health of Children. Selected data from the National Center for Health Statistics, U.S. Govt. Printing Office, Washington, D.C., 1970, p. 37.)

drift hypothesis (Goldberg and Morrison, 1963; Dunham, 1965), and Birtchnell (1971) found that downward mobility is not limited to schizophrenia but is generally true of all psychoses except depressive psychosis. Actually both these mechanisms may contribute to a social class gradient through a complex set of interrelations to which genetic susceptibility probably contributes. In addition, the association between low social class and schizophrenia may result from class-related differences in labelling, with such cases in the upper social classes more likely to be called "affective illness."

Social class is related to mental illness in other ways as well. In 1958, Hollingshead and Redlich published a study of the relationship between social class and treated mental illness in New Haven. Not only did they find the social class gradient previously described, but they also documented important differences by class in the setting and type of treatment provided. It is also likely that a person's social class will influence whether or not he receives care for psychiatric illness. The Midtown Study in New York City (Srole et al., 1962), which surveyed a sample of the general population, found that for persons severely impaired on a global rating of mental health, the proportion receiving treatment was 19 per cent for upper class, 4 per cent for middle class, but only 1 per cent for lower class subjects. It is clear from this that rates of mental illness based only on persons known to treatment facilities would be quite misleading.

Occupation

Since people spend a substantial portion of their lives at work under widely differing conditions, it is not surprising that occupationally related experiences can exert a profound effect on health and contribute to large differences in mortality (Maclure and MacMahon, 1980) and morbidity rates. This influence may occur through a variety of exposures— unfavorable physical conditions (heat, cold, changed atmospheric pressure), chemicals, noise, occupationally induced stress. On the other hand, rates of disease among occupational groups may differ not because of the work itself but because of differential selection into various occupations.

Epidemiologic investigation has related many specific diseases to occupational exposures. Among them are pulmonary fibrosis from exposure to free silica (SiO_2) (Trasko, 1958), mesothelioma and lung and gastrointestinal cancers in asbestos workers (Selikoff et al., 1968), bladder cancer in workers exposed to aniline dyes (Case et al., 1954), and lung cancer among chromate workers (Brinton et al., 1952).

Workers in mining, construction, and agriculture have high rates of injury and death from trauma. In another sense, however, the occupa-

tions that are associated with physical activity may be protective. There is some evidence (Morris and Crawford, 1958; Mann et al., 1965) that working in an occupation that demands physical exertion protects against coronary heart disease. Morris and co-workers (1973) have demonstrated that vigorous leisure-time physical activity can serve the same function.

The occupational milieu includes not only physical surroundings but also a social and psychologic climate, an important aspect of which is the degree of stress of the job. Except for extreme conditions, stress is difficult to quantify; a situation that is extremely stressful to one individual may be emotionally neutral for another. To test possible effects of stress on health, Cobb and Rose (1973) selected for study a group incontrovertibly subject to a high level of occupational stress, air traffic controllers. The work of this group is unusually stressful because of the constant vigilance required and the potentially disastrous effects of errors in judgment. When the health records of the controllers were compared with a control group, the controllers were found to have higher rates of hypertension, peptic ulcer, and possibly diabetes.

If specific occupational risks are identified and corrective programs instituted, then successive groups of workers can be followed to determine whether the risk has been eliminated. Seltser and Sartwell (1965) studied the mortality experience of several medical specialty groups to test whether occupational exposure to radiation shortens life. Three specialty groups were selected — radiologists, internists, and ophthalmologists-otolaryngologists — to provide a gradient of occupationally related exposure to radiation. Mortality was analyzed for two time periods, 1935 to 1944 and 1955 to 1958. It could be expected that the level of occupational exposure would have declined in the interval.

In the earlier period, the predicted gradient in mortality was noted in all age groups; radiologists had the highest death rates, the ophthalmologists and otolaryngologists the lowest. In the later period there was still a difference among the older physicians, but not among the younger ones. A follow-up study (Matanoski et al., 1975) confirmed the absence of excess mortality in radiologists. This study, which is basically analytic rather than descriptive, is cited here to illustrate the effects of occupational exposure on health and the way in which disease and death rates can be used to monitor health hazards.

In interpreting differences in morbidity and mortality among occupational groups, it must be remembered that state of health itself may determine entry into a specific occupation. Undemanding jobs may attract people in poor health, and demanding jobs selectively include only those in good health.

Occupational selection was demonstrated by Morris and his colleagues in studies done to test the hypothesis that physical activity at

work protects against coronary heart disease (CHD). In one study, coronary heart disease rates were compared for drivers and conductors of the London transport system (Morris et al., 1953). The drivers spend the day sitting; the conductors are much more active. The rate of CHD was found to be lower among the conductors. However, there was also evidence that the two groups differed initially. By obtaining indirect measures of physique through records of the sizes of uniforms issued to the men, an approach labelled "the epidemiology of uniforms," Morris demonstrated that drivers were more corpulent than conductors even in their twenties (Morris et al., 1956).

The subject of occupational epidemiology is now of such importance that a separate chapter has been devoted to it (see Chap. 12).

Marital Status

It has been observed repeatedly over the past hundred years that marital status is associated with level of mortality for both sexes. Death rates, for most specific diseases and from all causes combined, have generally been found to vary from lowest to highest in the following order: married, single, widowed, and divorced. Although better health of the married may be attributed in part to the psychologic and physical support provided by the spouse, the more favorable health record may not be due entirely to the effects of being married. Selective factors also influence marital status; people who get married may be more robust physically or emotionally than those who remain single. Misclassification of marital status on death certificates or in the census (Sheps, 1961; Berkson, 1962) may also contribute to the reported differences.

For women, marital status may also be related to health through differences in sexual exposure, pregnancy, childbearing, and lactation. These etiologic factors differ in relative importance in different diseases. For example, in cancer of the cervix, a disease more common in married than single women, early sexual experience and multiple partners appear to be decisive factors (Martin, 1967). In contrast, for carcinoma of the breast, which is more common among single than married women, hormonal balance is probably of crucial importance. Factors associated with *lower* risk of breast cancer are early age at first pregnancy (MacMahon et al., 1970a, b) and artificial menopause before the age of 40 years (Feinleib, 1968). Sexual activity probably is important only as it affects the risk of pregnancy.

The old idea that prolonged lactation protects against breast cancer was tested through an international collaborative study (MacMahon et al., 1970a, b). No support for this hypothesis was found. Large series of cases and controls in seven countries did not differ significantly with respect to history of lactation.

Pregnancy and childbearing also entail special risks aside from any possible effects on subsequent development of cancer. In early pregnancy, the woman is subject to various risks from abortion (either spontaneous or induced) and its complications and from rupture of an ectopic (extrauterine) pregnancy. Toward term toxemia, although decreasing in frequency, still accounts for some mortality. Parturition itself is associated with hazards that include hemorrhage and anesthetic accidents. Complications of the puerperium include sepsis and thromboembolic phenomena, as well as postpartum psychosis. Another aspect of pregnancy is its effect on preexisting disease. Pregnancy tends to exacerbate some conditions (hypertension and rheumatic heart disease) and to unmask certain latent problems (diabetes), while it often leads to remission of others (rheumatoid arthritis).

Family Variables

The preceding section dealt with differentials in death and disease associated with a person's own marital condition. In the terminology of the anthropologist, we have looked at the *family of procreation,* the family during the reproductive years when the person is the actual or potential head of a household. We move now to a consideration of the effects on health of the *family of origin or orientation,* the family into which a person is born or with which he spends his formative years. Numerous aspects of the family of orientation may be examined: the number of generations represented in the household; whether both parents are present; the number of children; the position of the "index person" in the sibship; the age of both parents at the child's birth; religion of the parents; presence of any marked discrepancy in age, religion, or social class of origin of the two parents, and so on. Although it is difficult to establish an etiologic significance for these variables separately because they tend to be interrelated, it is worth considering a few factors individually.

Family Size. Family size is associated with social class, large families being more common among the poor. In large families, especially if they are poor, children may be at a disadvantage, since many persons have to share the family's limited resources. The disadvantages to children from large families include higher rates of fetal, neonatal, and infant deaths, higher rates of childhood mortality, and a tendency to poorer intellectual performance. The current trend toward a lowered birth rate and smaller families has important implications for changes in lifestyle and hence changes in health.

Birth Order. A variety of findings relating to birth order have been reported, from an increased representation of first-borns among eminent and highly educated persons, to association of birth order with

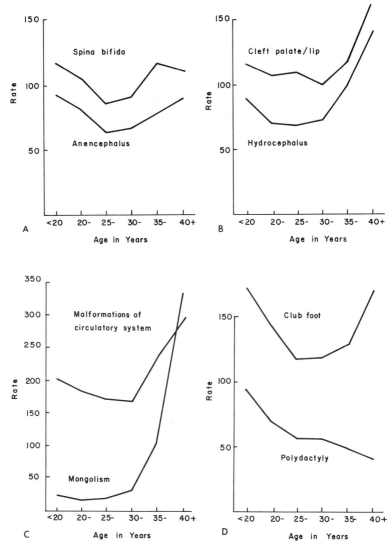

Figure 6–9 Incidence of selected congenital malformations by maternal age, upstate New York, 1950–1960 (cases per 100,000 total births). (From Gittelson, A. M., and Milham, S., Jr.: Vital record incidence of congenital malformations in New York State. In Neel, J. V., Shaw, M. W., et al. (eds.): Genetics and the Epidemiology of Chronic Diseases. USPHS Pub. No. 1163, U.S. Govt. Printing Office, Washington, D.C., 1965.)

diverse diseases — asthma, schizophrenia, peptic ulcer, and pyloric stenosis. There is no doubt that birth order does play a part in a person's life experiences. The first-born in particular receives a kind of attention from his family that is not duplicated for his younger sibs. However, studies of birth order are fraught with danger of bias. Schooler (1972) has stressed the biassing effects of trends in family size over time. Others have emphasized the errors inherent in studies based on incomplete sibships. For example, by reanalyzing the data from several widely quoted studies that had shown a predominance of first-borns among infants with pyloric stenosis, Huguenard and Sharples (1972) found no such excess.

Maternal Age. Maternal age is known to be of distinct etiologic importance in a number of congenital malformations. Figure 6 – 9 shows that several malformations have a J- or U-shaped incidence curve, with high rates at one or both extremes of maternal age, particularly the upper end of the age range. The outstanding example is Down's syndrome (trisomy 21). In European populations, the risk of this anomaly is less than 1 in 1000 births for women under the age of 30. It then increases. For women between 40 and 44 years of age it is close to 1 in 100, and at ages 45 and above it is about 1 in 50. While there is no evidence of change in the incidence of Down's syndrome over the years, there is no doubt that the prevalence of the disorder has increased as the survival of affected children has improved.

Parental Deprivation. Effective loss of one or both parents by death, divorce, or separation has been found to be particularly high among certain types of patients — those with psychiatric and psychosomatic disorders, persons with tuberculosis, those who have attempted suicide, and accident repeaters (Chen and Cobb, 1960). This suggests a particular need for intensified health supervision for children who have lost one or both parents. Unfortunately, this group is very large; the 1980 census revealed that almost one-quarter of all children under 18 in the United States were living with neither or only one parent. Compounding the problem is the fact that a large proportion of these children are concentrated in lower class families.

Other Personal Variables

Blood Type. ABO blood type is associated with several diseases. Persons with type A blood have an increased risk of gastric cancer (Aird et al., 1953), while those with type O are more likely to develop duodenal ulcer (Clarke et al., 1955). Sickle cell trait is associated with a decreased risk of malaria due to *Plasmodium falciparum* (Allison, 1954).

Environmental Exposures. Other attributes are primarily the result of past environmental exposures. Thus, one of the major components in resistance to infectious disease is *specific immunity,* a state of altered responsiveness to a specific substance acquired through immunization or natural infection. For certain diseases (e.g., measles, chickenpox), this protection generally lasts for the life of the individual.

Other types of environmental exposure are chemical in nature and may come from an individual's personal environment (as with cigarette smoking), from exposure at work (as to asbestos), or from more generalized air or water pollution.

Personality Traits. Personality is one host factor for which separation of intrinsic and extrinsic variables is difficult (Mischel, 1968). It is beyond our scope to explore systematically the relationship between personality and illness. However, we should note that personality variables do influence the course of illness, at least partly, through their effect on tendency to seek medical care and to comply with medical advice.

One well-documented association between personality traits and disease concerns coronary heart disease. Since the late 1950s, Rosenman and Friedman, two California cardiologists, have been exploring with their colleagues the relevance of behavior to the development of CHD (1970). Over the years they have produced evidence that a certain style of behavior is predictive of CHD. Their work, at first received with skepticism, is now widely accepted. The behavior they have identified, called Type A, is characterized by aggressiveness, competitiveness, ambition, restlessness, and a sense of time urgency. Type B individuals, who do not exhibit these characteristics, have lower rates of CHD.

PLACE AND TIME

In these considerations lie the germs of a science, which . . . will give: firstly, a picture of the occurrence, the distribution and the type of diseases of mankind, in distinct epochs of time, and at various points of the earth's surface; and secondly, will render an account of the relations of these diseases to the external conditions surrounding the individual and determining his manner of life (Hirsch, 1883).

Hirsch's statement, although written almost a century ago to define the science he called geographic and historical pathology, embodies current thinking about the importance of place and time to disease. It states explicitly that the frequency of disease often varies by geographic location and period of time. It implies that these variations in frequency provide etiologic clues. In this section we will explore some sources, manifestations, and implications of variations in frequency of disease by place and time.

Place

Frequency of disease can be related to place of occurrence in terms of areas set off either by natural barriers, such as mountain ranges, rivers, or deserts, or by political boundaries.

Natural Boundaries. Natural boundaries are likely to be more useful than political lines for understanding the etiology of disease. An area defined by natural boundaries may have a high or low frequency of certain diseases because it is characterized by some particular environmental or climatic condition, such as temperature, humidity, rainfall, altitude, mineral content of soil, or water supply. Moreover, the physical boundaries separating the region from neighboring areas may have led to the isolation of a population group distinguished by genetic inheritance or social custom. Natural contours also affect economic activities and patterns of transportation, including access to medical care facilities.

Characteristics of the physical and biological environment (Chap. 2) can cause certain diseases to be particularly prevalent in certain areas. Diseases that depend upon specific environmental conditions may be considered *place diseases*. Parasitic and other infectious diseases, which exhibit marked differences in occurrence between tropical and temperate areas, exemplify such place diseases. Other examples are endemic goiter in iodine-deficient inland regions and certain fungus diseases, or mycoses. One of the mycoses, coccidioidomycosis, also known as "San Joaquin Valley fever," is found in the hot, arid southwest portion of the United States.

Another example of "place" epidemiology is the irregular geographic distribution of persons with mottled dental enamel, a condition found to be related to the fluoride content of drinking water. Knowledge of this association led first to an identification of the role of fluoride in preventing dental caries, and subsequently to artificial fluoridation of drinking water supplies.

Some cancers show distinct geographic patterns. For example, Figure 6–10 shows a pattern of low rates of melanoma in the northern United States and high rates in the South. This pattern suggests that sunlight may play an important role in the pathogenesis of malignant melanoma.

Two other conditions with distinctive geographic distribution are Burkitt's lymphoma and multiple sclerosis. Burkitt's lymphoma (Burkitt, 1962) is a malignant neoplasm endemic to New Guinea and equatorial Africa. The localization of this neoplasm to specific low-lying areas of high temperature and rainfall, as well as its peak incidence in early childhood, suggested that a vector-borne organism could be the etiologic agent. Further evidence of an infectious etiology has been achieved by the repeated recoveries of a virus known as Epstein-Barr (EB) virus from cultures of Burkitt tumor cells and by the regular finding of high titers to EB virus in African patients with Burkitt's lymphoma (DeThé, 1979). Multiple sclerosis, a remitting but progressive neurologic disease that typically develops in young adults, shows a different

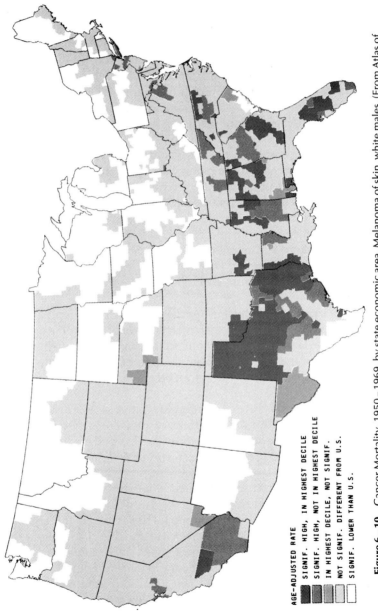

AGE-ADJUSTED RATE

SIGNIF. HIGH, IN HIGHEST DECILE

SIGNIF. HIGH, NOT IN HIGHEST DECILE

IN HIGHEST DECILE, NOT SIGNIF.

NOT SIGNIF. DIFFERENT FROM U.S.

SIGNIF. LOWER THAN U.S.

Figure 6–10 Cancer Mortality, 1950–1969, by state economic area. Melanoma of skin, white males. (From Atlas of Cancer Mortality For U.S. Counties, 1950–1969 (RC 261 U 55). DHEW Pub. No. (NIH) 75–780, p. 44.)

type of geographic pattern. The disease is rare between the equator and 30° to 35° latitude. It becomes more common with increasing distance from the equator in both northern and southern hemispheres.

Another disease localized to one area is kuru, a progressive, rapidly fatal neurologic disease localized to one section of New Guinea, mainly among members of one tribal group, the Fore natives. This condition apparently has resulted from cannibalistic practices that lead to exposure to an infective agent with a long latent period. As the area has come under control of the Australian government, various tribal practices, including cannibalism, have been discouraged and kuru has been disappearing. Incidentally, no sharp geographic boundaries delimit the kuru area; tribal membership appears to be the key factor in the distribution of the disease (Gajdusek and Zigas, 1957; Hornabrook and Moir, 1970).

Political Subdivisions. Despite the relation of natural boundaries and climate to occurrence of disease, it is often more convenient to deal with disease statistics by political units since data for these are more readily available. The political units may vary in size from entire nations to counties, towns, and boroughs. Not only do political subdivisions provide denominators for rates from census data, but local agencies often collect information on cases (numerator) because of their own administrative needs. For example, a city or county health department will need information on the number of persons with newly diagnosed, active tuberculosis residing in its area of jurisdiction, the number of premature infants who may require supervision by public health nurses, or the number of handicapped children unable to attend school.

Natural and political boundaries may be coterminous. Thus, the Mississippi River establishes state borders and the Andes mountains separate Argentina and Chile. Often, however, political boundaries are arbitrary, and either bisect homogeneous areas or join disparate ones. The latter problem is exemplified by the variation in health and socioeconomic indicators within almost any large city. In Philadelphia, for example, the infant mortality rate of 17.8 per 1000 in 1979 masked a substantial difference in rates, from 13.5 to 22.0, for different health districts of the city.

Where political boundaries join heterogeneous areas, it is necessary to examine the data by subdivisions in order to appreciate the distribution of disease and to plan appropriately for health services. Conversely, where political subdivisions separate units that perhaps should be joined, there is a great advantage in regionalization. This concept is coming to the fore increasingly as communities grapple with such problems as water supply, air pollution, vector control, and provision of emergency medical care. In accordance with the concept of providing statistics useful for regional planning, the census now presents data in terms of large urban conglomerates known as standard metropolitan statistical areas or SMSAs (Chap. 4).

For all large cities, geographic units called "census tracts" have been designated. At least initially, these were homogeneous in character. Over time some tracts have tended to become diversified in income, racial composition, and so on. Nevertheless, such heterogeneity has not significantly impaired the usefulness of census tracts as ecological units. Because of the wealth of socioeconomic data available from the United States census, classification by census tract continues to yield information on socioeconomic factors as well as on geographic distribution of disease. Of course, numbers of cases of disease for a census tract or other designated area must be converted to rates before the frequency of disease can be interpreted; without this information, differences in population density alone could make a disease appear prevalent or rare in a given area.

Mapping of Environmental Factors. To examine distribution of disease even more specifically, it is common practice to plot individual cases by census tract or block on maps. Superimposed representation of such environmental factors as water supply, milk routes, direction of prevailing winds, school buses, and so on may sometimes provide a clue about mode of spread.

The following example illustrates the usefulness of such environmental analysis. Early in the summer of 1960, an outbreak of hepatitis occurred in two small communities in Connecticut (Rindge et al., 1962). There were 21 cases in July of that year and 9 cases in August. Investigation revealed that all but one of the 20 children in the initial wave of cases attended a consolidated school. The school went from kindergarten through grade six, but illness was confined to grades three through six. There were no cases among children who attended a nearby parochial school.

Localization of the cases to grades three through six ruled out person-to-person spread on school buses as well as transmission by food and milk in the cafeteria, since all children shared such exposure. Study of the water supply (Fig. 6–11) provided an explanation. Ever since a valve had been shut a few months earlier, there were essentially two separate water supplies in the school. One well, the east well, supplied three fountains used by children in kindergarten through grade two; none of these children developed hepatitis. Water from the other two wells, which intercommunicated, supplied the upper grades. On examination during the subsequent school year, the west well repeatedly showed bacterial contamination.

Urban-Rural Differences. In describing trends in urban-rural distribution of the United States population, probably the central fact is the extensive migration from the farms to the cities over the past 100 years.

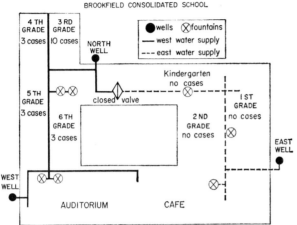

Figure 6–11 Diagram of water supply and cases of infectious hepatitis in a grade school in Connecticut, 1960. (From Rindge, M. E., Mason, J. O., et al.: Infectious hepatitis. Report of an outbreak in a small Connecticut school due to water-borne transmission, J.A.M.A., *180*:36, 1962.)

Underlying factors have been the mechanization of farm work and consequent decreased number of jobs on the farms, coupled with the availability of jobs and other attractions in the cities. Whereas 50 years ago the population was almost evenly split between rural and urban areas, today the population is largely urbanized (approximately 75 per cent in the 1980 census). A significant proportion of those who have remained in the rural areas are disadvantaged through illiteracy, lack of job opportunities, malnutrition, disease, and a shortage of medical personnel and facilities. Some rural areas in particular — Appalachia, the bayou country of Louisiana, the more remote Indian reservations — maintain an isolation that has kept their residents apart from many of the advances of the twentieth century.

There are a number of health problems peculiar to working farms. Farm accidents remain a serious cause of disability and death; they are the result of the use of mechanized equipment without the benefit of the training, supervision, and regulation that are standard in industrial operations. Other potential hazards related to agricultural work include silo-filler's disease, skin cancers from repeated exposure to ultraviolet radiation, and exposures to pesticides and to a variety of microorganisms (e.g., anthrax, tetanus, actinomyces).

One group found in rural areas in many parts of the country consists of migrant workers who shuttle from one community to another following the crops. Although the appalling circumstances in which they live have been publicized widely, their health problems remain serious. In

1972 a massive outbreak of typhoid fever (over 200 cases) occurred in a migrant labor camp in Florida because of pollution of the camp's water supply.

On the other hand, cities also pose a variety of hazards to health. One of the chief problems is air pollution. The concentration of industrial plants and large numbers of automobiles has led to a critical deterioration of the quality of air in urban areas. The Environmental Protection Agency and its counterparts in state and local governments have sketched in broad outline the extensive changes needed to reverse environmental deterioration. Despite some partial successes, translation of their proposals into a comprehensive program of action faces grave obstacles.

In addition to environmental problems, the big cities continue to be faced with the consequences of anomie and social disorganization, including homicide and other acts of violence, as well as patterns of behavior that favor the spread of venereal disease and drug abuse. As an incidental note, these problems are not limited to big cities. Smaller communities are experiencing similar troubles.

In earlier days the life patterns of rural and urban dwellers probably differed more than they do today. The isolation of rural residents has decreased because of improved transportation and communication. Similarly, rural areas have become more accessible to city dwellers. Further, with the development of extensive suburban areas around big cities, large numbers of working people are exposed to the hazards of an urban setting by day and then come home to an environment that holds some of the dangers typical of rural areas, such as exposure to rickettsial disease from tick bites, to mosquito-borne encephalitides, and, occasionally, to rabies from feral animals. Other factors have also reduced rural-urban differences in patterns of occupational disease. The programs to eradicate bovine tuberculosis and brucellosis in herds of animals have decreased the risk of these diseases for farm workers.

International Comparisons. One of the most important political boundaries for epidemiologic purposes is that between nations. Disease and death rates for each country provide information needed to monitor the country's health status. International comparisons of these health indices are widely used to assess relative progress in control of disease. (See, for example, the discussion in Chapter 5 on infant mortality rates.) They are also of interest because they may provide clues to causation of disease. Contrasts in the frequency of a particular disease can be utilized for studies of possible association with climatic and ecological factors as well as with socioeconomic indices, customs, and genetic constitution.

In making comparisons of disease frequency among countries, one should be aware that apparent differences can be created by factors such as variation in accuracy of diagnosis, in completeness of reporting, and in classification and statistical processing of data.

One example of differences in diagnostic labelling comes from the field of respiratory disease. For many years there was debate over apparently major differences in the nature of the chronic, obstructive respiratory disease seen in Great Britain and the United States, Great Britain having higher rates of bronchitis, the United States of emphysema. After conducting a study that applied a standardized questionnaire and examination protocol to "typical" patients in both countries, Fletcher and his collaborators (1964) concluded that "the distinction between British bronchitis and American emphysema is largely semantic."

Similarly, an extensive series of cross-national studies of psychiatric diagnosis (Cooper, 1970; Cooper et al., 1972) demonstrated differences in psychiatric labelling by psychiatrists in New York and London. This can explain in part the markedly higher rates of schizophrenia in the United States and of manic-depressive psychosis in the United Kingdom. The New York psychiatrists were found to apply the diagnosis of schizophrenia more broadly than their London counterparts (or their colleagues in other parts of the United States as well).

Many international differences are substantively large and exceed discrepancies that may be explained by artifacts. For example, for cancer of the breast and stomach, there is approximately a sixfold difference between the countries with the highest and lowest death rates (Figs. 6 – 12 and 6 – 13). Such marked contrasts provide opportunities to formulate and test etiologic hypotheses.

Study of Migrants. One type of study that attempts to separate genetic from environmental factors focusses on migrants. Comparison of disease and death rates for migrants with those for their kin who remained at home permits study of genetically similar groups under different environmental conditions. Comparison of migrants with residents of the new country or area provides information on genetically different groups living in a similar environment. While such studies are helpful in separating factors of place from those of person, selective factors in migration must always be kept in mind during interpretation of findings.

Several groups of migrants have been particularly valuable sources of epidemiologic information. Death rates of Japanese migrants to the United States have been studied intensively because the patterns of death from cancer and cardiovascular disease are very dissimilar in the two countries (Haenszel and Kurihara, 1968). Figures 6 – 12 and 6 – 13 illustrate differences observed in cancer of the breast and cancer of the stomach (see also page 126).

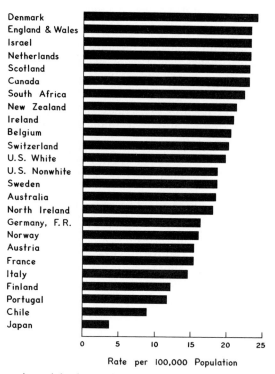

Figure 6–12 Age-adjusted death rates for breast cancer, 1966–1967. (From Segi, M., and Kurihara, M.: Cancer Mortality for Selected Sites in 24 Countries, No. 6, 1966–67. Japan Cancer Society, 1972.)

The great influx of Jews from all over the world to Israel has been useful for epidemiologic study (Modan, 1980). For example, the peculiar geographic distribution of multiple sclerosis was noted earlier in this chapter. When the rates of this disease were studied in immigrants to Israel (Alter et al., 1962), they were found to reflect the rates characteristic of the country of origin. Groups whose rates were high originally remained at high risk even years after migration. It is possible that this may reflect exposure to an infectious agent early in life.

Cancer of the colon provides an interesting contrast to the pattern described for multiple sclerosis. For reasons that are still obscure, death rates from cancer of the colon are higher in urban than rural areas in the United States and elsewhere. In evaluation of death rates by current and previous area of residence, Haenszel and Dawson (1965) found that death rates from cancer of the colon tend to reflect the type of residence (i.e., urban or rural) at death rather than residence in early life.

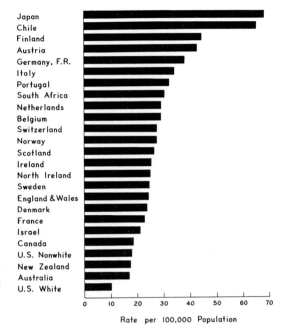

Japan
Chile
Finland
Austria
Germany, F.R.
Italy
Portugal
South Africa
Netherlands
Belgium
Switzerland
Norway
Scotland
Ireland
North Ireland
Sweden
England & Wales
Denmark
France
Israel
Canada
U.S. Nonwhite
New Zealand
Australia
U.S. White

0   10   20   30   40   50   60   70

Rate per 100,000 Population

Figure 6-13 Age-adjusted death rates for stomach cancer, 1966-1967. (From Segi, M., and Kurihara, M.: Cancer Mortality for Selected Sites in 24 Countries, No. 6, 1966-67, Japan Cancer Society, 1972.)

Time

Study of disease occurrence by time is a basic aspect of epidemiologic analysis. Occurrence is usually expressed on a monthly or annual basis. As mentioned earlier, decennial years (e.g., 1970, 1980) are particularly useful because they provide a census count rather than an estimated population for calculation of rates. If there are not enough cases of a particular disease annually for stable rates, cases for several years around a census may be combined (e.g., 1979 to 1981).

Three major kinds of change with time may be identified. The first consists of long-term variations called *secular trends*. The second are periodic fluctuations on an annual or other basis, *cyclic changes*. Finally, there are short-term fluctuations, such as are found in epidemics of infectious disease. Secular trends and cyclic changes will be discussed here. Short-term fluctuations will be discussed in Chapter 11.

Secular Trends. This term refers to changes over a long period of time, years or decades. Such trends may occur in both infectious and noninfectious conditions.

Secular trends in this century have occurred in death rates from cancer of several sites. In Figures 6-14 and 6-15, note the declining death rate from cancers of the stomach and uterus and the rise in cancers

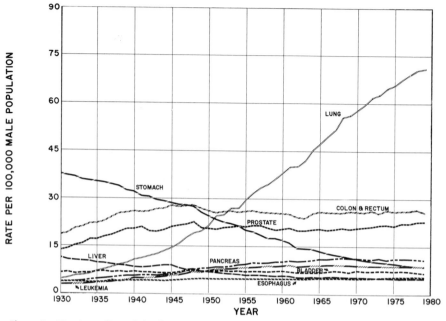

Figure 6–14 Age-adjusted death rates* per 100,000 male population, by selected sites of cancer, United States, 1930–1979. Rate for female population standardized for age on the 1970 U.S. population. (Data from National Vital Statistics Division and Bureau of the Census, United States. Epidemiology & Statistics Dept., American Cancer Society, 5-83.)
   * Rate standardized for age on the 1940 population.

of the lung and pancreas. In contrast, there has been little change in the death rate from breast cancer over this time.

In assessing secular trends in *deaths,* one must consider to what extent they reflect changes in *incidence* and how much they may reflect changes in *survival.* Death rates closely parallel incidence rates only if the disease is fatal and if death occurs shortly after diagnosis. For example, death rates from lung cancer are a good indication of the magnitude of incidence rates because lung cancer has a high and early fatality rate.

Further, apparent secular trends in morbidity or mortality may be due to artifacts, such as changes in physicians' index of suspicion, in diagnostic methods, and in rules for reporting and coding cause of death on death certificates (see Chap. 4).

In addition, apparent time trends may be related to changes over time in the accuracy of enumeration of the population by the Bureau of the Census.

In general, the larger an observed difference the more likely it is to

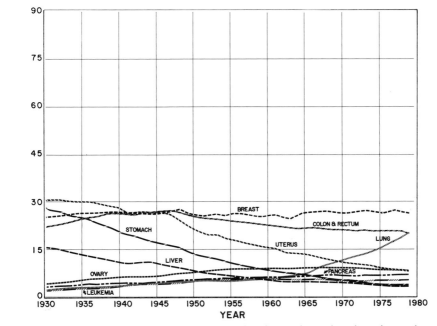

Figure 6–15   Age-adjusted death rates* per 100,000 female population, by selected sites of cancer, United States, 1930–1979. Rate for female population standardized for age on the 1970 U.S. population. (Data from National Vital Statistics Division and Bureau of the Census, United States. Epidemiology & Statistics Dept., American Cancer Society, 5-83.)
   * Rate standardized for age on the 1940 population.

be real. But even with substantial apparent change, such as that which occurred in mortality from stomach and lung cancer, improved diagnostic ability should be ruled out as a possible explanation. A study of the decrease in death rates from cancer of the stomach (Pedersen and Magnus, 1961) indicated that the change appeared to exceed the possible effect of a shift in diagnostic fashion from one form of abdominal cancer to another. Similarly, Gilliam (1955) found evidence for a true increase in lung cancer, although he concluded that early misdiagnosis of some lung cancer as tuberculosis probably inflated the apparent magnitude of the increase over time.

One consequence of marked secular trends is their effect on the age distribution of a disease at a given point in time. For full understanding of the dynamics underlying a secular change, it may, therefore, be necessary to analyze the disease in terms of the experience of *birth cohorts* (i.e., groups of people born within defined periods of time). This will be discussed at greater length in Chapter 13.

Cyclic.   *Cyclic* change refers to recurrent alterations in the frequency of disease. Cycles may be annual (seasonal) or have some other periodicity. For example, measles epidemics used to occur every two or three years (see Fig. 11 – 10). Influenza A epidemics tend to occur in two- to three-year cycles, whereas epidemics of influenza B are more widely spaced, recurring every four to six years.

Seasonal fluctuations in frequency of disease and death are observed in many conditions, both infectious and noninfectious. The overall death rate (all causes) fluctuates markedly by season, with rates higher in winter than summer. Figure 6 – 16 shows the mortality statistics associated with pneumonia and influenza over a three-year period. Note the seasonal peaks in incidence in winter and also the contrast between epidemic years (1979 and 1980) and a year with no epidemic (1981 – 1982).

Seasonal analysis has been particularly useful for evaluation of the possible role of insect vectors since temperature and humidity provide the limiting conditions for this kind of transmission. Seasonal variation in infectious diseases may also be related to differences in people's activity. For example, bathing and fishing provide exposure to Leptospira, a type of spirochete, in water contaminated with the urine of infected animals. However, the seasonal occurrence characteristic of many infections remains puzzling. Explanations such as congregation of children indoors with the opening of school (e.g., for influenza epidemics) and changes in host resistance due to drying of mucosal surfaces by central heating are not entirely satisfactory. The seasonal nature of some diseases spread largely by the enteric route has also not been explained fully.

In general, there is no seasonal pattern in the onset of cancer. However, a striking exception is seen in melanoma of the upper extremities. Several studies have demonstrated a marked seasonal pattern in this condition, with rates of onset much higher in the summer months than at other times of the year. It has been proposed that this pattern results from promotion of tumor by high-intensity ultraviolent radiation over short periods of time (Scotto and Nam, 1980). At this time it is clear that exposure to sunlight is related in some way to melanoma, but the nature of the relationship is unclear. It seems likely that other factors, such as age at exposure and outdoor activities, especially in youth, deserve further study.

Other presumably noninfectious conditions also show seasonal variation. The seasonal occurrence of drownings and skiing injuries could easily be predicted, but other seasonal relations remain relatively obscure.

Clusters in Time and Place. Over the past two decades, there has been considerable interest in "clusters" of disease, such as an apparent clustering of cases of leukemia in Niles, Illinois (Heath et al., 1963), and later of Hodgkin's disease in New York State (Vianna et al., 1971).

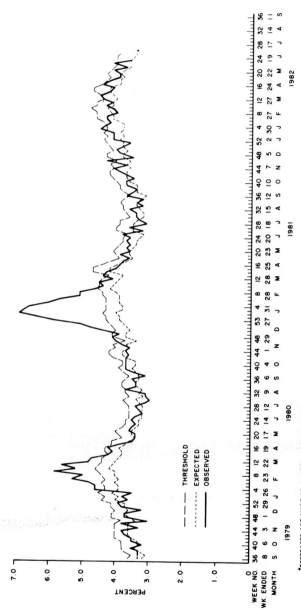

Figure 6-16 Observed and expected rates of deaths attributed to pneumonia and influenza in 121 cities, September 1979–August 1982. (From Morbidity and Mortality Weekly Report, 31:376, 1982.)

However, it has been impossible to determine the significance of the linkages between cases, because there is no defined denominator that could be used to calculate expected numbers of cases. Further advances in identification of infectious agents may make it feasible to study similar future outbreaks in a more satisfactory manner.

SUMMARY

Descriptive epidemiology is concerned with the study of the distribution of disease in population groups. Descriptive epidemiology summarizes in systematic fashion the basic data on health and the major causes of disease and death. The objectives are (1) to permit evaluation of trends in health and comparisons among countries and among subgroups within countries; (2) to provide a basis for the planning, provision, and evaluation of health services; and (3) to identify problems to be studied by analytic methods and to suggest areas that may be fruitful for investigation.

The major dimensions of descriptive epidemiology are person (host), place, and time. In this chapter, we reviewed a number of host characteristics that affect health status. Probably the most important are the attributes of age, sex, race, and socioeconomic status. Other factors pertinent to health are occupation (see Chap. 12), marital status, and other family variables.

Although the focus in this chapter was to a great extent on each host variable separately, it should be remembered that these factors do interact with each other and with environmental factors.

Further, population medicine requires that areas under study be well delineated. Implicit in the term "place" are such considerations as climatic conditions and natural as well as political boundaries. Political subdivisions are useful primarily for the planning and administration of health services, while classification by natural conditions tends to be more useful in the search for clues to etiology of disease. Whatever the objective of study, the concept of place, i.e., a clearly defined geographic area with its related population, is central to epidemiologic study.

Epidemiologic analysis also requires that cases be located in time. The major types of variation over time — secular, cyclic, and short-term fluctuations — were outlined and the first two discussed briefly. We also noted the value of studies of migrants for delineating the relative contributions of genetic inheritance and environment to the etiology of disease.

REFERENCES

Aird, I., Bentall, H. H., et al.: Relationship between cancer of the stomach and ABO blood groups. Br. Med. J., *1*:799, 1953.

Allison, A. C.: Protection afforded by sickle-cell trait against subtertian malarial infection. Br. Med. J., *1*:290, 1954

Alter, M., Halpern, L., et al.: Multiple sclerosis in Israel: Prevalence among immigrants and native inhabitants. Arch. Neurol., *7*:253, 1962.

Antonovsky, A.: Social Class, Life Expectancy and Overall Mortality. *In* Jaco, E. G. (Ed.): Patients, Physicians and Illness. A Source Book in Behavioral Science and Health, 2nd Ed. The Free Press, New York, 1972.

Baker, S. P.: Motor Vehicle Occupant Deaths in Young Children Pediatrics, *64*:860, 1979.

Berkson, J.: Mortality and marital status. Am. J. Public Health, *52*:1318, 1962.

Birtchnell, J.: Social class, parental social class, and social mobility in psychiatric patients and general population controls. Psychol. Med., *1*:209, 1971.

Brinton, H. P., Frasier, E. S., et al.: Morbidity and mortality experience among chromate workers. Public Health Rep., *67*:835, 1952.

Buell, P., and Dunn, J. E., Jr.: Cancer mortality among Japanese Issei and Nisei of California. Cancer, *18*:656, 1965.

Burkitt, D.: A tumor syndrome affecting children in tropical Africa. Postgrad. Med. J., *38*:71, 1962.

Case, R. A. M., Hosker, M. E., et al.: Tumors of the urinary bladder in workmen engaged in the manufacture and use of certain dyestuff intermediates in the British chemical industry. Br. J. Ind. Med., *11*:75, 1954.

Chen, E., and Cobb, S.: Family structure in relation to health and disease. J. Chronic Dis., *12*:544, 1960.

Clarke, C. A., Cowan, W. K., et al.: Relationship of ABO blood groups to duodenal and gastric ulceration. Br. Med. J., *2*:643, 1955

Cobb, S., and Rose, R. M.: Hypertension, peptic ulcer, and diabetes in air traffic controllers. J.A.M.A., *224*:489, 1973.

Cooper, J. E.: The use of a procedure for standardizing psychiatric diagnosis. *In* Hare, E. H., and Wing, J. K. (Eds.): Psychiatric Epidemiology. Proceedings of the International Symposium held at Aberdeen University, July, 1969. Oxford University Press, London, 1970.

Cooper, J. E., Kendall, R. E., et al.: Psychiatric diagnosis in New York and London: A comparative study of mental hospital admissions (Maudsley Monographs, No. 20). Oxford University Press, London, 1972.

Davis, J. P., Chesney, P. J., Wand, P. J., LaVenture, M., and the Investigation and Laboratory Team: Toxic shock syndrome. Epidemiologic features, recurrence, risk factors and prevention. N. Engl. J. Med., *303*:1429, 1980.

DeThé, G.: The epidemiology of Burkitt's lymphoma. Evidence for a causal association with Epstein-Barr virus. Epid. Rev., *1*:32, 1979.

Dunham, H. W.: Community and Schizophrenia; An epidemiological analysis. Wayne State University Press, Detroit, 1965.

Eaton, W. W., and Kessler, L. G.: Rates of symptoms of depression in a national sample. Am. J. Epidemiol., *114*:528, 1981.

Faris, R. L., and Dunham, H. W.: Mental Disorders in Urban Areas: An Ecological Study of Schizophrenia and Other Psychoses. University of Chicago Press, Chicago, 1939. Reprinted by Hafner Publishing Company, New York, 1965.

Feinleib, M.: Breast cancer and artificial menopause: A cohort study. J. Nat. Cancer Inst., *41*:315, 1968.

Fletcher, C. M., Jones, N. L., et al.: American emphysema and British bronchitis. A standardized comparative study. Am. Rev. Respir. Dis., *90*:1, 1964.

Gajdusek, D. C., and Zigas, V.: Degenerative disease of the central nervous system in New Guinea. The endemic occurrence of "Kuru" in the native population. N. Engl. J. Med., *257*:974, 1957.

Gilliam, A. G.: Trends of mortality attributed to carcinoma of the lung: Possible effects of faulty certification of deaths due to other respiratory diseases. Cancer, 8:1130, 1955.

Goldberg, E. M., and Morrison, S. L.: Schizophrenia and social class. Br. J. Psychiatry, 109:785, 1963.

Guralnick, L.: Mortality by occupation and industry among men 20 to 64 years of age, United States, 1950. Vital Statistics Special Reports 52:2, U.S. Govt. Printing Office, Washington, D.C., 1962.

Haenszel, W., and Dawson, E. A.: A note on mortality from cancer of the colon and rectum in the United States. Cancer, 18:265, 1965.

Haenszel, W., and Kurihara, M.: Studies of Japanese migrants. I. Mortality from cancer and other diseases among Japanese in the United States. J. Nat. Cancer Inst., 40:43, 1968.

Heath, C. W., Jr., Greenspan, I., and Brown, E.: Leukemia among children in a suburban community. Am. J. Med., 34:796, 1963.

Hirsch, A.: Handbuch der historisch geographischen pathologie, 1883.

Hollingshead, A. B., and Redlich, F. C.: Social Class and Mental Illness: A Community Study. John Wiley & Sons, Inc., New York, 1958.

Hornabrook, R. W., and Moir, D. J.: Kuru. Epidemiologic trends. Lancet, 2:1175, 1970.

Huguenard, J. R., and Sharples, G. E.: Incidence of congenital pyloric stenosis in birth series. J. Chronic Dis., 25:727, 1972.

Karwacki, J. J., and Baker, S. P.: Children in motor vehicles. Never too young to die. J.A.M.A., 242:2848, 1979.

Maclure, K. M., and MacMahon, B.: An epidemiologic perspective of environmental carcinogenesis. Epidemiol. Rev., 2:19, 1980.

MacMahon, B., Cole, P., et al.: Age at first birth and breast cancer risk. Bull. WHO, 43:209, 1970a.

MacMahon, B., Lin, T. M., et al.: Lactation and cancer of the breast. A summary of an international study. Bull. WHO, 42:185, 1970b.

Mann, G. V., Shaffer, R. D., et al.: Physical fitness and immunity to heart disease in Masai. Lancet, 2:1308, 1965.

Martin, C. E.: Marital and coital factors in cervical cancer. Am. J. Public Health, 57:803, 1967.

Matanoski, G. M., Seltser, R., Sartwell, P. E., Diamond, E. L., and Elliott, E. A.: The current mortality rates of radiologists and other physician specialists: Deaths from all causes and from cancer. Am. J. Epidemiol., 101:188, 1975.

Mischel, W.: Personality and Assessment. John Wiley & Sons, Inc., New York, 1968.

Modan, B.: Role of migrant studies in understanding the etiology of Cancer. Am. J. Epidemiol., 112:289, 1980.

Morris, J. N., Chave, S. P. W., et al.: Vigorous exercise in leisure-time and the incidence of coronary heart-disease. Lancet, 1:333, 1973.

Morris, J. N., and Crawford, M. D.: Coronary heart disease and physical activity of work. Br. Med. J., 2:1485, 1958.

Morris, J. N., Heady, J. A., et al.: Coronary heart-disease and physical activity of work. Lancet, 2:1053, 1111, 1953.

Morris, J. N., Heady, J. A., et al.: Physique of London busmen. Epidemiology of uniforms. Lancet, 2:569, 1956.

National Center for Health Statistics. National Health Interview Survey. Current Estimates, United States, 1981. U.S. Govt. Printing Office, Washington, D.C.

Pedersen, E., and Magnus, K.: Gastro-intestinal cancer in Norway. Acta Un. Int. Cancer, 17:373, 1961.

Rindge, M. E., Mason, J. O., et al.: Infectious hepatitis. Report of an outbreak in a small Connecticut school due to water-borne transmission. J.A.M.A., 180:33, 1962.

Rosenman, R.H., Friedman, M., et al.: Coronary heart disease in the Western Collaborative Group Study. J. Chronic Dis., 23:173, 1970.

Schooler, C.: Birth order effects: Not here, not now. Psychol. Bull., 78:161, 1972.

Scotto, J., and Nam, J-M.: Skin melanoma and seasonal patterns. Am. J. Epidemiol., 111:309, 1980.

Selikoff, I. J., Hammond, E. C., et al.: Asbestos exposure, smoking and neoplasia. J.A.M.A., 204:106, 1968.

Seltser, R., and Sartwell, P. E.: The influence of occupational exposure to radiation on the mortality of American radiologists and other medical specialists. Am. J. Epidemiol., *81*:2, 1965.

Sheps, M. C.: Marriage and mortality. Am. J. Public Health, *51*:547, 1961.

Snyder, C. R.: Alcohol and the Jews. A Cultural Study of Drinking and Sobriety. Free Press, Glencoe, Ill., 1958.

Srole, L., Langner, T. S., et al.: Mental Health in the Metropolis, the Midtown Manhattan Study. Vol. I. McGraw-Hill, Inc., New York, 1962.

Trasko, V. M.: Silicosis, a continuing problem. Public Health Rep., *73*:839, 1958.

Vianna, N. J., Greenwald, P., and Davies, J. N. P.: Extended epidemic of Hodgkin's disease in high school students. Lancet, *1*:1209, 1971.

ANALYTIC
STUDIES
7

EPIDEMIOLOGIC STUDY CYCLES

In earlier chapters, we indicated the dimensions used in describing the distribution of disease in population groups by person, place, and time. A logical question is: what is the ultimate purpose of such efforts at description? Aside from their value for the planning and programming of health services, descriptive data provide a first step in elucidating the causes of disease by identifying groups with high or low rates of a specific disease. Once such identification has been made, the next step is to determine why the rate is high or low in a particular group. Observations of differences in occurrence of disease between populations lead to the formulation of *hypotheses*, i.e., testable propositions, which can then be accepted or rejected through more searching epidemiologic studies. In turn, the results of these analytic (i.e., hypothesis-testing) studies generate ideas for additional descriptive studies as well as new hypotheses. This sequence of events may be schematized as a feedback system or an *epidemiologic study cycle* (Fig. 7 – 1).

In determination of etiology, the usual progression is from identification of groups with unusual rates of disease through descriptive studies, to study of the association between a suspected risk factor and disease in populations, to study of this association in individuals with specific characteristics. For example, on the basis of international differences in death rates from lung cancer, tobacco consumption in different countries might be studied for its relation to death rates from lung cancer. If one were to find a correlation in rates for population groups, an appropriate next step would be to compare the proportion of smokers in countries with high and low rates of disease. (Studies that are based on the characteristics of groups rather than individuals are referred to as *ecologic studies*.) If the rate of smoking were found to be higher in the country with the higher disease rate, then one might further test the hypothesized etiologic link between smoking and lung cancer by studies that examine the smoking habits of individuals within a population. This

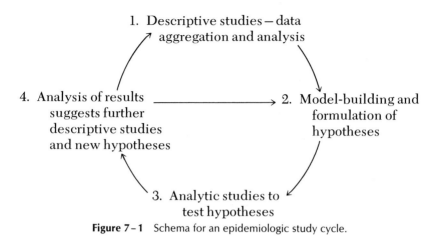

Figure 7–1 Schema for an epidemiologic study cycle.

final step would clarify whether it was in fact the smokers and not the nonsmokers in that country who were contributing to the high rate of death from lung cancer.

In addition to hypotheses that arise from international differences, in a number of instances a hypothesis has originated from the observations of an alert clinician. For example, many studies of the relationship between cigarette smoking and lung cancer were initiated following Ochsner's observations in 1936: (1) that he, as a chest surgeon, was noticing an increase in the number of lung cancer cases, and (2) that all of the cases occurred among heavy smokers.

These clinical observations and descriptive analyses act as leads to the formulation of hypotheses. These hypotheses are then tested in sequence by retrospective (case-control) studies, and, if these are positive, by prospective (cohort) studies (see page 186). Risk factors are then identified, and an intervention trial may be designed to ascertain whether modification of such factors in patients is followed by reduction in amount of disease.

OBSERVATIONAL VERSUS EXPERIMENTAL STUDIES

Bascially there are two approaches to testing hypotheses about etiology: experimental and observational. The experimental approach is perhaps more familiar, since it provides the basic model for investigation in other sciences. In an *experiment* the investigator studies the impact of varying some factor that he controls. For example, he may take a litter of rats, expose one of two randomly selected halves to a supposedly carcinogenic agent, and then record the frequency with which cancer develops in the two groups. The translation of this animal experiment into a study of the etiology of disease in human beings would entail selecting a number of individuals alike in specified characteristics, subjecting a randomly chosen subgroup to a hypothesized disease-producing factor, and then comparing the occurrence of disease in this subgroup with the control group. Patently, this is not possible in human subjects except in certain circumstances. (See Chapter 8 for a discussion of controlled trials in epidemiology.)

In the more usual approach the investigator can only observe the occurrence of disease in people who are already segregated into groups on the basis of some experience or exposure (e.g., married versus single or smoker versus nonsmoker). In this kind of study, allocation into groups on the basis of exposure to a factor is not under the control of the investigator. The study is *observational,* because contrasts between study groups in outcome are observed and analyzed, not created experimentally.

The difficulty with observational studies is that the observed groups usually differ in some characteristics in addition to the specific factor under study. Thus, people in various occupations differ not only in exposure to occupational hazards but also in prior life experiences: different occupations may recruit different kinds of people. In part this may be a matter of self-selection, but it can also reflect prior education as well as fitness for a particular occupation and the selective effects of hiring practices. Because of these confounding and often unmeasurable factors, the role of a specific factor under investigation is more difficult to demonstrate.

While experimentation can establish the causal association of a factor with a disease more conclusively than observation, observational studies have provided and continue to provide the major contribution to our understanding of many diseases.

ANALYTIC STUDIES

Retrospective and Prospective Studies

Two major analytic methods are available for observational studies of etiology — one retrospective, the other prospective.

The purpose of both kinds of study is to produce a valid estimate of a hypothesized cause-effect relationship between a suspected risk factor and a disease. In a **retrospective study** people diagnosed as having a disease (cases) are compared with persons who do not have the disease

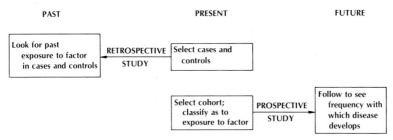

Figure 7–2 Schematic diagram of time factor in epidemiologic studies.

(controls). The purpose is to determine if the two groups differ in the proportion of persons who had been exposed to a specific factor or factors (Fig. 7–2). Such a study is retrospective because it compares cases and controls with regard to the presence of some element in their past experience. The term "case-control method" can also be applied to this kind of study to indicate the way in which the study group is assembled. The risk factors being investigated are not limited to exogenous factors but may include host characteristics, such as genetic constitution and hormonal levels.

In contrast, a **prospective study** starts with a group of people (a cohort) all considered to be free of a given disease, but who vary in exposure to a supposed noxious factor (Fig. 7–2). The cohort is followed over time in order to determine differences in the rate at which disease develops in relation to exposure to the factor.

The difference between retrospective and prospective studies can be further illustrated by a diagram (Fig. 7–3) in which each person is classified simply as "exposed" or "not exposed" and as "diseased" or "not diseased." The classification of each person according to both variables yields a fourfold table.

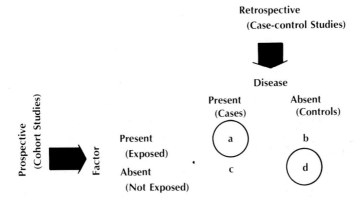

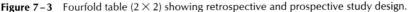

Figure 7–3 Fourfold table (2 × 2) showing retrospective and prospective study design.

Figure 7–3 emphasizes that the essential difference between the two types of studies lies in the way the study groups are assembled. In retrospective studies, diseased and nondiseased groups (cases and controls) are selected and compared for presence or absence of an antecedent factor. In prospective studies, we begin with individuals who are free of the disease under consideration. Information is gathered about their exposure to a suspected risk factor, and the individuals are classified as having been exposed or not exposed to the factor of interest. The two groups are then followed over time to compare rates of disease.

With either method of study, if there is a positive association between the factor and the disease (Fig. 7–3), those exposed will tend to develop the disease (group a), while those not exposed will tend not to develop it (group d). Thus, there will be a disproportionate aggregation of study subjects in groups a and d as compared with b and c.

We should note that the model presented in Figure 7–3 is the simplest possible one. It is often desirable to analyze a factor in terms of level of exposure (e.g., number of cigarettes smoked, estimated person-years of contact with an industrial hazard, and so on) or it may also be desirable to divide a disease into several subcategories. For example, coronary heart disease (CHD) may be subdivided according to its manifestations — angina pectoris, myocardial infarction, fatal CHD, and sudden death. Figure 7–4 will show that the morbidity ratio for heavy smokers as compared with nonsmokers is much greater for sudden death than for the other manifestations of CHD.

Prior to conducting a study, it is necessary to calculate the sample size required in order to achieve statistically meaningful results.

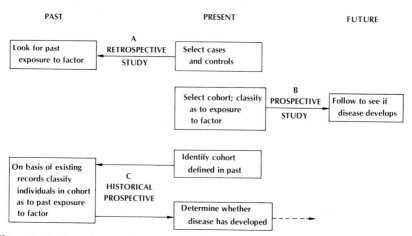

Figure 7–4 Comparison of three study designs — A, Retrospective; B, Prospective; C, Historical prospective.

Chapter 13 outlines the considerations relevant to calculating sample size for observational and experimental studies (p. 348).

RETROSPECTIVE STUDIES

Selection of Cases and Controls

Cases. In a retrospective study, the nature of the study group must be delineated precisely. Definite criteria should be established so that there is no ambiguity about types of cases and stages of disease to be included in, or excluded from, the study. The choice of case and control groups should be guided more by concern for validity than for generalizability. For example, in a study of breast cancer one might learn more about etiology by limiting the cases to premenopausal women with lobular breast cancer than by studying a sample of women of all ages with all forms of breast cancer. The ability to generalize results to an entire population is less important than establishing an etiologic relationship, if only for a narrow segment of the population.

Several guidelines may be cited regarding the selection of cases for a retrospective study. Optimally, selection should consist of all *newly diagnosed* (incident) cases with specified characteristics during a specified period of time in a defined population. Incident rather than prevalent cases are preferred, because prevalent cases represent a selected subgroup of all the incident cases. That is, prevalent cases do not include patients with a short course of disease, the result of either rapid cure or rapid demise (see p. 49 in Chapter 3.) This could produce biased results, as different sets of risk factors may be important for induction and for maintenance of disease. An additional protection against bias is to include in the series the deceased cases as well as those who are alive at the time the study is undertaken.

Cases may be ascertained from a variety of sources, such as hospital records, death certificates, records of physicians or employers, and prepaid medical plans. Information may be gathered about cases from the cases themselves (or from a respondent by proxy), from medical records, or from a combination of these. In addition, some studies are based exclusively on records and do not involve personal contact.

Controls. Controls may also be drawn from a variety of sources, including the general population, cases with different diseases diagnosed at the same hospital(s), and the cases' relatives and friends.

An important assumption underlying the validity of retrospective studies is that controls are representative of the general population in terms of probability of exposure to the risk factor, and they should also have had the same opportunity to be exposed as the cases have. That is not to say that cases and controls should have been equally exposed, simply that both groups should have had the same opportunity for exposure. Another important consideration is that the source(s) and method(s) of data collection should be similar for cases and controls.

Let us assume that the cases in a given study are from a defined population (e.g., all the newly diagnosed cases of childhood cancer in the five counties that contribute to a regional cancer registry). Controls for these cases would appropriately be drawn from the population of the same area in the same age-sex groups. Unfortunately, it is generally expensive and time-consuming to draw controls from a random sample of the general population. A list of all eligible subjects or households must be available, and the general public may not be inclined to participate, which leads to serious problems related to nonresponse. However, population controls do have an advantage in that (1) they are generally healthy and (2) they reflect well the population living in the area.

Random-digit dialing on the telephone is a good approach to identifying controls from the general population, if a high proportion of people in the area under study have telephones. This method involves selecting controls on the basis of their phone numbers. The phone numbers selected for the study may be randomly generated by computer. In designating individuals for the sample, one frequently retains the area code and exchange (i.e., first three numbers) and matches control to case on these, with the last four digits chosen at random. This process yields case and control groups similar in area of residence. However, randomness still prevails in the selection of specific controls.

Often used are hospitalized controls from the same hospital in which the cases were diagnosed. There are many selective factors that bring people to hospitals (e.g., financial standing, area of residence, ethnicity, religious affiliation). Selecting controls from the same pool of patients that gave rise to the cases duplicates these selective factors, and thereby nullifies their effects. Another point about selection of hospital controls is that they are often selected from a variety of diagnostic groupings. This means that if risk factors are associated with specific diseases, this effect can be diluted by other patient groups.

A major problem with using hospitalized patients as controls is that they are not typical of the general population. Hospitalized patients tend to possess more risk factors for disease and often represent the extremes of a distribution.

However, hospitalized controls have several advantages. They are generally easily identified, available for interview, and they tend to be cooperative. In addition, since they have also experienced illness and hospitalization, they may resemble the cases with respect to their tendency to give complete and accurate information, thus reducing potential differences in recall and salience between cases and controls. A

TABLE 7-1 Expected and Observed Deaths for Smokers of Cigarettes*
Compared to Nonsmokers, with Mortality Ratio; Seven Prospective Studies
Combined, for Selected Causes of Death†

Underlying Cause of Death	Expected Deaths (E)	Observed Deaths (O)	Mortality Ratio (O/E)
Cancer of lung	170.3	1,833	10.8
Bronchitis and emphysema	89.5	546	6.1
Cancer of larynx	14.0	75	5.4
Cancer of esophagus	37.0	152	4.1
Stomach and duodenal ulcer	105.1	294	2.8
Cancer of bladder	111.6	216	1.9
Coronary artery disease	6430.7	11,177	1.7
General arteriosclerosis	210.7	310	1.5
Cancer of the rectum	207.8	213	1.0
All causes of death	15,653.9	23,223	1.7

*Excludes those who smoked pipes or cigars in addition to cigarettes.

†Adapted from Smoking and Health. Report of the Advisory Committee to the Surgeon General of the Public Health Service, U.S. Dept. of Health, Education, and Welfare. USPHS Pub. No. 1103, U.S. Govt. Printing Office, Washington, D.C., 1964, p. 102.

major disadvantage of a control group selected from diseased individuals is that some of their illnesses may share risk factors with the disease under study. For example, Table 7-1 shows the number of different diseases associated with smoking. If people with one of these diseases (e.g., bronchitis and emphysema) were chosen as controls for a study of lung cancer, the result would be an association much smaller than that which truly exists. One can see that if the relative risk for smoking and lung cancer were not very large the association might be totally masked by the association between smoking and disease in the control group.

Controls may also be selected from close associates of the case, such as friends and relatives. Although little effort is required to identify these controls and obtain their cooperation, there is a danger that they will be too similar (overmatched) to cases in terms of exposures and other characteristics.

Because each source of controls has its own merits and limitations, it is sometimes desirable to form two or more distinct control series from different sources and to compare results among them.

The Problem of Confounding Variables

In designing studies of the relationship between a suspected risk factor and a disease, it is important to consider how to remove the influence of "confounding variables," i.e., factors known to be associated both with the exposure of interest and causally with the disease under study. Confounding factors are important to control, because they may lead to a spurious or biased relationship between the risk factor of interest and the disease. For example, age, educational level, and socioeconomic status are common confounding variables because each is often related to the exposure and disease under study. There are two major ways to control for confounding: (1) by designing the study through a process known as matching, and (2) by using statistical techniques such as stratification or regression.

Matching cases and controls with respect to a confounding factor is the most common method employed to control confounding. *Matching* is the selection of controls so that they are similar to the cases in specified characteristics. Cases and controls may be individually matched to each other. Age, sex, and race are the most common matching variables. Thus, if a case is a 26-year-old black female, her matched control would be a black female aged 26 years (or perhaps 26 ± 2 or 3 years, if it is not possible to match exactly by year of age). Alternatively, cases and controls may be group matched. According to this process, the matching factor is divided into strata and the control group chosen so that their distribution is similar to that for the cases. For example, if group matching is to be done by 10-year age groups, cases and controls will be similar in the proportion of the two groups in each age stratum.

When controls are matched to cases, the pairing should be maintained in analysis of the data (Breslow and Day, 1980). Sartwell (1971) has demonstrated that if the analysis ignores the fact that matching has been done, an underestimate of relative risk may be obtained.

Care must be taken to match only on a factor (or factors) that clearly leads to confounding, and to match only on the most important confounding variables. Obviously, one cannot investigate the effect of a variable on which cases and controls are matched. Thus, if one matches on a factor, its etiologic role cannot be evaluated. For example, suppose that we did not know that breast cancer rates are higher among single than among married women. A study to identify risk factors in breast cancer that incorporated matching on marital status could not detect any difference between cases and controls with respect to that factor. However, once the role of a factor has been established, an investigator might then choose to match cases and controls on that factor while investigating other variables.

Matching on too many variables has several disadvantages. For one thing, it can lead to matching of case and control groups on the risk factor under study. In addition, the cost of matching may be high, particularly if there are several matching variables and if matches are hard to locate. Further disadvantages are that cases may have to be eliminated if matches cannot be found, and the need to identify suitable matches may prolong the time required to collect data.

Matching is part of the design of the study. To avoid some of the problems caused by matching, it is possible to control confounding factors statistically after all the data have been collected. With this approach, controls are not matched to cases but are chosen without regard for predetermined characteristics.

Statistical approaches that remove the effect of confounding variables include *stratification* of the case and control groups by the confounding variables (Fleiss, 1981; Kleinbaum et al., 1982; Breslow and Day, 1980), and regression techniques that can control for several variables simultaneously (Anderson et al., 1980).

An advantage of adjusting the data as compared with controlling variation in the design phase by matching is that data may be analyzed for a greater range of associations and relationships without concern that the study groups have been made unnecessarily similar. The problem with depending on statistical adjustment is that a larger sample must be studied than if matching were employed, in order to analyze all the various categories of interest.

There is a tradeoff in benefits from the two methods. Matching of controls requires time to identify controls, whereas statistical control of confounding requires that one collect data from a larger number of subjects. There are excellent discussions of the pros and cons of matching in Breslow and Day (1980) and in Schlesselman (1982).

Advantages of Retrospective Studies

Retrospective studies are rather inexpensive to carry out, at least compared with prospective studies. The number of subjects can be small since the study is initiated by the identification of cases, which are often compared with a like number of controls. Even when two or three controls are selected for each case, the number of persons studied is small in comparison with the numbers needed for prospective studies. This is particularly important for etiologic study of rare diseases for which a retrospective study may be the only feasible way to accumulate cases. Further, the results of a retrospective study can be obtained relatively quickly, whereas results from a prospective study are not available until enough time has elapsed for the disease to develop, which may require months or years. An additional advantage of retrospective studies is that they can identify more than one risk factor in the same set of data.

All these advantages of the retrospective method are illustrated by the demonstration of transplacental carcinogenesis (Herbst et al., 1971).

Between 1966 and 1969, seven cases of adenocarcinoma of the vagina were seen in young women (aged 15 to 22 years) in one Boston hospital. This was a most unexpected occurrence. Not only is carcinoma of the vagina a rare disease, but also the usual victim is past 50 years of age and the histologic type is generally different (i.e., epidermoid).

The cause of this puzzling occurrence was investigated by a retrospective study that drew on four controls for each of the eight cases of adenocarcinoma of the vagina (the seven cases mentioned above plus one other treated at another hospital). The controls were matched to the cases by sex, date of birth, hospital of birth, and type of hospital service (private versus ward). As shown in Table 7 – 2 the cases differed dramatically from the controls in past history. All but one of the cases, and none of the controls, had been exposed to an estrogenic substance, diethylstilbestrol (DES), in fetal life. This drug had been given to the mother because of bleeding, or prior pregnancy loss, or both. Since this study, additional cases have been reported; these have confirmed the association with DES.

In addition to illustrating the usefulness of the retrospective study method for investigating a rare disease, this particular outbreak has profound significance because it provided the first example of transplacental carcinogenesis. It serves to remind us that ill effects from thera-

TABLE 7–2 Comparison of Cases of Adenocarcinoma of the Vagina and Controls for Specified Variables

Case No.	Maternal Age (years) Case	Maternal Age (years) Mean of 4 Controls	Maternal Smoking Case	Maternal Smoking Control	Bleeding in This Pregnancy Case	Bleeding in This Pregnancy Control	Any Prior Pregnancy Loss Case	Any Prior Pregnancy Loss Control	Estrogen Given in This Pregnancy Case	Estrogen Given in This Pregnancy Control
1	25	32	Yes	2/4	No	0/4	Yes	1/4	Yes	0/4
2	30	30	Yes	3/4	No	0/4	Yes	1/4	Yes	0/4
3	22	31	Yes	1/4	Yes	0/4	No	1/4	Yes	0/4
4	33	30	Yes	3/4	Yes	0/4	Yes	0/4	Yes	0/4
5	22	27	Yes	3/4	No	1/4	No	1/4	No	0/4
6	21	29	Yes	3/4	Yes	0/4	Yes	0/4	Yes	0/4
7	30	27	No	3/4	No	0/4	Yes	1/4	Yes	0/4
8	26	28	Yes	3/4	No	0/4	Yes	0/4	Yes	0/4
Total			7/8	21/32	3/8	1/32	6/8	5/32	7/8	0/32
Mean	26.1	29.3								
χ^2 (1 df)°°				0.53		4.52		7.16		23.22
p value	(N.S.)†			0.50 (N.S.)		<0.05		<0.01		<0.00001

°Adapted from Herbst, A. L., Ulfelder, H., et al.: Association of maternal stilbestrol therapy with tumor appearance in young women. N. Engl. J. Med., 284:878, 1971.

°°Matched control χ^2 test as described by Pike and Morrow.

†Standard error of difference 1.7 years (paired t-test); NS, not statistically significant.

peutic procedures may not become manifest until years after exposure has occurred.

This study of the epidemic occurrence of carcinoma of the vagina illustrates the usefulness of case-control studies in detecting adverse drug reactions (Jick, 1977; Jick and Vessey, 1978). Case-control studies are particularly appropriate to the study of drug-induced illness, because if a drug is suspected of producing serious side effects, it is important to investigate this immediately. It would be unwise to wait for the results of a prospective study, and randomized trials in the face of possible adverse effects would be unethical.

Disadvantages of Retrospective Studies

The first problem with a retrospective study is that needed information about past events may not be available from routine records or may be inaccurately recorded. If information is sought by an interview or questionnaire, the informant (patient, relative, or physician) may have inadequate information about, or recall of, events in the distant past.

Further, information supplied by an informant may be biased. At the time of the study, the disease has already been diagnosed in the cases. As a result, patients or the informant for the patient may have a different recall of past events than informants for controls have. People may be more likely to search for explanations for the disease in the cases and, therefore, may assign more significance to past events. The more severe the disease (e.g., leukemia, cancer, or severe congenital defect), the greater may be the likelihood of such bias.

At times it may be possible to test for the presence of bias. For example, in one of the early retrospective studies of cigarette smoking and lung cancer (Doll and Hill, 1950), after the cases and controls had been interviewed it was discovered that some patients had erroneously been thought at time of interview to have lung cancer. The fact that the smoking histories of these patients were subsequently found to resemble those of controls rather than cases was reassuring evidence that the difference between cases and controls in smoking could not be attributed to interviewer bias.

However, the most serious problems associated with the use of the retrospective method are perhaps those related to the selection of an appropriate control group, the "Achilles' heel" of any retrospective study (Kannel and Dawber, 1973). The selection of controls from hospital or clinic rosters can readily introduce serious bias. If the disease among the controls is affected (either positively or negatively) by the factor being investigated, a true association may be partially masked or a spurious association found. For example, in a retrospective study (Jick et al., 1973) an association between coffee drinking and coronary heart disease was found that had not emerged from prospective studies. One possible explanation is that the hospitalized control group might contain individuals who had been advised against coffee drinking for medical reasons, such as peptic ulcer. As a result, consumption of the coffee in the control group might be unrepresentative of the patterns of consumption in the general population.

The opposite effect, that of minimizing a positive association, occurred in some early retrospective studies of the role of cigarette smoking in lung cancer (Wynder, 1950). Because the association of smoking with chronic pulmonary disease was not known at that time, patients with this disease were included among the controls for the lung cancer patients.

For these reasons it is often advisable to select more than one control series, including a general population control (see discussion of the Oleinick study on p. 182). If several control series all show a much lower frequency of exposure to the factor than do the cases, then this is good evidence for the validity of the association of the factor with the disease under study. Alternatively, if other types of patients are to serve as the control group, it may be possible to elicit items of information (e.g., marital status, distribution of occupations, and smoking habits) for which general population values are known. Comparison of the population and the control group for these variables would then provide some measure of the extent to which the controls were representative of the population.

Further discussions of issues related to retrospective studies may be found in Mantel and Haenszel (1959) and Cornfield and Haenszel (1960) and, more recently, an entire issue of the *Journal of Chronic Diseases* was devoted to this subject (Ibrahim, 1979). Other recommended references are Breslow and Day (1980) and Schlesselman (1982).

PROSPECTIVE STUDIES

Selection of the Study Group, or Cohort

In a prospective study, healthy cohorts are assembled and followed forward in time for the development of disease. A *cohort* is a group of persons who share a common experience within a defined time period. For example, a birth cohort consists of all persons born within a given period of time. A marriage cohort would consist of all persons married within a certain period of time. (Note that a marriage cohort that included 20- and 30-year-old brides would be derived from different birth cohorts.) An occupational cohort would include, for example, all the persons employed in a shipyard in a given time period for a specified minimum period of time.

It is essential that individuals be correctly classified with regard to exposure to the hypothesized risk factor. Basic assumptions in this method are that exposed individuals in the study are representative of all exposed persons with respect to risk of disease and that unexposed persons are likewise representative of all unexposed persons in the population.

In prospective studies several approaches to selection of a cohort are possible. A particular group may be chosen for study because it is accessible (e.g., volunteers), or because its medical records or history of exposure are readily available (e.g., armed forces), or because the group is known to have experienced some particular exposure, such as that arising during the course of work.

The cohort may thus be heterogeneous with respect to some previous exposure or may be restricted to a group of either high or low exposure. Examples of heterogeneous cohorts can be found in studies of lung cancer, in which each study population included both smokers and nonsmokers.

When the study group is essentially homogeneous in exposure, comparison can be made with another cohort differing in previous exposure or with rates derived from vital statistics. The latter type of comparison was utilized by Selikoff and his colleagues (1968) in studies of the frequency of cancer among asbestos workers. By setting up comparisons with general population values, they were able to demonstrate a marked excess of deaths among the asbestos workers from cancer of the lung, stomach, and colon, as well as several deaths from a rare tumor, mesothelioma of the pleura and peritoneum.*

Advantages of Prospective Studies

A major advantage of prospective studies is that the cohort is classified in relation to exposure to the factor before the disease develops. Therefore, this classification cannot be influenced by knowledge that disease exists, as may be true of retrospective studies. Of course, knowledge of exposure to the factor could introduce bias into the ascertainment of disease, but this is less likely to be a serious problem.

Prospective studies also permit calculation of incidence rates among those exposed and those not exposed. Therefore, the absolute difference

---

* This is actually an example of a historical prospective study to be described later. The principles in selection of cohorts for study are the same in both types of investigations.

in incidence rates between groups (attributable risk) and also the true relative risk can be measured.

Further, prospective studies permit observation of many outcomes. For example, although prospective studies of smokers and nonsmokers were originally designed to detect association of smoking with lung cancer, they also showed that smoking is associated with the development of a host of additional ailments: emphysema, coronary heart disease, peptic ulcer, and cancers of the larynx, oral cavity, esophagus, and urinary bladder.

Disadvantages of Prospective Studies

The main disadvantage of such a study is that it is usually a long, expensive, and large-scale undertaking. A large cohort must be followed, particularly if the disease has a low incidence. For example, in seven major prospective studies of smoking and lung cancer, the 1833 deaths from lung cancer in cigarette smokers came from follow-up data for more than one million persons. The larger the number of factors or variables to be studied (race, area of residence, and so on), the larger the cohort must be.

In addition, the need to follow a cohort over a long period of time (longitudinal study) results in special obstacles. Perhaps the outstanding problem is attrition, the loss of patients from follow-up due to lack of interest, migration, or death from other causes. Other difficulties arise from change in the status of subjects with respect to variables of interest (e.g., the subject may change area of residence, occupation, or smoking habits) leading to error in classification of exposure. There may also be changes in diagnostic criteria and methods over time affecting the classification of individuals as diseased or not diseased. Administrative problems include loss of staff, loss of funding, and the high costs of the extensive record-keeping required. For all these reasons, prospective studies even more than retrospective should not be undertaken without careful planning.

The advantages and disadvantages of retrospective and prospective study methods are summarized in Table 7–3.

Analysis of Results

Analytic studies are designed to determine whether an association exists between a factor (or exposure) and a disease and, if so, to determine the strength of the association. An important measure of association that relates the incidence rates of the disease under study among those with and without the factor is called the relative risk. *Relative risk*

TABLE 7-3 Retrospective and Prospective Studies: Summary of Advantages and Disadvantages

	Advantages	Disadvantanges
Retrospective Study	Relatively inexpensive	Incomplete information
	Smaller number of subjects	Biased recall
	Relatively quick results	Problems of selecting control group and matching variables
	Suitable for rare diseases	Yields only relative risk
Prospective Study	Lack of bias in factor	Possible bias in ascertainment of disease
	Yields incidence rates as well as relative risk	Large numbers of subjects required
	Can yield associations with additional disease as byproduct	Long follow-up period
	Efficient for studying rare exposures	Problem of attrition
		Changes over time in criteria and methods
		Very costly

is defined as the ratio of the incidence rate for persons exposed to a factor to the incidence rate for those not exposed:

$$\text{Relative risk} = \frac{\text{Incidence rate among exposed}}{\text{Incidence rate among unexposed}}$$

Prospective studies permit direct calculation of the incidence rate of disease for the populations exposed and not exposed. This is because both groups represent defined populations at risk that are followed for development of disease. Therefore, the excess risk caused by exposure to a given factor can be calculated directly. (See Table 7-4 for an example.)

In a retrospective study, incidence rates cannot be derived directly because there are no appropriate denominators (populations at risk). Because of the way the study group is assembled in retrospective studies, groups (a + b) and (c + d) in such studies (see Fig. 7-3) do not represent the total populations exposed and not exposed to the factor.

Nevertheless, even though the magnitude of the two rates (incidence) cannot be determined from a retrospective study, the ratio of these rates (e.g., is one rate five times the other?) can usually be estimated.

The relative risk can be estimated from a retrospective (case-control) study if the assumptions can be made that (1) the controls are

TABLE 7-4 Comparison of Relative Risk and Attributable Risk in Mortality from Lung Cancer and from Coronary Heart Disease for Heavy Smokers and Nonsmokers*

	Annual Death Rates per 100,000 Persons	
Exposure Category	*Lung Cancer*	*Coronary Heart Disease*
Heavy smokers	166	599
Nonsmokers	7	422
Measure of Excess Risk		
Relative risk:	$\dfrac{166}{7} = 23.7$	$\dfrac{599}{422} = 1.4$
Attributable risk:	$166 - 7 = 159$	$599 - 422 = 177$

*Doll, R., and Hill, A. B.: Lung cancer and other causes of death in relation to smoking. A second report on the mortality of British doctors. Br. Med. J., 2:1071, 1956.

representative of the general population; (2) the assembled cases are representative of all cases; and (3) the frequency of the disease in the population is small. If these assumptions are satisfied, a term known as the *odds ratio* or *risk ratio* can be used as an estimate of the relative risk. An abbreviated derivation follows. (See Cornfield and Haenszel, 1960, for a fuller explanation.)

A total population may be divided by proportions as follows:

	Disease		
	Present	Absent	Total
Exposed to Factor	P_1	P_2	$P_1 + P_2$
Not Exposed to Factor	P_3	P_4	$P_3 + P_4$
Total	$P_1 + P_3$	$P_2 + P_4$	

The ratio of incidence rates (relative risk) would be

$$\frac{P_1}{P_1 + P_2} \div \frac{P_3}{P_3 + P_4}$$

If, as is often true, the proportion of diseased persons is small, then P_1 is small in relation to P_2, and P_3 is small in relation P_4. The denominators then reduce to P_2 and P_4 yielding

$$\frac{P_1}{P_2} \div \frac{P_3}{P_4}, \text{ or } \frac{P_1 P_4}{P_2 P_3},$$

as an approximation of the relative risk.

$$\frac{A}{c} : \frac{B}{D} = \frac{AD}{cB} \quad or \quad \frac{P_1\,P_4}{P_2\,P_3}$$

The expression $\dfrac{P_1}{P_2} \div \dfrac{P_3}{P_4}$ is called the odds ratio because the quantities can be considered as the odds in favor of having the disease with the factor present and with the factor absent, respectively.

The above analysis of relative risk is applicable to prospective studies. However, under the assumptions mentioned previously, in a retrospective (case-control) study the formula $\dfrac{ad}{bc}$ (using the symbols for frequencies in Fig. 7–3) can be substituted for $\dfrac{P_1P_4}{P_2P_3}$, yielding a reasonable approximation of relative risk. The odds ratio can thus be obtained easily by multiplying diagonally in the fourfold table (cross-products).

For an example of the calculation of the odds ratio, consider the data from a study to determine whether tonsillectomy is associated with subsequent development of Hodgkin's disease (Vianna et al., 1971). The 109 cases of Hodgkin's disease and 109 disease-free controls were found to have the following histories of tonsillectomy:

		Cases	Controls
	Yes	67(a)	43(b)
Prior Tonsillectomy	No	34(c)	64(d)
	Unknown	8	2
		109	109

Ignoring the unknowns, the odds ratio from the formula $\dfrac{ad}{bc} = \dfrac{(67)(64)}{(43)(34)} = 2.9$. This study thus yielded an estimate that the relative risk of developing Hodgkin's disease was about three times greater for those with a prior tonsillectomy than for persons with intact tonsils.

The methods just presented for calculating the relative risk and odds ratio are applicable to studies in which cases and controls have not been matched. When matching is employed, a somewhat different method of calculating the relative risk is required, because in a matched study the cases and controls are more similar than if the controls were chosen at random, and this similarity must be incorporated into the analysis.

In a matched study, the unit of analysis is the matched pair. For example, let E be the exposed, NE the nonexposed, and N the total number of case-control pairs. There are four possible outcomes, shown for both retrospective and prospective studies:

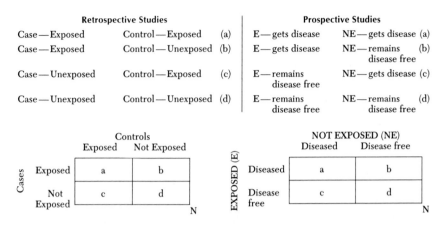

Retrospective Studies		
Case—Exposed	Control—Exposed	(a)
Case—Exposed	Control—Unexposed	(b)
Case—Unexposed	Control—Exposed	(c)
Case—Unexposed	Control—Unexposed	(d)

Prospective Studies		
E—gets disease	NE—gets disease	(a)
E—gets disease	NE—remains disease free	(b)
E—remains disease free	NE—gets disease	(c)
E—remains disease free	NE—remains disease free	(d)

In these tables, a and d represent concordant pairs and therefore do not contribute to the results. A matched analysis is based solely upon discordant pairs, as represented by cells b and c. The matched relative risk or odds ratio is given by $\frac{b}{c}$. The test of significance of the matched relative risk commonly employed is McNemar's test (Fleiss, 1981).

An example of a matched analysis can be found in the report by Antunes and colleagues of a large case-control study done to test the hypothesis that an association exists between the use of estrogens and cancer of the endometrium (Antunes et al., 1979). This study, which was carried out at a number of Baltimore hospitals between 1973 and 1977, enrolled 451 cases and 888 controls. Controls were matched to cases according to hospital, race, age (within five years), and date of admission (within six months). For stage I, grade I tumors, the odds ratio was found to be 7.6, obtained from the following matched analysis:

	Controls	
	Estrogen use +	Estrogen use −
Cases Estrogen use +	17	76
Estrogen use −	10	111

$$(N = 214)$$

$$\text{Odds ratio} = \frac{b}{c} = \frac{76}{10} = 7.6$$

In addition to knowing the relative risk of disease for exposed as compared to unexposed individuals, one might also be interested in the extent to which the incidence of disease can be attributed to the risk factor. Such a measure, known generally as the attributable risk, can be defined either for the entire population or for exposed persons only.

The original concept of attributable risk, introduced by Levin in 1953, indicates the proportion of all cases in a general population that can be ascribed to a specific factor. The proportion of disease occurring in the total population attributable to the exposure (population attributable risk, or PAR) may be calculated by the following ratio:

$$\frac{\text{(Incidence in total population)} - \text{(Incidence in unexposed group)}}{\text{(Incidence in total population)}}$$

For example, if the incidence of disease X in the total population is 2.5 per 1000 and the incidence in unexposed persons is 1 per 1000, then the proportion of disease incidence attributable to exposure is $\dfrac{2.5 - 1}{2.5}$, or 0.6. This means that 60 per cent of cases may be ascribed to the factor in question.

An algebraically identical way to calculate the PAR from prospective studies is Levin's formula (1953):

$$\frac{p\,(r - 1)}{p\,(r - 1) + 1}$$

where p is the proportion of the population with the characteristic or exposure and r is the relative risk of disease for the exposed group.

The PAR may also be estimated from case-control studies using Levin's formula. The odds ratio may be substituted for the relative risk, and p, the proportion of the population exposed, may be estimated by the proportion of controls exposed (b/b + d), assuming controls are representative of the population with respect to exposure.

Another application of attributable risk is for an exposed group. This is calculated from a prospective study and can be defined as the arithmetic or absolute difference in incidence rates between an exposed and an unexposed group, as is illustrated in Table 7–4.

The data from a classic report on the mortality experience of British doctors (Doll and Hill, 1956) illustrates the contrast between relative and attributable risk. Table 7–4 shows annual death rates from lung cancer and from coronary heart disease for heavy smokers and for nonsmokers, along with the two measures of excess risk (relative risk and attributable risk).

In this example, the very high relative risk for heavy smokers as compared to nonsmokers (about 24) is evidence of a strong association between heavy smoking and lung cancer. The relative risk of coronary heart disease for heavy smokers is much smaller, only 1.4. This suggests that prevention of coronary heart disease would require alteration of other factors in addition to smoking. Nevertheless, because death from coronary heart disease is so common among the unexposed (annual death rate of 422 per 100,000 persons), even a fairly small relative increase in this rate attributable to smoking can create an absolute increase in death rate that is as large as that for lung cancer (177 per 100,000 for coronary heart disease versus 159 for lung cancer).

In contrast, the population attributable risk indicates the proportion of all cases in a total defined population that can be ascribed to a factor. This measure, which has also been called the *population attributable risk proportion,* is a compound measure which reflects both relative risk and frequency of the factor in the population. This measure would show, for example, that a large proportion of the deaths from lung cancer in the total population are due to smoking, not only because of the high relative risk associated with smoking, but also because of the large proportion of the population that smoke. Thus, it has been estimated that 80 to 85 per cent of lung cancer deaths in the United States can be attributed to smoking. If a smaller proportion of the population smoked, there would be fewer lung cancer deaths attributable to smoking even if the relative risk due to smoking remained constant.

In summary, then, relative risk is the critical measure for assessing the etiologic role of a factor in disease. Both measures of attributable risk have utility from a public health standpoint. Lilienfeld (1973) has suggested that population attributable risk deserves more attention from epidemiologists than it has received heretofore. The various definitions and formulas for attributable risk given by several authors have been summarized by Kleinbaum et al. (1982).

HISTORICAL PROSPECTIVE STUDIES

One additional type of study deserves mention because it combines the advantages of both the retrospective and the prospective study designs. This type of study, called *historical prospective,* is like a prospective study in that it involves following healthy exposed and unexposed cohorts for the development of disease. However, these cohorts are constructed retrospectively through existing records that permit correct classification of the exposure status of individuals. Study subjects are traced to the present time, and sometimes into the future as well, to ascertain whether they have developed the disease of interest since the inception date of the study (Fig. 7 – 4). The analysis of this kind of study parallels that of a prospective study in which one can directly calculate incidence rates of disease, and relative risk.

To conduct such a study it must first be possible to identify from records the membership of some previously existing group, such as all the employees of a given industry or all the students in a certain school at a specific date in the past. Second, it is necessary that the factors of interest had been recorded adequately at that time, or can be reconstructed from other sources. Third, it must be possible to obtain the needed information about outcome (i.e., disease or death) for almost all the cohort. This may be accomplished through routine records maintained by the organization itself, or it may be possible to obtain the necessary follow-up information through death certificates, hospital records, disability pensions, and so on. Figure 7 – 4 illustrates the time sequence of this kind of study in relation to the two study designs presented earlier, the purely retrospective and prospective studies.

Conceptually, despite the fact that it utilizes previously assembled data, the historical prospective study is essentially longitudinal. It is more akin to a cohort (prospective) study than to a case-control (retrospective) approach. Unlike the purely prospective cohort study, the longitudinal information covers a time interval extending from past to present rather than present to future. However, it is also possible to set up a cohort study retrospectively and then continue it forward prospectively (dotted lines in Fig. 7 – 4), adding contemporaneous data to that assembled retrospectively.

Several studies have taken advantage of previously assembled data on cohorts to examine the biological effects of radiation. Court-Brown and Doll (1965) and Smith and Doll (1978) examined the deaths over 34 years (1935 – 1969) among some 14,000 patients who had received large doses of radiation for treatment of rheumatoid arthritis of the spine (ankylosing spondylitis). They found that the death rate from aplastic anemia and leukemia in this cohort was substantially higher than that of the general population. The investigation by Seltser and Sartwell of the mortality of groups of physicians in relation to their probable exposure to radiation (page 131) is another example. We have also mentioned the study by Selikoff (1968) (page 130) in which the hazards associated with occupational exposure to asbestos were estimated in a retrospectively identified cohort of asbestos workers.

Paffenbarger and co-workers (1966a, b; 1967) have applied this approach to the identification of precursor factors for coronary heart disease, suicide, stroke, and other conditions in former students at the University of Pennsylvania (1931 to 1940) and Harvard (1916 to 1950). His studies have utilized the detailed personal and health histories recorded for college students and the routine follow-up information maintained over the years by the alumni offices of the two institutions.

An increasing number of studies are being based on already assembled cohorts as large numbers of people come under medical care in organizations, such as Kaiser-Permanente and the Health Insurance Plan of Greater New York, which utilize uniform and mechanized methods for recording, storing, and retrieving data about health. When institutions such as the universities in Paffenbarger's studies have an independent need to maintain current information on the status and location of their members, this eases the burden and expense of follow-up.

CHOICE OF STUDY METHODS

It should be apparent that each type of study can make a distinctive contribution to elucidating etiologic factors in disease. Any one of the available study methods may be the most appropriate strategy, depending on such factors as the state of existing knowledge about a disease, its incidence, the interval between exposure and development of disease, and the nature of the factors to be studied for possible etiologic significance.

In general, when there is relatively little information about etiologic factors, the first step is a retrospective study to search for statistical associations. If a factor has proved important in one or two retrospective studies, replication with another group of subjects might seem the procedure of choice. However, once there is consistent evidence of an association between a factor and a disease from retrospective studies, the limitations of the retrospective method generally lead to prospective investigation whenever feasible, in order to confirm an etiologic link. On the whole, prospective studies have tended to confirm associations uncovered by the retrospective method.

The incidence of the disease is a crucial factor in determining the choice of study methods. If the disease is rare, a very large number of persons would have to be observed prospectively to yield an adequate number of affected individuals. Thus, a high proportion of the efforts and resources would be devoted to the study of persons who do not develop the disease. Fortunately, it is precisely in rare disease that relative risk can be estimated through retrospective study. Conversely, the more common a disease, the more feasible is a prospective study, since fewer individuals need be followed.

In addition, the shorter the timespan between exposure to the suspected factor and a discernible outcome, the more practical is a prospective study. Thus, it would be easier to study prospectively the relation between events during pregnancy and an outcome observable at birth than to determine possible carcinogenic hazards manifest only after a 20-year latent period.

Another factor in choice of method is the nature and availability of the desired information. If the information is both objective and uniformly available for most or all study subjects, a retrospective study can be satisfactorily and economically carried out. For example, if one wished to study the relationship between prematurity and subsequent scholastic performance, it would be quite feasible to obtain birth weights for most, if not all, potential subjects, since this information is routinely recorded at time of birth.

The need to design a special questionnaire or form for recording past information of interest does not rule out a retrospective investigation. However, in such circumstances, if there are likely to be problems with memory or bias about crucial information without the possibility of checking its validity, a prospective study may be preferable. The historical prospective approach combines the advantages of both methods and should be used if possible.

As a concluding note, we would emphasize that in all types of studies, retrospective and prospective, it is necessary to evaluate carefully the comparability of the groups being surveyed with respect to any other variables (e.g., age, socioeconomic status) that could affect the findings. If such differences between groups are found, they should be eliminated in the analyses through statistical techniques, such as age-adjustment, analysis by subgroups, or analysis of covariance.

CROSS-SECTIONAL STUDIES

For the sake of completeness we should mention an additional form of observational study called a *cross-sectional study* (or a survey). In this type of study, both risk factor(s) and disease are ascertained at the same time. For example, in examinations carried out by the National Health Survey, the prevalence of CHD and the level of serum cholesterol were determined at the same visit. The fact that those with CHD had a higher mean cholesterol level than those without CHD does not necessarily lead to the conclusion that elevated serum cholesterol increases the risk of CHD. This may well be so, but it is only by demonstrating increased CHD in people with *previously* elevated cholesterol that a causal inference about the relationship may be drawn. Thus cross-sectional surveys, while easy and rapid to accomplish, do not establish the temporal sequence of events necessary for drawing causal inferences.

PROBLEMS IN ETIOLOGIC INVESTIGATION OF DISEASE

Several aspects of the natural history of chronic diseases create special problems for investigation of causality.

Absence of a Known Agent

The absence of a known agent is a troublesome feature of many chronic diseases because it makes diagnosis difficult. In most infectious diseases, one is able to confirm or rule out the presence of disease by identification of the organism, by skin test, or by serologic reaction. Similarly, in acute intoxications, such as lead poisoning, one can demonstrate the agent in body tissues. Since there is no diagnostic test of comparable specificity for many chronic diseases, the distinction between diseased and nondiseased persons may be more difficult to establish.

Multifactorial Nature of Etiology

Although infectious diseases involve host resistance and other factors in addition to the infectious agent, the operation of multiple factors is particularly important in chronic diseases. The pertinent factors may be both environmental and constitutional (e.g., ABO blood type and oral contraceptives as risk factors for thromboembolism). The interaction of factors may be purely additive or it may be synergistic (i.e., multiplicative). For example, smoking and occupational exposure were found to have an additive effect as risk factors for bladder cancer (data of Cole, cited in MacMahon, 1972). The risk for persons with a history of both exposures is similar to that which would be predicted by summing the individual effects of each factor. In contrast, smoking appears to act synergistically with occupational exposures to asbestos (Berry et al., 1972; Selikoff et al., 1968) and uranium ore (Lundin et al., 1969). The lung cancer risk in the presence of smoking and either of these occupational exposures far exceeds that predicted from the sum of the risks.

Such interactions must be taken into account in the design of etiologic studies. They also have implications for the control of disease. For example, knowledge of a synergistic interaction makes it particularly urgent for asbestos and uranium workers to abstain from smoking.

Long Latent Period

Many chronic diseases have a long latent period during which host and environmental factors interact before the disease becomes manifest.

The latent period is the equivalent of the incubation period in infectious disease, except that it is generally much longer. The long duration of the latent period makes it difficult to link antecedent events with outcomes. It is easy to identify the common exposure to staphylococcal enterotoxin of a group of students or military personnel who develop gastrointestinal illnesses within a few hours. It is much more difficult to investigate a possible relation between patterns of food consumption in youth (i.e., diet high or low in saturated fats) and the occurrence of coronary heart disease in middle age, or between suspected aspects of parent-child relationships and various mental disorders in adult life.

Indefinite Onset

Many chronic conditions are characterized by an indefinite onset. Examples are the arthritides and mental illness. In other chronic diseases an apparently sudden onset may be merely a dramatic episode in a longstanding process, such as acute occlusion in coronary vessels that have been undergoing atherosclerotic change for many years. Problems in pinpointing the time of onset make incidence data difficult to collect.

Differential Effect of Factors on Incidence and Course of Disease

Finally, another difficulty is that a factor may be related differently to the initial development of disease than to its later course. For example, cancer of the breast develops more frequently in women of upper than of lower socioeconomic class. However, studies from the California Tumor Registry (Linden, 1969) have shown that, within stage, survival of patients with breast cancer was better for more advantaged women (i.e., those treated in private rather than county hospitals). Thus, social class gradient seems to favor lower class women with lower incidence, but upper class women with better prognosis. This emphasizes that attempts to identify etiologic factors on the basis of prevalence data or mortality rates may be difficult.

Another example can be given to show how factors may act differently at various stages of disease. The Framingham study cited previously has shown that the association between smoking and coronary heart disease varies with manifestations of the disease (Fig. 7–5). That is, smoking is more strongly associated with sudden death from coronary heart disease than with less fatal forms of the disease. It follows from this that discrepant results may arise if studies do not differentiate among different stages or categories of a disease.

Chronic diseases provide our major health challenges today. Many patients with these diseases seek medical help at a stage when cure is not

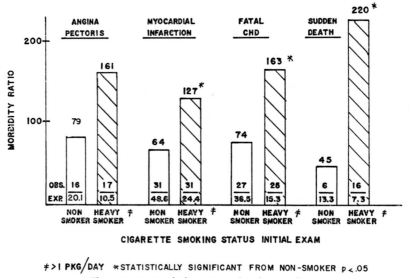

Figure 7-5   Morbidity ratios related to smoking.

possible and symptomatic treatment (tertiary prevention) over a protracted period of time is all that can be offered. Attempts to intervene earlier in the natural history of a chronic disease include not only screening for early detection (secondary prevention) but also focus on primary prevention. The necessity for primary prevention makes it imperative that we identify the etiologic factors underlying these conditions. Thus, we need to consider the methods available for unravelling the antecedents of the so-called chronic diseases.

THE CONCEPT OF CAUSALITY AND STEPS IN THE ESTABLISHMENT OF CAUSAL RELATIONSHIPS

The determination of the cause of a disease through either natural or manipulated experiments may be fairly straightforward. The problem of identifying causal relations in the more usual observational studies is much more difficult. Nevertheless, it is of central importance. Detection of causal associations may indicate key points at which a chain of disease production can be interrupted. On the other hand, it is important not to mislabel an association as causal if it is not, since that could initiate fruitless control efforts and deflect attention from more profitable approaches to prevention. Therefore, before any association is accepted as causal, all alternative explanations should be considered. How then do we decide if a factor is causally linked to a disease? What chain of logic can we follow to determine whether a specific exposure is related to a specific disease entity?

Let us say, for example, that each year a certain proportion of the general population develops a certain disease. If there were no difference in risk for subgroups in the population, one would expect that essentially the same proportion of any subgroup would develop the disease in a given time period. However, if a higher proportion of a subgroup evidenced disease in an observational study, one could not conclude from this alone that there is a causal relation between some factor in the subgroup and the disease. Several questions must be considered and answered first.

The first question to ask about a difference between groups in frequency of disease is whether it is statistically significant. If it is not, the problem may either be dismissed or pursued further through studies on a larger sample. If the difference is significant, a *statistical association* is said to exist. This may be positive or negative. It is positive if the proportion of individuals with both the factor and the disease is higher than expected, negative if the proportion is lower.

Another question is whether the subgroup with the high (or low) rate of disease has any characteristics (e.g., age distribution) other than the one being studied that might influence this rate. If there are evidences of such "noise" in the system, analytic procedures can be employed to determine the effect of such factors and to neutralize them. Of course, one cannot ensure that all relevant variables have been considered, merely those judged to be important on the basis of existing knowledge.

Let us assume, then, that a statistical association between a factor and a disease has been demonstrated in groups that are similar or for whom differences have been erased by adjustment. Such an association may be of three types: (1) artifactual (or spurious), (2) indirect, or (3) causal.

Artifactual (Spurious) Association

As the name implies, an *artifactual association* is a false or fictitious association that can result from chance occurrence or from some bias in study methods. One implication of decision theory based on concepts of probability is that in a certain proportion of trials an outcome will be declared statistically significant even though it actually results from random fluctuation (so-called type I error). In order not to be misled into premature acceptance of an association, one should attempt to confirm a positive finding by replication. One can suspect that an association is spurious if it does not hold up on such attempts.

Bias can also give rise to artifactual association through flaws in study design, in the methods used to collect the data, or in the way the study group is selected. Biases due to inadequacies of study design are difficult to detect and control in the analysis of a study, and great care must therefore be exercised in the planning stages of a study. Bias may also result from failure to control for important confounding variables.

First, we will give an example of bias arising from a defect in methods. Let us assume that a study is being conducted to test whether a given disease (X) is associated with alcohol intake. If an interviewer knew whether he were dealing with a case (i.e., a person with disease X) or a control and if he believed in the hypothesis linking alcohol and disease, he might probe more intensively for a history of drinking for a case than for a control. Even if one were to guard against this by holding the interviewer to a fixed interview schedule, there might still be subtle differences in facial expression or tone of voice that could influence the replies. The solution to this kind of problem is to keep the interviewer unaware of the status of his respondent as case or control (i.e., blind interview).

Another source of bias lies in the selection of the study group. The group chosen for comparison with the cases, the *controls,* can easily be a source of bias, particularly if they consist of patients attending a treatment facility for some disease other than the one under study. When this is true, there may be characteristics peculiar to the control group that would not be present if it were truly representative of the population.

The following illustrates the importance of choice of control group. In a study of the role of early socialization experiences and intrafamilial environment in the development of mental illness in children (Oleinick et al., 1966), two controls were selected for each case seen in a psychiatric clinic. One was a *hospital control,* a child who had attended the pediatric or ophthalmology (refraction) clinic or had had an appendectomy or a tonsillectomy during the same time period. The other was a *population control* drawn from Baltimore public school children.

The cases consistently showed more problem behavior and symptoms than the controls. However, the two control groups differed on a number of factors. Hospital controls had more fears, problems with temper, and more frequent nightmares than the population controls. The hospital controls also were intermediate (as compared with cases and population controls) with regard to possible etiologic factors, such as frequency of disruption of the parents' marital relationship and separation of father and child. This finding is not surprising when we consider that emotional problems could lead to hospitalization and various types of operative procedures.

If only hospital controls had been used, the results would have been misleading. In this example, the study would have understated the difference between cases and controls. It is also possible for differences to be exaggerated as, for example, when more medical information is available about the cases than about the controls.

Thus, whenever a statistically significant association is found, it must be scrutinized carefully to be sure that it is not attributable to some artifact or bias.

Noncausal (Indirect) Association

Noncausal (indirect) association means that a factor and a disease are associated only because both are related to some common underlying condition. Alteration in an indirectly associated factor will not produce alteration in the frequency of disease unless the change affects the common underlying condition as well. Many associations that at first appeared to be causal in nature have been found upon further study to be due to indirect association, as in the following example.

Altitude and Cholera. In studying the statistics on cholera in nineteenth-century England, William Farr, the Registrar General, noted an inverse relation between altitude and deaths from cholera. He interpreted this as support for the then popular theory that miasma, i.e., bad air, was responsible for causing the disease. According to this theory, one would expect high cholera rates in areas of low altitude because the air is more dangerous and, conversely, low rates in regions with pure air. Indeed, the observed mortality (Fig. 7–6) is remarkably close to that predicted on the basis of the miasma theory. According to current knowledge, however, cholera death rates were high in areas of fetid air because they were areas of low altitude where water supplies were also less pure. It was the impure water, not the fetid air, that led to the high death rate from cholera. Figure 7–6 demonstrates that classes of events that are indirectly, rather than causally, related can nonetheless yield an impressive correlation.°

Without the artificial conditions of a rigidly controlled experiment, it is generally not easy to determine that a causal relationship exists. In real life any relationship is likely to be obscured by a large number of confounding variables. Since decisions about causality can have far-reaching practical consequences, a rigorous set of criteria for evaluation of evidence about causality is needed. Such criteria will be presented in the next section of this chapter.

° Parenthetically, it may be noted that the nineteenth-century studies of cholera draw heavily on *mortality* statistics. At the time mortality closely paralleled incidence because the case fatality rate was so high, probably over 50 per cent. With current practices of rapid rehydration, fatalities can be virtually eliminated if treatment is initiated promptly.

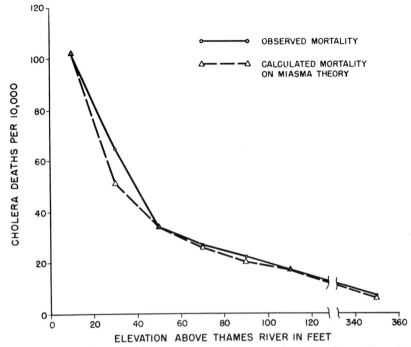

Figure 7–6 Correlation of cholera mortality and elevation above the Thames River, London, 1849. (From Langmuir, A. D.: Epidemiology of airborne infection. Bacteriol. Rev., 1961.)

Causal Association

Although the word "cause" is part of everyday speech, it is, nonetheless, difficult to define. Over the years, different philosophers have assigned different meanings to the term. These philosophical differences have had practical consequences for the formulation of criteria for the determination of causality.

We will define cause by saying that A causes B if, and only if, (1) A is prior to B, (2) change in A is correlated with change in B, and (3) this correlation is not itself the consequence of both A and B being correlated with some prior C.

A set of rules known as Koch's postulates was set forth in the late nineteenth century, after the importance of bacteria in the causation of disease had been established. These postulates represented an attempt to develop criteria for establishing causal relations for one class of agents, microorganisms. These rules, as translated in Susser (1973), require that the following conditions be fulfilled before an organism is accepted as the agent of a disease.

. . . first, the organism is always found with the disease, in accord with the lesions and clinical stage observed; second, the organism is not found with any other disease; third, the organism, isolated from one who has the disease and cultured through several generations, reproduces the disease (in a susceptible experimental animal). . . . Even where an infectious disease cannot be transmitted to animals, the "regular" and "exclusive" presence of the organism proves a causal relationship.

Thus, satisfaction of the first two postulates was considered sufficient evidence of a causal association.

Upon close inspection these postulates are somewhat less helpful than one might wish. Even when all three postulates are fulfilled, animal studies provide only indirect evidence that the organism can be introduced and propagated in a human host. Further, the existence of inapparent infection interferes with a one-to-one relationship between the presence of the organism and the existence of disease. An additional and most important limitation of the postulates is that they do not make reference to the need for a control or comparison group.

Further Criteria for Judging Whether an Association Is Causal

The following formal criteria are widely used to evaluate the likelihood that an association is causal.

STRENGTH OF THE ASSOCIATION. This criterion refers to the ratio of disease rates for those with and without the hypothesized causal factor, that is, the relative risk. The larger the ratio, the greater the likelihood that the factor is causally related to the outcome.

DOSE-RESPONSE RELATIONSHIP. Closely related to the strength of the association is the demonstration of a dose-response relationship. The likelihood of a causal relation is strengthened if a dose-response effect (gradient) can be demonstrated. That is, with increasing levels of exposure to the factor, a corresponding rise in occurrence of disease is found.

CONSISTENCY OF THE ASSOCIATION. This criterion requires that an association uncovered in one study persist on testing under other circumstances, with other study populations, and with different study methods. The more often the association appears under diverse circumstances, the more likely it is to be causal in nature. One should be aware, however, that the same bias (i.e., systematic error) occurring in multiple studies could produce an apparent but spurious consistency.

TEMPORALLY CORRECT ASSOCIATION. Exposure to the suspected factor must antedate the onset of disease and allow for any necessary period of induction and latency. Temporal relations between environmental factors and outcomes are easy to demonstrate for events such as a food-borne epidemic or the London fog of 1952. They are more difficult to establish in many chronic conditions, especially those with a long latent interval.

SPECIFICITY OF THE ASSOCIATION. This criterion refers to the extent to which the occurrence of one variable can be used to predict the occurrence of another. To quote Susser (1973):

> . . . the ideal is a one-to-one relationship, where a cause is both necessary and sufficient. The more closely the relationship meets these conditions, the more specific it will be. Specificity is complete where one manifestation follows from only one cause.

Examples of specificity are provided by rare tumors that can be attributed to one causal factor, such as angiosarcoma of the liver resulting from exposure to vinyl chloride and adenocarcinoma of the vagina in female offspring resulting from DES ingestion by the mother during pregnancy.

The requirement of specificity is less satisfactory than the first four criteria for two reasons. The first is that a single factor can cause more than one disease (Fig. 7–7).

The second derives from the multifactorial nature of disease. Two models of multifactorial causation are shown in Figure 7–8. In one model (**A**) there are alternative causal factors; in the other (**B**) the causal factors act cumulatively. None of the factors alone is sufficient to produce disease.

While one-to-one specificity is strong evidence for causal association, lack of specificity is of less significance. This will be illustrated later in the chapter by reference to the role of cigarette smoking in producing lung cancer.

COHERENCE WITH EXISTING INFORMATION (BIOLOGICAL PLAUSIBILITY). Finally, additional support for the causal nature of an association exists if a causal interpretation is plausible in terms of current knowledge about the factor and the disease (e.g., its pathology, natural history, and so on). This, of course, is dependent upon the state of scientific information at a given time. Certainly a proposed explanation that conflicted with the existing body of knowledge would have to be examined with particular care.

On the other hand, major advances in knowledge have resulted from findings that could not be incorporated into the existing body of knowledge and therefore were regarded at the outset with extreme skepticism. Apparently Minot's Nobel prize-winning work on the use of

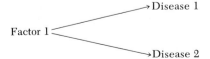

Figure 7–7 Model of etiology of disease in which one factor is shown to lead to more than one disease.

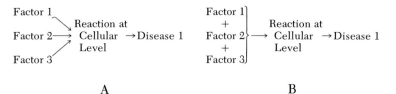

Figure 7–8 Two models of multifactorial etiology of disease. (Adapted from Lilienfeld, A. M., Pedersen, E., et al.: Cancer Epidemiology: Methods of Study. Johns Hopkins University Press, Baltimore, 1967.)

liver to treat pernicious anemia was accomplished in the face of repeated dissuasion from people who felt that liver had already been "proven" ineffective for that condition (Williams, 1954).

There is a general moral to be drawn from this example. The development of biological knowledge often introduces new factors that previous studies have not taken into account. In the existing studies, the major causal factors may have been missed because their importance was not appreciated.

Application to a Specific Problem: Cigarette Smoking and Lung Cancer

Let us now apply these six criteria to a specific problem, the nature of the relationship between cigarette smoking and lung cancer. In doing this we will cover territory explored in depth in the early 1960s by an official committee composed of experts from various biomedical fields. The report of this committee is widely known as the Surgeon General's Report (Smoking and Health, 1964).

For illustration we will draw on data from several major epidemiologic studies that were used by the Surgeon General's committee in their deliberations. In the section on biological plausibility we will also cite evidence that has been developed since publication of the report. Table 7–5 summarizes the major facts from three so-called prospective studies. In each study the mortality experience of nonsmokers was set at 1.0 and the experience of smokers compared to that of the nonsmokers. This is an indirect method of adjustment (see page 341).

STRENGTH OF THE ASSOCIATION. Table 7–5 shows that in all three studies the death rates from lung cancer were higher for smokers than for nonsmokers. The mortality ratio for heavy smokers was approximately 20 to 1 in two of the studies and 40 to 1 in the third.

DOSE-RESPONSE RELATIONSHIP. Furthermore, there is a dose-response effect. Death rates from lung cancer are higher with each successive increment in amount smoked. Thus the criterion of dose-response relationship is fulfilled.

TABLE 7–5 Lung Cancer Mortality Ratios for Current Smokers of Cigarettes*
by Amount Smoked from Three Prospective Studies†

Study	Doll and Hill (1956)	Hammond and Horn (1958)	Dorn (1958)
Types of subjects	British doctors	United States men, nine states	United States veterans
Number of subjects	34,000	188,000	248,000
Age range	35–75 and over	50–69	30–75 and over
Months followed	120	44	78
Mortality Ratios			
Nonsmokers	1.0	1.0	1.0
Smokers (cigarettes per day)			
Less than 10	4.4	5.8	5.2
10–20	10.8	7.3	9.4
21–39	43.7	15.9	18.1
40 and over		21.7	23.3

*Excludes persons who smoked pipes or cigars in addition to cigarettes.
†Adapted from Smoking and Health. Report of the Advisory Committee to the Surgeon General of the Public Health Service, U.S. Dept. of Health, Education, and Welfare. USPHS Pub. No. 1103, U.S. Govt. Printing Office, Washington, D.C., 1964, pp. 83, 164.

CONSISTENCY OF THE ASSOCIATION. The association between cigarette smoking and lung cancer has been found in several countries among diverse study groups. Moreover, the association was demonstrated by studies that followed different designs, retrospective and prospective studies. In the *retrospective* studies, patients with lung cancer and controls were identified and then compared for smoking history. In the *prospective* studies (Table 7–5), people were classified with respect to smoking habits and then were followed to observe the occurrence of lung cancer and other diseases. These various studies were consistent not only with respect to the existence of an association, but also, in general, with regard to the magnitude and gradient of the effect.

It is true that the mortality ratio was higher in the Doll and Hill studies of British doctors (1956, 1964) than in the studies done in the United States. This may be explained by factors in addition to the number of cigarettes smoked—greater air pollution or other differences in smoking habits, such as starting age, or differences in the proportion of smokers who use filtered cigarettes or who inhale. It is known that the British tend to smoke cigarettes down to a tiny stub.

TEMPORALLY CORRECT ASSOCIATION. This criterion too is satisfied by the known facts about cigarettes. Lung cancer tends to develop late in life, many years after the inception of cigarette smoking. This is compatible with the known, long latent period characteristic of carcinogenesis.

Another type of temporal evidence is found in the Hammond and Horn study (1958) (Table 7 – 6). For both light and heavy smokers (i.e., less than and more than one pack per day, respectively), the death rate from lung cancer decreases with increasing duration of time off cigarettes. The rate for heavy smokers remains elevated even years after cessation of smoking, but is appreciably reduced in comparison with the rate for those who continue to smoke.

SPECIFICITY OF THE ASSOCIATION. Most of the controversy over the cigarette-cancer hypothesis has centered on this criterion. One statistician, Berkson (1958), cited the wide range of diseases (Table 7 – 1) claimed to be associated with smoking as evidence against the causal role of cigarette smoking in lung cancer.

Actually this argument is not tenable. It is true that smoking is associated with many diseases other than lung cancer. This is not surprising since tobacco smoke is a complex substance containing not only benzypyrene and other known carcinogens but also nicotine, particulates, carbon monoxide, and other ingredients. Its different components might be expected to relate independently to different disease states. Moreover, there is specificity in the *strength* of the association, as shown in Table 7 – 1. For cancer of the lung, the difference in death rates for smokers and nonsmokers far exceeds that found in any other condition. The ratio in lung cancer is about 10 to 1, whereas in coronary heart disease, for example, it is 1.7 to 1.

Under the heading of specificity two further observations require comment: (1) not everyone who smokes develops lung cancer; (2) not everyone who develops this kind of cancer has smoked. The first apparent paradox is related to the multifactorial nature of disease. It may well

TABLE 7-6   Death Rates from Lung Cancer among Current Smokers and Ex-smokers by Length of Time since Smoking Had Stopped and by Heaviest Consumption*

	Age Standardized Death Rates per 100,000	
	Less than 1 Pack a Day	1 or More Packs a Day
Still smoking in 1952	57.6	157.1
Stopped smoking less than 1 year	56.1	198.0
Stopped smoking 1–10 years	35.5	77.6
Stopped smoking 10 or more years	8.3	60.5

*From Hammond, E. C., and Horn, D.: Smoking and death rates—report on forty-four months of follow-up on 187,783 men. II. Death rates by cause. J.A.M.A., *166*:1294, 1958.

be that there are other factors as yet unidentified that must be present in conjunction with smoking for lung cancer to develop. As for lung cancer in nonsmokers, we know that there are factors other than smoking that increase the risk of lung cancer, including occupational exposure to chromates, asbestos, nickel, chloromethyl methyl ether (Figueroa et al., 1973), and, possibly, exposure to air pollution. Deviations from a one-to-one relationship between cigarette smoking and lung cancer therefore cannot be said to rule out a causal relationship.

COHERENCE WITH EXISTING KNOWLEDGE. This criterion is amply met by cigarette smoking. First, cigarette smoke, as noted, contains a number of carcinogens. Inhalation draws hot smoke into the lungs, bringing these carcinogens into intimate contact with tissues. Second, the temporal trends in lung cancer are consistent with what is known of cigarette consumption in the population. The increase in use of cigarettes preceded by about 30 years the increase in death rates from lung cancer. Male-female differences in trends of lung cancer death rates are also consonant with the more recent adoption of cigarette smoking by women. Death rates rose first in males, but are now increasing relatively more rapidly in females.

Finally, there is coherence in terms of anatomic evidence of tissue changes. In extensive autopsy studies, Auerbach and co-workers (1961) identified epithelial change (i.e., loss of cilia, increase in number of cell rows, and presence of atypical cells) in the tracheobronchial trees of smokers; these changes were present to a much lesser extent in non-smokers. A series of ex-smokers (Auerbach et al., 1962) showed epithelial changes intermediate in extent between those of smokers and nonsmokers.

The anatomic evidence includes the induction of pulmonary tumors similar to those of human beings in beagle dogs trained to smoke through tracheostomy tubes (Auerbach et al., 1970) and in hamsters and rats treated by intratracheal instillation of components of cigarette smoke condensate (Health Consequences of Smoking, 1973).

In summary, the association between cigarette smoking and occurrence of lung cancer essentially meets all the criteria proposed for judging such relations. Nevertheless, we must also ask if an alternative hypothesis could be invoked to explain these findings. We can rule out a spurious association on the basis of the massive and generally consistent evidence. The association does not appear to be an artifact. However, could the explanation be an indirect association? Is there a common factor underlying both cigarette smoking and lung cancer that might produce the results shown? The opponents of the cigarette hypothesis have adopted this position. They have posited constitutional differences between smokers and nonsmokers to explain these apparent effects of cigarette smoking (Fisher, 1958; Seltzer, 1968). Against this hypothesis is the convergence of the several lines of evidence already cited.

As we have noted before, the only indisputable way to settle this matter would be to put the effect of smoking to experimental test in human beings. Since this is impossible we cannot disprove the constitutional hypothesis. However, the weight of evidence for a causal role of cigarettes is so massive that most scientists find it totally persuasive. In their report (1964), the Surgeon General's committee concluded that:

> . . . cigarette smoking is causally related to lung cancer in men; the magnitude of the effect of cigarette smoking far outweighs all other factors. The data for women, though less extensive, point in the same direction.

As we have pointed out, the rate of lung cancer in women is now increasing more rapidly than it was at the time of the initial report. Since the 1964 report, the causal relationship between cigarette smoking and lung cancer has been strengthened and confirmed by evidence in thousands of additional studies.

This brings us to the critical point. When should one make a decision that a causal relationship has been established? It is unlikely that we will ever have incontrovertible experimental proof that cigarette smoking is a causal factor in lung cancer in human beings. If a causal relation can be considered established, then its implications for practice need to be evaluated through the assessment of costs and benefits of alternative courses of action. With respect to smoking, health officials must make practical decisions (e.g., support of antismoking programs, control over cigarette advertising) based on acceptance or rejection of the cigarette hypothesis. There is no absolute rule to guide such decisions; rather, they must be based on review of the totality of evidence in accordance with the criteria that have just been outlined.

Each factor under scrutiny as being causally linked to a health problem deserves evaluation so that responsible decisions can be reached. In the matter of cigarette smoking, the Surgeon General's committee summarized their judgment as follows:

> On the basis of prolonged study and evaluation of many lines of converging evidence, the Committee makes the following judgment: Cigarette smoking is a health hazard of sufficient importance in the United States to warrant appropriate remedial action.

On a more general level, Bradford Hill (1965) has summed up the problem of the evaluation of evidence in this way:

> All scientific work is incomplete—whether it be observational or experimental. All scientific work is liable to be upset or modified by advancing knowledge. That does not confer upon us a freedom to ignore the knowledge we already have, or to postpone the action that it appears to demand at a given time.

SUMMARY

Analytic studies are a necessary extension of descriptive epidemiology for searching out factors that affect the risk of disease. Preliminary clinical observations, descriptive studies, and ecological approaches (to determine rates of disease in groups) lead to analytic studies based on individuals. Since a temporal sequence is implied in studies of causality, the putative risk factor and resulting disease cannot be observed simultaneously. If one initiates the study by first identifying a diseased group and then a nondiseased control group, this becomes a case-control or retrospective study. If one starts with a healthy cohort and follows it forward in time, this becomes a prospective or cohort study. A variant of the cohort study is the use of a historic cohort, in which the investigator identifies individuals at some time in the past and follows them to the present time (or into the future) to determine development of disease. These basic types of study have different advantages and disadvantages, which were discussed in some detail.

Further discussion centered on control of confounding, either through matching or stratification. Analysis of results was discussed in terms of relative risk, odds ratio, and attributable risk, with the heaviest emphasis on relative risk.

We then took note of some of the major factors causing difficulties in etiologic investigations. Chief among them were absence of a known agent, multifactorial nature of etiology, long latent period, indefinite onset, and differential effect of factors on the onset and progression of disease.

Three types of association were noted to exist: (1) artifactual, (2) noncausal, or indirect, and (3) causal. Having discussed each of these in turn, we focussed on causal relationships and on the major criteria used to judge whether a given association is causal. The criteria include: (1) strength of the association, (2) the existence of a dose-response relation, (3) consistency of the association, (4) the temporal correctness of the association, (5) biological plausibility, and (6) specificity of the association.

Finally, these criteria were applied to the evidence indicating cigarette smoking to be causal in the development of lung cancer.

REFERENCES

Anderson, S., Auquier, A., Hauck, W. W., Oakes, D., Vandaele, W., Weisberg, H. I.: Statistical Methods for Comparative Studies. John Wiley and Sons, N.Y., 1980.

Antunes, C. M. F., Stolley, P. D., Rosenshein, N. B., Davies, J. L., Tonascia, J. A., Brown, C., Burnett, L., Rutledge, A., Pokempner, M., and Garcia, R.: Endometrial cancer and estrogen use: Report of a large case-control study. N. Engl. J. Med., *300*:9, 1979.

Auerbach, O., Hammond, E. C., et al.: Effects of cigarette smoking on dogs. II. Pulmonary neoplasms. Arch. Environ. Health, *21*:754, 1970.

Auerbach, O., Stout, A. P., et al.: Changes in bronchial epithelium in relation to cigarette smoking and in relation to lung cancer. N. Engl. J. Med., *265*:253, 1961.

Auerbach, O., Stout, A. P., et al.: Bronchial epithelium in former smokers. N. Engl. J. Med., *267*:119, 1962.

Berkson, J.: Smoking and lung cancer: Some observations on two recent reports. J. Am. Stat. Assoc., *53*:28, 1958.

Berry, G., Newhouse, M. L., et al.: Combined effect of asbestos exposure and smoking on mortality from lung cancer in factory workers. Lancet, *2*:476, 1972.

Breslow, N. E., and Day, N. E.: Statistical Methods in Cancer Research. Vol. 1, The Analysis of Case-Control Studies. International Agency for Research on Cancer. Lyon, 1980.

Cornfield, J., and Haenszel, W.: Some aspects of retrospective studies. J. Chronic Dis., *11*:523, 1960.

Court-Brown, W. M., and Doll, R.: Mortality from cancer and other causes after radiotherapy for ankylosing spondylitis. Br. Med. J., *2*:1327, 1965.

Doll, R., and Hill, A. B.: Smoking and carcinoma of the lung. Preliminary report. Br. Med. J., *2*:739, 1950.

Doll, R., and Hill, A. B.: Study of aetiology of carcinoma of lung. Br. Med. J., *2*:1271, 1952.

Doll, R., and Hill, A. B.: Lung cancer and other causes of death in relation to smoking. A second report on the mortality of British doctors. Br. Med. J., *2*:1071, 1956.

Doll R., and Hill, A. B.: Mortality in relation to smoking. Ten years' observations of British doctors. Br. Med. J., *1*:1399, 1964.

Dorn, H. F.: The mortality of smokers and non-smokers. Proc. Soc. Stat. Sect. Am. Stat. Assoc., *34*, 1958.

Figueroa, W. G., Raszkowski, R., et al.: Lung cancer in chloromethyl methyl ether workers. N. Engl. J. Med., *288*:1096, 1973.

Fisher, R. A.: Lung cancer and cigarettes? Nature, *182*:108, 1958.

Fleiss, J. L.: Statistical Methods for Rates and Proportions, 2nd Ed. John Wiley and Sons, N.Y., 1981.

Hammond, E. C., and Horn, D.: Smoking and death rates — report on forty-four months of follow-up on 187,783 men. II. Death rates by cause. J.A.M.A., *166*:1294, 1958.

Health Consequences of Smoking. U.S. Dept. of Health, Education, and Welfare. Pub. No. 73–8704, U.S. Govt. Printing Office, Washington, D.C., 1973, pp. 79–80.

Herbst, A. L., Ulfelder, H. et al.: Association of maternal stilbestrol therapy with tumor appearance in young women. N. Engl. J. Med., *284*:878, 1971.

Hills, A. B.: The environment and disease: Association or causation? Proc. R. Soc. Med., *58*:295, 1965.

Ibrahim, M. A. (Ed.): The Case-Control Study. Consensus and Controversy. Pergamon Press, Oxford, 1979. (Also published as a special issue of J. Chronic Dis., *32*, Nos. 1 and 2.)

Jick, H.: The discovery of drug-induced illness. N. Engl. J. Med., *296*:481, 1977.

Jick, H., and Vessey, M. P.: Case-control studies in the evaluation of drug-induced illness. Am. J. Epidemiol., *107*:1, 1978.

Jick, H., Miettinen, O. S., et al.: Coffee and myocardial infarction. N. Engl. J. Med., *289*:63, 1973.

Kannel, W. B., and Dawber, T. R.: Coffee and coronary disease. (Editorial) N. Engl. J. Med., *289*:100, 1973.

Kleinbaum, D. G., Kupper, L. L., and Morganstern, H.: Epidemiologic Research: Principles and Quantitative Methods. Lifetime Learning Publications, Belmont, CA, 1982.

Levin, M. L.: The occurrence of lung cancer in man. Acta Unio. Int. Contra Cancrum, *19*:531, 1953.

Leviton, A.: Definitions of attributable risk. Am. J. Epidemiol., *98*:231, 1973.

Lilienfeld, A. M.: Epidemiology of infectious and non-infectious disease: Some comparisons. Am. J. Epidemiol., *97*:135, 1973.

Linden, G.: The influence of social class on the survival of cancer patients. Am. J. Public Health, *59*:267, 1969.

Lundin, F. E., Lloyd, J. W., et al.: Mortality of uranium miners in relation to radiation exposure, hard-rock mining and cigarette smoking—1950 through September 1967. Health Phys., *16*:571, 1969.

Mantel, N., and Haenszel, W.: Statistical aspects of the analysis of data from retrospective studies. J. Natl. Cancer Inst., *22*:719, 1959.

MacKinley, S. M.: Pair matching—A reappraisal of a popular technique. Biometrics, *33*:725, 1977.

MacMahon, B.: Concepts of Multiple Factors. *In* Multiple Factors in the Causation of Environmentally-Induced Disease, Lee, D. H., and Kotin, P. (Eds.). Academic Press, New York, 1972.

Miettinen, O. S.: Matching and design efficiency in retrospective studies. Am. J. Epidemiol., *91*:111, 1970.

Ochsner, A., and Debakey, M.: Primary pulmonary malignancy. Treatment by total pneumonectomy. Analysis of 79 collected cases and presentation of 7 personal cases. Surgery, Gynecology and Obstetrics *68*:435, 1939.

Oleinick, M. S., Bahn, A. K., et al.: Early socialization experiences and intrafamilial environment. A study of psychiatric outpatient and control group children. Arch. Gen. Psychiatry, *15*:344, 1966.

Paffenbarger, R. S., Jr., and Asnes, D. P.: Chronic disease in former college students. III. Precursors of suicide in early and middle life. Am. J. Public Health, *56*:962, 1966a.

Paffenbarger, R. S., Jr., Notkin, J., et al.: Chronic disease in former college students. II. Methods of study and observations on mortality from coronary heart disease. Am. J. Public Health, *56*:962, 1966b.

Paffenbarger, R. S., Jr., and Williams, J. L.: Chronic disease in former college students. V. Early precursors of fatal stroke. Am. J. Public Health, *57*:1290, 1967.

Palta, M., and McHugh, R.: Planning the size of a cohort study in the presence of both losses to follow-up and non-compliance. J. Chronic Dis., *33*:501, 1979.

Pike, M. C., and Morrow, R. H.: Statistical analysis of patient control studies in epidemiology. Factor under investigation and all-or-none variable. Br. J. Prev. Soc. Med., *24*:42, 1970.

Sartwell, P. E.: Oral contraceptives and thromboembolism: A further report. Am. J. Epidemiol., *94*:192, 1971.

Schlesselman, J. J.: Case-Control Studies. Design, Conduct, Analysis. Oxford University Press, New York, 1982.

Selikoff, I. J., Hammond, E. C., et al.: Asbestos exposure, smoking and neoplasia. J.A.M.A., *204*:106, 1968.

Seltser, R., and Sartwell, P. E.: The influence of occupational exposure to radiation on the mortality of American radiologists and other medical specialists. Am. J. Epidemiol., *81*:2, 1965.

Seltzer, C. C.: Morphological constitution and smoking. A further validation. Arch. Environ. Health, *17*:143, 1968.

Smith, P. G., and Doll, R.: Age- and Time-Dependent Changes in the Rates of Radiation-Induced Cancers in Patients With Ankylosing Spondylitis Following a Single Course of X-Ray Treatment. *In* Late Biological Effects of Ionizing Radiation, Vol. 1, International Atomic Energy Agency, Vienna, 1978, pp. 205–218.

Smoking and Health. Report of the Advisory Committee to the Surgeon General of the Public Health Service. U.S. Dept. of Health, Education, and Welfare, USPHS Pub. No. 1103, U.S. Govt. Printing Office, Washington, D.C., 1964.

Susser, M.: Causal Thinking in the Health Sciences. Concepts and Strategies in Epidemiology. Oxford University Press, New York, 1973.

Vianna, N. J., Greenwald, P., et al.: Tonsillectomy and Hodgkin's disease: The lymphoid tissue barrier. Lancet, *1*:431, 1971.

Williams, R. H.: The clinical investigator and his role in teaching, administration, and the care of the patient. J.A.M.A., *156*:127, 1954.

Wynder, E. L. and Graham, E. A.: Tobacco smoking as a possible etiologic factor in bronchogenic carcinoma. A study of six hundred and eighty-four proved cases. J.A.M.A., *143*:329, 1950.

PROPHYLACTIC AND THERAPEUTIC TRIALS: EXPERIMENTAL STUDIES

8

Although experiments provide the strongest evidence for testing any hypothesis, they are rarely possible in human populations. However, experiments to reduce the frequency of disease or death are possible and form an important part of epidemiology. These can consist of trials to prevent disease (*prophylactic trials*) or trials to treat established disease processes (*therapeutic trials*). They may involve whole communities or selected groups of individuals.

We will begin by outlining the principles that should govern the conduct of trials and will then cite several examples of experimental trials conducted with individual subjects and with whole communities. Finally, we will discuss some ethical issues related to human experimentation.

PRINCIPLES OF CONDUCTING EXPERIMENTAL TRIALS

The experiment must begin with a clearly formulated *hypothesis*. This may be defined as "a supposition or conjecture put forth to account for known facts . . . which serves as a starting point for further investigation by which it may be proved or disproved and the true theory arrived at" (Oxford English Dictionary).

An example of a hypothesis is that cigarette smoking is associated with risk of lung cancer. Once this hypothesis has been formulated, the next step is to develop strategies to measure cigarette smoking, to measure the rates of lung cancer, to establish temporal relationships, and to determine whether cigarette smoking and lung cancer are indeed associated. In epidemiologic work, the factors that influence disease generally form the independent variable. We are interested in the impact of the constellation of independent variables on the dependent, or outcome variable — the disease under study. When the investigator controls the assignment of subjects to the independent variable(s), the resulting study is an *experiment.*

Prerequisite to any experimental trial is the development of a standard study protocol that defines the question or questions to be answered and specifies all details of the selection of subjects and of procedures. The protocol should include an explicit statement of the characteristics of the subjects to be recorded at the start of the trial. The characteristics to be recorded should be selected with careful attention to the issues in the study. In therapeutic trials, for example, staging of the disease is of crucial importance. The protocol must also include clear specification of such matters as the allocation of subjects to treatment groups, whether the total group is to be subdivided (stratified), how compliance is to be measured, the frequency of follow-up, the circumstances under which patients will be withdrawn from the trial, and the times at which data from the study will be analyzed.

Reference and Experimental Populations

Studies are generally carried out only if the results can be applied to a larger group than the one actually studied. There would be little interest in carrying out a test of pertussis vaccine, for example, if one could not apply the findings of the trial to subsequent groups of children. The group of ultimate interest is called the *reference population,* the group actually studied, the *experimental population.*

The steps in the conduct of a typical experimental trial are outlined in Figure 8–1 (adapted from MacMahon and Pugh, 1970).

Note that assignment of the experimental population to study and control groups is done after those who have agreed to participate have been identified. That is, the nonparticipants should be eliminated from the pool of potential subjects before experimental and control groups are formed.

Having selected an experimental population, the investigator must then recruit its members for the study. The issues of informed consent and other rights of subjects have recently received a great deal of attention as absolute prerequisites to ethically sound research. Many professional organizations and all medical institutions have adopted codes of ethics to guide human experimentation. The National Institutes of Health have a firm rule that no research supported by them may be funded until a disinterested committee in the investigator's institution has studied and approved the procedures proposed for protecting the rights of subjects.

Random Allocation

Once subjects have been recruited and have signed an informed consent form, they are divided into treatment groups preferably by random allocation, usually through the use of a table of random numbers. *Randomization* has been defined by Byar (1976) as

. . . a procedure for assigning treatments to patients in such a way that all possible assignments of treatments to patients are equally likely within the constraints of the experimental design.

In other words, random allocation permits chance to determine the assignment of subjects to various groups. Compared to other methods of allocating subjects, randomization has three major advantages: (1) it eliminates selection bias on the part of the participants and investigators; (2) it tends to create groups that are comparable in all factors that influence prognosis, whether these be known or unknown; and (3) it gives validity to the statistical treatment of data.

In the simplest form of randomization, two groups are formed. One, the *experimental* or *study group,* receives a drug, vaccine, or other procedure. The other group, often referred to as the *control group,* receives no treatment, a placebo (dummy) procedure, or a standard form of therapy.

Variants of this scheme are possible. The unit of randomization may be an individual, a family unit, an existing group such as a school class or military unit, a hospital, or even a community. In addition, when response to treatment is likely to differ markedly for subgroups in the study population (e.g., patients of different ages or with different stages of disease), the population may be stratified according to relevant variables either before or after random allocation.

With random allocation, the groups formed can be expected to be generally alike at the beginning of the trial. This should be true for risk factors as well as other characteristics, all within the limits of sampling variability. However, when analyzing the results of the trial, a first step is to compare the groups to verify that they are basically similar in composition.

In Table 8–1, which comes from the Hypertension Detection and Follow-up Program (HDFP), it is shown how randomization can create groups that resemble each other on a variety of different attributes.

TABLE 8-1 Comparability of Stepped Care (SC) and Referred Care (RC) Participants at Entry by Selected Characteristics, and Total

Characteristic	Total SC	RC
No.	5,485	5,455
Average age, yr	50.8	50.8
White men, %†	34.5	34.1
White women, %†	21.6	21.2
Black men, %	19.4	19.9
Black women, %	24.5	24.8
Systolic blood pressure (BP), mean mm Hg	159.0	158.5
Diastolic BP, mean mm Hg	101.1	101.1
Pulse rate, mean beats per minute	81.7	82.2
Serum cholesterol, mean mg/dL	235.0	235.4
Smoking more than 10 cigarettes per day, %	25.6	26.2
Percent of desirable weight, mean	124.4	125.0
Serum creatinine, mean mg/dL	1.1	1.1
Plasma glucose (1 hr post-load), mean mg/dL	178.5	178.9
Left ventricular hypertrophy on ECG, %‡	4.8	5.1
History of stroke, %	2.5	2.5
History of myocardial infarction, %	5.1	5.2
History of diabetes, %	6.6	7.5
Receiving antihypertensive medication, %	26.3	25.7

*DBP indicates diastolic blood pressure.
†Includes less than 1% others, eg, Asians.
‡Based on combined R wave and ST-T segment changes: tall R wave (Minnesota code 3.1) and major ST segment depression (Minnesota code 4.1-4.3) or major T wave inversion (Minnesota code 5.1-5.3).

(Adapted from Hypertension Detection and Follow-Up Program Cooperative Group. Five-Year Findings of the Hypertension Detection and Follow-Up Program 1. Reduction in Mortality of Persons with High Blood Pressure, Including Mild Hypertension. J.A.M.A., 242, No. 23, 1979.

Here, two randomized groups resemble each other on 27 variables. None of the differences are statistically significant.

It should be remembered that even in a randomized controlled trial the participants are a group of volunteers and may therefore differ from the general population. These differences may restrict one's ability to apply the findings to groups other than that of the participants.

Blinding or Masking

An important consideration in any trial is the possible introduction of bias in assessment of outcomes from the expectations of either the investigator or the participant. The best protection against this source of bias is to have neither experimenter nor subject know the group to which the subject has been assigned. Such a trial is called *double blind*. If only the experimenter knows the assignment, it is said to be *single blind*. A further protection against bias has been the introduction of *triple blind* studies, in which not only the subject and the investigator but those responsible for data analysis are also blind to the assignments of individuals in the trial. With this triple-blind approach, the code is broken only after the entire study, including the analysis of data, is complete. This guards against bias in such matters as the assignment of equivocal cases, or the interpretation of outcomes.

A double-blind (or triple-blind) trial provides the best protection against bias, but it may not always be feasible. For one thing, the active substance being used may produce side effects that are not mimicked by the placebo. In addition, the setting in which care is given (e.g., home versus hospital) may be the crucial experimental variable. Lastly, the physician may need information about the patient's assignment in the trial to monitor his clinical status. At times the latter problem can be circumvented if a physician not involved in the evaluation of results can take over the management of the patient's condition. When the study is not conducted "blind," it is important that the experimental and control groups be followed with equal intensity for evaluation of the outcome.

Blinding is of greatest importance when the outcome is subjectively determined. If death or stroke is the outcome measure, blinding is less essential.

Sample Size (Statistical Power)

An important step in designing a trial is determining the sample size required in order to answer the study questions. The process of determining sample size is discussed in Chapter 13, on p. 348. It is recommended that the reader review that section carefully before planning a study, regardless of the design.

Sometimes it would take too long to enroll the desired study group if the investigation were limited to one institution or one area. Under these circumstances, it is usual to set up a multicenter trial such as the trial of therapy for diabetes known as the University Group Diabetes Program (Klimt et al., 1970; Meinert et al., 1970). Other advantages of a multicenter trial include the opportunity for greater variety in the types of subjects enrolled and the fact that it may be easier to keep the results unknown to the investigators. In trials in which a number of investigators are cooperating to carry out the study, it is especially important that a rigorously defined protocol be developed and adhered to. Obviously, maintaining standard procedures under such circumstances is far from easy.

Figure 8–1 also serves to emphasize that attrition may occur throughout the study. In addition to those who do not enter the study

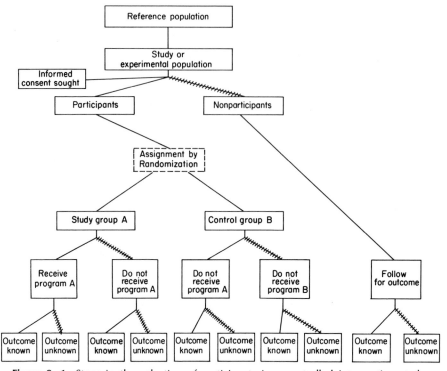

Figure 8-1 Steps in the selection of participants in a controlled intervention study. (Adapted from MacMahon, B., and Pugh, T. F.: Epidemiology: Principles and Methods, Little Brown & Co., Boston, 1970.

initially, some of those assigned to the study and control groups do not complete the study protocol. Also, not all of those who complete the program may be available for the final evaluations. The required sample size that one calculates should include a correction for estimated losses due to loss to follow-up and noncompliance.

An important assumption underlying the validity of any follow-up study is that drop-outs experience the same risk of the various outcomes as do individuals who remain under observation. If there are substantive biases from nonparticipation and attrition, it may be difficult to generalize from the results of the trial to the total experimental population. Generalization to the reference population may be even more hazardous.

To evaluate current practices in the conduct of clinical trials, Freiman, Chalmers, and their co-workers (1978) reviewed 71 "negative" randomized controlled trials and calculated for each the number of subjects that would be required to draw conclusions. They found that most of the studies had an insufficient number of subjects to allow detection of a difference between treatment and control groups (i.e., inadequate power) and that the results of many "negative" trials were really inconclusive. This points out the potential wastefulness of conducting expensive trials that do not enroll a sufficient number of individuals to test the study hypothesis.

Natural Experiments

On rare occasions, by chance, groups may exist that are similar in every respect save for degree of exposure to a specific environmental factor. In such circumstances the conditions for drawing conclusions about the cause of disease may be so favorable that a *natural experiment* is said to exist.

Perhaps the most famous natural experiment is that reported by John Snow (1855), a British physician, over a hundred years ago. On the basis of extensive studies on the epidemiology of cholera, Snow had formulated the hypothesis that cholera could be transmitted by discharge of fecal wastes into water supplies. Some preliminary analyses by the Registrar General during an outbreak of cholera in 1853 suggested that among people living in the same area of London, those served by one water company, the Lambeth Company, had a lower death rate from cholera than those served by another company, Southwark and Vauxhall. The latter received water drawn from the Thames River at points where the water was already contaminated by sewage from London. Snow reported that nature had devised an

. . . experiment, . . . on the grandest scale (in that) no fewer than three hundred thousand people of both sexes, of every age and occupation, and of every rank and station, from gentlefolks down to the very poor, were divided into two groups without their choice, and, in most cases, without their knowledge; one group being supplied with water containing the sewage of London, and, amongst it, whatever might have come from the cholera patients, the other group having water quite free from such impurity.

To turn this grand experiment to account, all that was required was to learn the supply of water to each individual house where a fatal attack of cholera might occur.

Snow's subsequent investigations, which showed an eightfold difference in the death rates for the households supplied by the two companies (Table 8–2), gave clear evidence of an association between cholera death rate and source of water supply to the household.

More recently, the close juxtaposition of areas quite similar except for the fluoride concentration in the drinking water provided another fortuitous experiment. Contrasts in the amounts of dental mottling and dental caries in these areas led to a series of actual experiments that will be described later in this chapter.

TABLE 8-2 Deaths from Cholera by Company Supplying Water to the Household[°]

Water Company	Number of Houses	Deaths from Cholera	Deaths in Each 10,000 Houses
Southwark and Vauxhall Company	40,046	1263	315
Lambeth Company	26,107	98	37
Rest of London	256,423	1422	59

[°]From Snow, J.: On the Mode of Communication of Cholera (2nd ed.). Churchill, London, 1855. Reproduced in Snow on Cholera, Commonwealth Fund, New York, 1936. Reprinted by Hafner Publishing Company, New York, 1936.

Another natural experiment was afforded by the atomic bombing of Japan in World War II. Beebe (1979) has written an excellent summary of the chronology of the Atomic Bomb Casualty Commission formed in 1950 to investigate the effects of the atomic bombs dropped on Hiroshima and Nagasaki in August of 1945.

Historic Controls

Another alternative to the randomized controlled trial is a trial in which the controls are historic; that is, the data for the controls are based on the experiences of recently seen patients or data recorded in the literature. Obviously, the possibility of a variety of biases entering such studies is great.

For example, suppose one wanted to compare the effects of medical and surgical treatment of carcinoma of the cervix. Let us suppose further that it was possible to assemble two study groups from the same institution, one that had been treated surgically and the other medically. By carrying out this procedure, if one were to find that the survival rate was higher in those treated surgically, this would not necessarily be evidence of the superiority of surgical treatment. Since only low-risk patients are accepted for surgery, the medical group would probably include more seriously ill patients who would have a poorer prognosis. If one wished to compare the efficacy of these two methods of treatment, the solution would be to assign medical or surgical treatment at random, drawing patients from a common pool of individuals. The trial would, of course, be limited to studying subjects who were suitable for either treatment. Note that this would restrict the reference population of the study.

Not surprisingly, when Sacks and co-workers (1982) compared results from randomized controlled trials (RCTs) and trials with historical controls (HCTs), they found that a higher proportion of the HCTs showed significant differences, with the results favoring the experimental over the control group. If dependable data are required, the need for randomized controls remains inescapable.

EXAMPLES OF EXPERIMENTAL TRIALS

By now there have been numerous trials of a variety of prophylactic and therapeutic measures that have contributed to our knowledge of the effectiveness of therapy. Control of infectious diseases has depended heavily on vaccines of tested effectiveness and safety. Generally, vaccines, once tested and licensed, have found ready acceptance in practice. For example, virtual elimination of poliomyelitis in the United States was achieved within a decade of the introduction of vaccine against the disease (Fig. 8 – 2). On the other hand, it has been a struggle to gain complete success in eliminating other diseases such as measles, which are not seen by the general public as significant hazards to children despite the morbidity and mortality they still cause.

Chemoprophylaxis has also been studied experimentally. Since 1955, the United States Public Health Service conducted a series of trials of isoniazid in the prophylaxis of tuberculosis. The efficacy of this drug has been demonstrated in a variety of populations.

In addition to the trials we have mentioned, there have been trials of chemotherapeutic agents in tuberculosis, of antimetabolites for ulcerative colitis, of steroids and immunosuppressive agents for chronic active hepatitis, and of different modes of surgery for portal hypertension.

The recent reports of large-scale trials for prevention of cardiovascular disease have been noted (p. 198). Trials that involve changes in lifestyle are becoming increasingly difficult to carry out. The general level of knowledge in the population and the necessity to have potential subjects give their informed consent lead the controls as well as the treated patients to alter their behavior in the direction desired, thereby reducing the difference between the two groups. This effect was clearly seen in the Multiple Risk Factor Intervention Trial (MRFIT) (Multiple Risk Factor Intervention Trial Research Group, 1982), in which the control group showed substantial changes in behavior over the course of the trial.

Oncology is a particularly suitable field for clinical trials. Participation, compliance, and follow-up rates tend to be good and the outcome measure (i.e., survival or death) is well-defined. In addition, in the face of serious illness, the ethical constraints are somewhat less limiting than they would be, for example, in a trial related to the management of pregnancy.

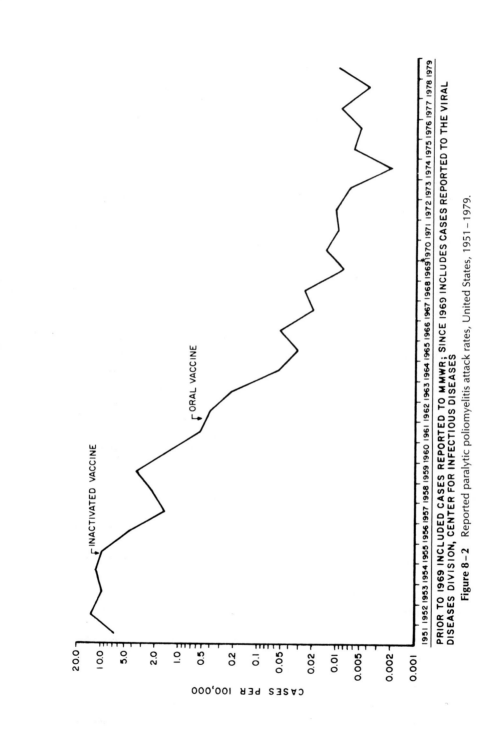

Figure 8-2 Reported paralytic poliomyelitis attack rates, United States, 1951–1979.

For mental illness, the effectiveness of psychoactive drugs has been demonstrated through controlled trials, mainly in institutional settings. In a unique clinical trial, Pasamanick and his associates (1967) evaluated the feasibility of home care for psychiatric patients. They randomly assigned acutely ill schizophrenics to one of three alternative forms of care: hospital treatment, home care on drugs, or home care on a placebo. The study demonstrated that when there was a family member or other person willing to provide supervision at home, drug therapy together with adequate attention from public health nurses reduced the frequency of hospitalization. Unfortunately, the trial was terminated after two-and-a-half years. In a follow-up study at the end of five years (Davis et al., 1972), it was found that the previous differences between groups had been gradually erased. Thus, the ultimate potential of a continued aggressive program of home care in combination with psychoactive medication is not known.

Clinical Trials

Clinical trials can often be used to evaluate policies that have become enshrined in clinical management. An example is the practice of providing special prehospital and hospital care to reduce mortality among patients with uncomplicated myocardial infarction (MI). In the late 1960s Mather and his colleagues (Mather et al., 1976) attempted to assess the relative benefit of home versus hospital care for acute MI. The patients were males under 70 years of age who had suffered, within the previous 48 hours, a myocardial infarction (or in whom myocardial infarction was suspected). Criteria for entrance included specific EKG changes and, if the patient died, autopsy evidence of MI. Patients who did not fulfill the diagnostic criteria were subsequently excluded.

Patients considered suitable for management either at home or in the hospital were accepted into the study and were randomly assigned to either home care or hospital care. Those randomized to home care were treated in their own homes. Diagnostic criteria were equally strict in both groups. Surprisingly, the results of this trial indicated that after approximately one year the mortality rate for patients treated at home was lower than for those treated in the hospital (20 per cent versus 27 per cent.) However, a major criticism of the trial was that only 31 per cent of all patients with MI were eligible for randomization. Because of the small proportion of patients who were randomized and because of other problems in the design of the study, Mather's findings were generally dismissed.

The question of home versus hospital care was studied further by another group of investigators. In this study (Hill et al., 1978), 76 per cent of the 349 eligible patients were randomized, a much larger proportion than in the earlier trial. General practitioners who examined the patients potentially eligible for the trial contacted a hospital-based team that went to each patient's home, gave emergency care, and evaluated the patient's cardiac status. If the patient was considered medically and socially suitable to enter the study, the team consulted a sealed envelope that gave the patient's assignment to an experimental group.

Mortality after six weeks in the group randomized to home care (20 per cent) did not differ significantly from the rate in the hospital care group (18 per cent). In addition, the mortality rate was higher (37 per cent) for individuals not eligible for randomization than for any other group, demonstrating that a high-risk group was identifiable at the time of initial examination. It was concluded that specialized coronary care in the hospital does not confer any benefit on patients with uncomplicated MI.

Recently, some cancer trials have sought to determine whether the amount of treatment could actually be reduced without impairing the ability to cure patients. These trials have been prompted by the known hazards of cancer therapy, which include disfigurement, impairments of growth, development, reproduction and intellectual functioning, and development of additional malignant neoplasms (Meadows, 1980). An example of such a trial can be found in studies of the treatment of Wilms' tumor in children.

Wilms' tumor is one of the most common tumors of early childhood; more than half develop before the age of four years. The tumor occurs with increased frequency in children who also have aniridia (lack of an iris) and other specific congenital defects associated with the genetic form of the disease.

In the late 1940s the radiosensitivity of Wilms' tumor was noted and irradiation was routinely added to surgical treatment (Abeshouse, 1957). Effective chemotherapeutic agents were identified and added to the treatment regimen. Survival improved, but severe disturbances in growth and muscle fibrosis were observed to occur, as did second neoplasms.

A cooperative multicenter trial called the National Wilms' Tumor Study (NWTS) was organized to address these points (D'Angio, 1981). Patients were stratified by extent of disease and entered randomly into treatment groups. The NWTS showed that patients with tumor limited to the kidney (so-called Group I) who received actinomycin D and vincristine after removal of the affected kidney did not require radiation therapy. The trial also showed that six months of chemotherapy was just as effective as a 15-month course. The search for further reductions in effective therapy continues.

Community Trials

In most trials, allocation to treatment groups is carried out on an individual basis. However, at times the unit of allocation may be an entire community or political subdivision, as in the trials of artificial fluoridation.

Fluoridation Trials. A number of years ago, it was observed that residents of areas with water naturally high in fluoride had considerably less dental caries than residents of low-fluoride areas (Dean, 1942). Shortly thereafter, trials to test the prophylactic effectiveness of artificial fluoridation of water were proposed. Several pairs of neighboring cities were chosen, all with a naturally low level of fluoride in the drinking water. Following baseline measurements of fluoride content and of dental caries, the water of one city in each pair was left unchanged, the other treated by the addition of approximately 1 part per million (ppm) of fluoride.

All the trials gave evidence of protection against caries by fluoride. For example, Figure 8–3 shows data from the Kingston-Newburgh trial in New York State 11 years after the start of fluoridation. Children aged 6 to 12 years in Newburgh, the city with fluoridated water, were found to have approximately 50 per cent fewer caries than did children in Kingston. When the analysis was refined to exclude the older children who had not been exposed to fluoridated water in their earliest years, even greater evidence of protection was found; the amount of caries in Newburgh was 60 per cent less than that in Kingston.

Over the years, studies in various parts of the world have demonstrated that adding 1 ppm of fluoride to the drinking water is both safe and effective in preventing dental caries (Rogot, 1978). Overall, fluoridation leads to approximately a 50 per cent reduction in caries. The possibility of harmful effects was studied carefully, because in 1977 a report was published implicating fluoride compounds as a cause of cancer. However, further analysis indicated no such association; the apparent increase was shown to be due to differences in the age-sex-race composition of the major fluoridated and nonfluoridated communities.

Despite the evident value of this procedure as a preventive for caries, a vigorous antifluoridation movement has impeded the widespread acceptance of this public health measure. It is estimated that even now almost half of the United States population who live in low-fluoride areas with central water supplies do not have fluoridated water.

Three-Community Survey. Attempts to lower the incidence and mortality from cardiovascular disease were exemplified by the Stanford Three-Community survey. In this study, three communities were se-

1944-1955

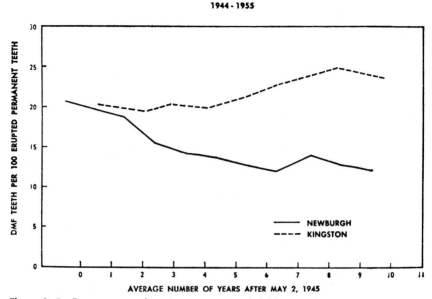

Figure 8-3 Permanent tooth caries experience of children aged 6-12 years, based on clinical examinations only, Newburgh and Kingston, New York, 1944-1955. Sodium fluoride was added to Newburgh's water supply beginning May 2, 1945. The DMF index, a count of decayed, missing and filled teeth, is used as a measure of the impact of caries experience, especially in children. (From Ast, D. B.: Dental public health. *In* Sartwell, P. E.: (ed.): Maxcy-Rosenau Preventive Medicine and Public Health. Appleton-Century-Crofts, New York, 1965, p. 571.)

lected: two were experimental communities, the third a control community. A profile including age, plasma cholesterol concentration, systolic blood pressure, smoking history, relative weight, and EKG findings was the basis for classifying individuals as "high risk." One of the two experimental communities received personal counselling for high-risk individuals; the other community received only messages through public media. Findings showed significant reduction in consumption of saturated fat and cholesterol for both communities, with a greater amount of change in the population that received intensive individual instruction (Stern et al., 1976).

THE NEED FOR EXPERIMENTALLY DERIVED INFORMATION: ETHICAL ISSUES

Although the experimental approach has been employed in the evaluation of prophylactic and therapeutic intervention only since about 1950, it is now widely accepted as the preferred method for evaluating new modalities. Despite this, the majority of published clinical trials have not used this method (Fletcher and Fletcher, 1979; Chalmers and Schroeder, 1979).

The need for sound, experimentally derived data on which to base public health programs and the medical care of individual patients cannot be emphasized too strongly. The medical literature is a virtual graveyard for inadequately tested preparations that die ignominiously after a brief moment of glory. Williams (1954) has aptly charted the life history of the typical introduction of a drug into clinical use (Fig. 8–4). After initial skepticism, uncontrolled trials lead to uncritical acceptance by hopeful investigators and desperate patients; this then gives way to a period of equally unbalanced negativism as the "miracle" drug proves to have its quota of complications and side effects. Finally, an equilibrium position is reached in which the drug achieves a level of acceptance appropriate to the benefits and risks associated with its use. At least part of this seesaw effect could be eliminated if a controlled trial were set up to test the drug at the outset.

Many standard medical and surgical practices used currently antedate the development of controlled trials and now enjoy an acceptance not supported by decisive evidence of their superiority over other forms of treatment. For example, only recently has the evaluation of drugs for effectiveness received adequate attention. The Food, Drug, and Cosmetic Act of 1938 required that drugs be proven safe before they were marketed, but not until 1962 did amendments to that act mandate that efficacy be demonstrated as well. This led to extensive review first of prescription drugs, then of preparations sold over the counter.

In the study of prescription drugs, all drugs were placed into one of five categories: effective, effective with reservations, probably effective, possibly effective, and ineffective. (Drugs in the last category were

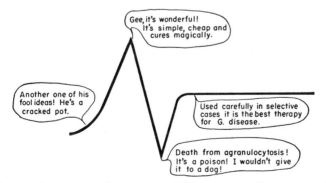

Figure 8–4 Oscillations in the development of a drug. (From Williams, R. H.: The clinical investigator and his role in teaching, administration, and the care of the patient. J.A.M.A., 156:131, 1954.)

required to be removed from the market.) The panels found that fully one-third of the prescription drugs were ineffective or only possibly effective; only two-thirds were effective or probably effective. In addition to evaluating over 3000 products, the FDA study contributed to public policy by barring anecdotal evidence of efficacy in favor of "substantial evidence," which was defined as

> . . . evidence consisting of adequate and well-controlled investigations . . . by experts qualified to evaluate the effectiveness of the drug involved, on the basis of which it could fairly and responsibly be concluded that the drug will have the effect it purports . . . to have under the conditions of use prescribed, recommended or suggested in the labelling thereof.

The FDA's criteria for an adequate, well-controlled study included careful selection of subjects and random assignment to test groups, comparison of results with those from a control group, and assurances that the study results were objective and statistically valid (Bryan, 1974).

With the growing emphasis on "scientific" medicine in the past two decades, one might expect that drugs introduced during this period would all have been subjected to careful clinical trials to evaluate their effectiveness and dangers. Unfortunately, this has not been true.

Similarly, a number of surgical procedures introduced without adequate testing through controlled trials have become the "accepted" or standard treatment for certain diseases. In this country, for almost 100 years through the mid 1970s, thousands of women were subjected to radical mastectomy each year for breast cancer despite the fact that it was not known whether any subgroup of the entire number might be treated more effectively by less radical surgery or by another modality. In 1973, a randomized trial was initiated to compare radical mastectomy with less extensive surgery, either with or without additional radiation. Eight years later, there were no differences among the treatment groups, leading to the consensus that radical mastectomy should be abandoned for the treatment of early breast cancer (Veronesi et al., 1981). Studies since then both in the United States and in Europe have supported the effectiveness of conservative treatment for this disease. Further studies are underway to evaluate the outcome of newer surgical techniques, of chemotherapy, and of postoperative irradiation.

Another procedure that has been widely employed with limited evidence of benefit has been tonsillectomy. In 1969, Bolande noted that 20 to 30 per cent of the children in most communities undergo this operation. More recently, the number of these operations performed has been drastically reduced (Moore and Pratt, 1981), as physicians and the general public have become aware of the limited benefits and possibly deleterious long-term effects of this procedure, and as tonsillectomy has increasingly become the province of board-certified ENT specialists rather than of general practitioners and general surgeons.

It is worth emphasizing that experimental trials can detect evidence of harm as well as benefit. There is usually no reason to assume a priori that a new form of prophylaxis or therapy can have only positive effects. Several of the examples we have cited illustrate this point. This reasoning applies equally to surgical therapy and to drugs. Since lymphoid tissues participate in immunologic defenses, their removal by tonsillectomy or radical mastectomy should be considered carefully to ensure that the benefits outweigh the disadvantages.

In summary, while ethical problems in experimental trials must not be brushed aside, the basic question would seem to be not **whether** experimental trials with human subjects are needed but rather **how** they should be conducted. As Bradford Hill has noted (1971), the ethical problems underlying a decision about undertaking a clinical trial are "eased more often than not by the state of our ignorance. (If) we have no acceptable evidence that a particular established treatment does benefit patients . . . whether we like it or no, we are then experimenting upon them." The problem then is to determine under what safeguards trials should be conducted in order to yield a maximum amount of information from the minimum number of study subjects.

One technique developed to minimize the ethical problems of withholding possibly beneficial agents is the *sequential trial*. The essence of this type of trial is an ongoing monitoring of results; the study is continued and new patients admitted to the trial only until statistical significance is achieved. In this way the number of patients in the trial is held to a minimum.°

SUMMARY

This chapter outlined the principles underlying the conduct of prophylactic and therapeutic trials. An experimental trial requires that there be a carefully designed protocol that specifies the criteria for selection of subjects, the procedures for allocation into study and control groups, the use of blind techniques, and any other measures to reduce bias in the collection and analysis of the data. Random allocation is essential to ensure that study and control groups are comparable. The

---

° For a discussion of the difficulties in deciding when to call a halt to a controlled trial and of other scientific and ethical issues related to clinical trials, see Chalmers, T. C., Block, J. B., et al.: Controlled studies in clinical cancer research. N. Engl. J. Med., 287:75, 1972.

danger of relying on historical rather than randomized controls was stressed.

Natural experiments were mentioned as rare occurrences that create groups similar in every way except for exposure to one factor. Such phenomena should be exploited for their epidemiologic value. Several examples of natural experiments were cited.

A variety of examples of randomized trials were given. These included home care for psychiatric patients, home versus hospital care for patients with myocardial infarction, trials of cancer therapy, trials of fluoridation of public water supplies, and a trial of cardiovascular disease in three communities.

The chapter concluded with a discussion of some of the ethical issues inherent in trials on human subjects. The need for experimentally derived data to provide a scientific basis for choosing among alternative modes of prevention and therapy was emphasized.

REFERENCES

Abeshouse, B. J.: The management of Wilms' tumor as determined by national survey and review of the literature. J. Urol., 77:792, 1957.

Beebe, G. W.: Reflections on the Work of the Atomic Bomb Casualty Commission in Japan. Epidemiol. Rev., 1:184, 1979.

Bolande, R. P.: Ritualistic surgery—circumcision and tonsillectomy. N. Engl. J. Med., 280:591, 1969.

Bryan, P. A.: Keeping Prescription Drugs Safe and Effective. Am. Fam. Physician, 10:189, 1974.

Byar, D. P., Simon, R. M., et al.: Randomized clinical trials—Perspectives on some recent ideas. N. Engl. J. Med., 295:74, 1976.

Chalmers, T. C., and Schroeder, B.: Controls in journal articles. N. Engl. J. Med. 301:1293, 1979.

Chalmers, T. C., Block, J. B., et al.: Controlled studies in clinical cancer research. N. Engl. J. Med., 287:75, 1972.

D'Angio, G. J., Evans, A., et al.: The treatment of Wilms' tumor: Results of the second national Wilms' tumor study. Cancer, 47:2302, 1981.

Davis, A. E., Dinitz, S., et al.: The prevention of hospitalization in schizophrenia: Five years after an experimental program. Am. J. Orthopsychiatry, 43:375, 1972.

Dean, H. T., Arnold, F. A., Jr., et al.: Domestic water and dental caries. Public Health Rep., 57:1155, 1942.

Ferebee, S. H.: United States Public Health Service trials of isoniazid prophylaxis. Bull. Int. Union Tuberc., 35:108, 1964.

Fletcher, R. H., and Fletcher, S. W.: Clinical research in general medical journals. A 30-year perspective. N. Engl. J. Med. 30:180, 1979.

Freiman, J. A., Chalmers, T. C., Smith, H., Jr., and Kuebler, R. R.: The importance of beta, the Type II error and sample size in the design and interpretation of the randomized control trial. N. Engl. J. Med. 299:690, 1978.

Hill, A. B.: Principles of Medical Statistics, 9th Ed. Lancet Ltd., London, p. 245, 1971.

Hill, J. D., Hampton, J. R., and Mitchell, J. R. A.: A randomized trial of home-versus-hospital management for patients with suspected myocardial infarction. Lancet, 1:837, 1978.

Hypertension Detection and Follow-up Program Cooperative Group: Five-year Findings of the Hypertension Detection and Follow-up Program: I. Reduction in mortality of persons with high blood pressure, including mild hypertension. II. Mortality by race, sex, and age. J.A.M.A., *242*:2562, 2572, 1979.

Klimt, C. R., et al.: A study of the effects of hypoglycemic agents on vascular complications in patients with adult-onset diabetes. I. Design, methods and baseline results. Diabetes, *19*(suppl.):747, 1970.

Mather, H. G., Morgan, D. C., Pearson, N. G., Read K. L. Q., Shaw, D. B., Steed, G. R., Thorne, M. G., Lawrence, C. J., and Riley, I. S.: Myocardial infarction: A comparison between home and hospital care for patients. Br. Med. J., *1*:925, 1976.

McMahon, B., and Pugh, T. F.: Epidemiology Principles and Methods. Little, Brown, and Co., Boston, 1970.

Meadows, A. T., D'Angio, G. J., Mike, V., Banfi, A., Harris, C., Jenkin, R. D. T. and Schwartz, A.: Patterns of Second Malignant Neoplasms in Children. Cancer, *40*:1903, 1977.

Meadows, A. T., Krejmas, N. L., and Belasco, J. B. for the late effects study group. The medical cost of cure: sequelae in survivors of childhood cancer. In Status of the Curability of Childhood Cancers, edited by J. van Eys and M. P. Sullivan. Raven Press, New York, pp 263–275. 1980.

Meinert, C. L., et al.: A study of the effects of hypoglycemic agents on vascular complications in patients with adult-onset diabetes. II. Mortality results. Diabetes, *19* (Suppl.):789, 1970.

Moore, F. D., and Pratt, L. W.: Tonsillectomy in Maine. Regulation versus education as modulators of medical care. Ann. Surg., *194*:232, 1981.

Multiple Risk Factor Intervention Trial Research Group: Multiple Risk Factor Intervention Trial. Risk factor changes and mortality results. J.A.M.A., *248*:1465, 1982.

Pasamanick, B., Scarpitti, F., et al.: Schizophrenics in the community: An experimental study in the prevention of hospitalization. Appleton-Century-Crofts, New York, 1967.

Rogot, E., Sharrett, A. R., Feinleib, M., and Fabsitz, R. R.: Trends in urban mortality in relation to fluoridation status. Am. J. Epidemiol., *107*:104, 1978.

Sacks, H., Chalmers, T. C., and Smith, H.: Randomized versus historical controls for clinical trials. Am. J. Med., *72*:233, 1982.

Snow, J.: On the Mode of Communication of Cholera, 2nd Ed. Churchill, London, 1855. Reproduced in Snow on Cholera, Commonwealth Fund, New York, 1936.

Stern, M. P., Farquhar, J. W., Maccoby, N. and Russell, S. H.: Results of a two-year health education campaign on dietary behavior. The Stanford Three-Community Study. Circulation, *54*:826, 1976.

Veronesi, U., Saccozzi, R., Del Vecchio, M., et al.: Comparing radical mastectomy with quadrantectomy, axillary dissection, and radiotherapy in patients with small cancers of the breast. N. Engl. J. Med. *305*:6, 1981.

Williams, R. H.: The clinical investigator and his role in teaching, administration, and the care of the patient. J.A.M.A., *156*:127, 1954.

SCREENING
IN THE
DETECTION
OF
DISEASE

━━━━━━━━━━━━━━━━ 9

Obviously, whenever primary prevention is possible, it provides the best approach to the prevention of disease. When primary prevention is not possible, early detection and treatment may serve as a secondary line of defense against diseases that are not currently susceptible to primary prevention. There are two possible approaches to early diagnosis: One depends on prompt attention to the earliest symptoms of disease, the other attempts to detect disease in asymptomatic individuals.

Early investigation of incipient symptoms or signs of disease requires the education of physicians and the public so that they can learn to respond promptly to clues indicative of disease. The efforts of the American Cancer Society to publicize "the seven signs of cancer" (unusual bleeding or discharge, a lump, a sore that does not heal, and so on) are an example of this approach.

Delays in response occur all too frequently. Studies of the sequence of events in the diagnosis of cancer have repeatedly shown that many patients delay appropriate action even if they are aware that a problem exists. Most of this delay is attributed to patient neglect, particularly in those of lower social class (Hackett et al., 1973), but physicians may also contribute to delay.

Rather than covering early response to signs or symptoms of disease, this chapter will focus on active detection of disease in *asymptomatic, apparently healthy individuals.*

The importance of the path by which disease is brought to diagnosis is illustrated by Figure 9–1. Currently (Fig. 9–1A), disease is diagnosed primarily because people refer themselves to medical care for the investigation of specific symptoms. Only a few cases of disease are

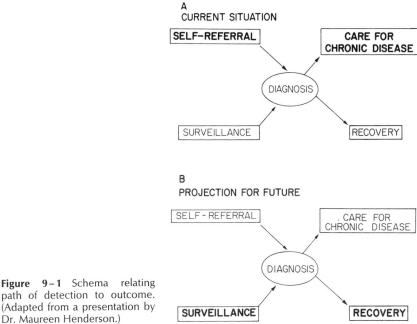

Figure 9-1 Schema relating path of detection to outcome. (Adapted from a presentation by Dr. Maureen Henderson.)

detected in the asymptomatic state because of participation in an ongoing surveillance program. Since many patients come to medical attention relatively late, the proportion of cases cured is small compared with the proportion that require protracted care, for conditions in which treatment can lead to cure.

It would be far better if most diseases could be detected in the course of regular surveillance (Fig. 9-1*B*) rather than through self-referral for symptoms. Theoretically, at least, it should always be more effective to detect disease in its preclinical stage than after it has started to produce symptoms and the threshold of clinical disease (Fig. 1-3) has been crossed. This generalization may not be true for all diseases. But, at least in the abstract, detection of disease before symptoms develop should improve the chances of preventing death and disability.

DEFINITION OF SCREENING

Screening was defined some years ago as

. . . the *presumptive* identification of *unrecognized* disease or defect by the application of tests, examinations, or other procedures which can be applied *rapidly* to sort out apparently well persons who *probably* have a disease from those who *probably do not*. A screening test is *not* intended to be diagnostic. Persons with positive or suspicious findings must be referred to their physicians for diagnosis and necessary treatment. (Commission on Chronic Illness, 1951. Italics added for emphasis.)

Figure 9–2 presents this definition of screening in the form of a flow diagram. Note that essentially two patient groups are formed by the screening procedure. Those negative on screening are presumed to be well, those positive to require further diagnostic tests. Of course, there may be some individuals whose results are so clearly abnormal that the screening test may be virtually diagnostic.

In addition to identifying persons who already have a disease, some newer screening programs are designed to identify individuals at high risk for developing the disease in the future. Figure 9–2 reflects this more inclusive concept of screening.

Screening may have one of several aims. It may be undertaken as part of an epidemiologic survey to determine the frequency or natural history of a condition (e.g., the Framingham study of coronary heart disease). Its primary purpose may also be prevention of contagion and protection of the public's health, as was true of the mass x-ray surveys formerly carried out to detect pulmonary tuberculosis. However, at this point we are concerned with *prescriptive screening*, i.e., the detection of disease, or precursors of disease, as a guide to the management of individuals.

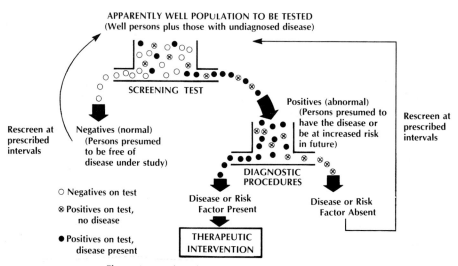

Figure 9–2 Flow diagram for a mass screening test.

PRINCIPLES UNDERLYING SCREENING PROGRAMS

The Screening Test

The screening test is the basic tool of the screening program and must, therefore, be thoroughly understood. Important characteristics include its *validity*, determined by measures of sensitivity and specificity; its *reliability* (that is, repeatability); and its *yield*, or amount of disease detected in the population. It is perhaps superfluous to note that since screening is designed to be applied to large groups of people, screening tests should be innocuous, rapid, and inexpensive; they should also be able to be carried out largely by technicians.

Validity

A screening test should provide a good preliminary indication of which individuals actually have the disease and which do not. This is referred to as the *validity* of the test. Validity has two components: sensitivity and specificity. *Sensitivity* is defined as the ability of a test to identify correctly those who have the disease. *Specificity* is defined as the ability of a test to identify correctly those who do **not** have the disease. These components are determined by comparing the results obtained by the screening test with those derived from some definitive diagnostic procedure. The extent to which the screening results agree with those derived by the more definitive tests provides a measure of sensitivity and specificity. For simplicity, we will assume that there is no error in the final diagnosis reached by the more definitive procedure.

An ideal screening test would be 100 per cent sensitive and 100 per cent specific. In practice this does not occur; sensitivity and specificity are usually inversely related. That is, one usually achieves high sensitivity at the expense of low specificity, and vice versa. This can be demonstrated readily with tests that measure a continuously distributed variable (e.g., hemoglobin, blood pressure, serum cholesterol, and intraocular pressure). For such tests, it is possible to vary the sensitivity and specificity by changing the level at which the test is considered positive. The determination of intraocular pressure as a screening test for glaucoma will be used as an example.

Determination of Sensitivity and Specificity: An Example. Glaucoma is an abnormality of the eyes in which increased intraocular pressure causes damage to the optic nerve and defects in the visual fields. In general, for the unequivocal diagnosis of glaucoma, three factors must be present: increased intraocular pressure, optic nerve atrophy, and typical defects in the visual fields.

The level of intraocular pressure on any one examination is not an infallible indication of glaucoma. Intraocular pressure varies during the day, and the variability is greater in persons with glaucoma than in others. In addition, people vary in the extent to which pathologic changes occur at a given level of pressure. Therefore, although persons with elevated intraocular pressure on casual examination are more likely to have glaucoma than those with lower pressure, further studies are needed for a definitive diagnosis. In addition to examining for changes in the optic nerve and defects in the visual field, the ophthalmologist may also conduct provocative tests (e.g., have the person drink a large quantity of water within a few minutes), which create a significant rise in intraocular pressure in persons with glaucoma.

How do the results of screening by determination of intraocular pressure relate to the presence or absence of glaucoma? The following discussion derives largely from a monograph by Thorner and Remein (1961). These authors suggest that screening tests may be understood in terms of overlapping distributions of an attribute for a diseased and a nondiseased group.* For some values of the test the distributions overlap, and it is not possible to assign persons with these values to the normal or diseased group on the basis of the screening test alone. When the screening value is clearly outside the normal range its interpretation poses less of a problem.

This situation is illustrated in Figure 9–3. Note that there are two groups, those without the disease (A) and those with the disease (B). The nonglaucomatous group (A) is much larger than group B and has a lower average intraocular pressure, with values ranging from approximately 14 to 27 mm Hg. Intraocular pressure in group B partially overlaps that in group A, lying between 22 and 42 mm Hg. The range from approximately 22 to 27 mm Hg thus includes both glaucomatous and nonglaucomatous eyes.

Now let us consider screening for glaucoma carried out by determination of intraocular pressure. If the screening level is set at 27 mm Hg, all of the nonglaucomatous eyes will be called negative, or normal. In other words, the test will be 100 per cent specific. However, since all of the glaucomatous eyes in which pressure levels lie between 22 and 27 mm Hg will also be called negative, the sensitivity of the test will be low. When diseased persons are labelled negative, or normal, the test results are referred to as *false negatives.*

On the other hand, if the screening level were set at 22 mm Hg, all eyes that are truly glaucomatous will be positive, or abnormal, on the

---

* Wilson and Jungner (1968) cite studies that do not support the existence of two overlapping distributions of intraocular pressure. Nevertheless, the model is presented because it is helpful for understanding of sensitivity and specificity.

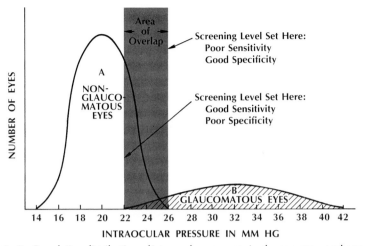

Figure 9 – 3 Population distribution of intraocular pressures in glaucomatous and non-glau-comatous eyes, as measured by tonometer (hypothetical data) (modified from Thorner & Remein, 1961).

test. That is, the test will now be 100 per cent sensitive. However, since the nonglaucomatous eyes with pressures between 22 and 27 mm Hg will also be called positive, the test will have poor specificity. Such test results are referred to as *false positives.*[*]

Of course, the level may be set anywhere between 22 and 27 mm Hg. The decision about where to set this level will be determined by a number of considerations — the cost of diagnostic testing of false positives, the importance of not missing a possible "case," the likelihood that the population will be rescreened at a reasonable interval, and the prevalence of the disease.

From what has been said so far, it can be seen that each person falls into one of the four groups labelled a, b, c, and d, (Fig. 9 – 4), depending on whether or not the disease is present and whether or not the person is positive on the screening test. Note that the percentage of false negatives is the complement of sensitivity, and the percentage of false positives the complement of specificity.

Naturally, we want a *sensitive* test, one that will identify a high proportion of those who actually have a disease and will thus create *few false negatives.* At the same time, we would like the test to be *specific* for

---

[*] Note the analogy between the selection of the screening level and of the significance (α) level in statistical decision making. The inverse relationship between false positives and false negatives is comparable to the inverse relationship between the risk of type I (α) and type II (β) errors.

Disease State

Disease	*No Disease*
True Positives (a)	False Positives (b)
False Negatives (c)	True Negatives (d)

$$\text{Sensitivity}^\circ = \frac{\text{True Positives}}{\text{True Pos} + \text{False Neg}} \qquad\qquad \text{Specificity}^\circ = \frac{\text{True Negatives}}{\text{True Neg} + \text{False Pos}}$$

$$= \frac{\text{True Positives}}{\text{All With Disease}} \qquad\qquad\qquad\quad = \frac{\text{True Negatives}}{\text{All Without Disease}}$$

° Often expressed as per cent.

Figure 9–4 Results of a screening test.

the disease; positive reactions should be limited largely to the group that is truly diseased and there should be *few false positives*.

Determination of the sensitivity and specificity of a test requires that a diagnosis of disease be established or ruled out for *every person* tested by the screening procedure, *regardless of whether he screens negative or positive*. This diagnosis must be established by techniques independent of the screening test. For example, if a urine test for diabetes is to be evaluated, the diagnosis of diabetes may be established on the basis of a blood sugar or glucose tolerance test, but not on the basis of the urine test.

It is important to be aware that the validity of a test is affected not only by characteristics of the test but also by host factors, such as stage or severity of the disease and presence of other conditions. For example, false negatives may occur early in a disease (e.g., a negative serologic test for syphilis [STS] in the first weeks after syphilitic infection is acquired) or late in disease, as in some cases of tertiary syphilis. Patients with overwhelming tuberculous infection, sarcoidosis, and Hodgkin's disease, or those taking immunosuppressive drugs may produce negative responses on a tuberculin test.

Conversely, the presence of one disease may cause a positive reaction to a screening test used to identify another condition. For example, malaria, leprosy, systemic lupus erythematosus, and other collagen diseases may cause false-positive results on screening tests for syphilis.

Predictive Value of a Screening Test

In practice, the ability to predict the presence or absence of disease from test results is dependent on the *prevalence* of the disease in the population tested, as well as on the sensitivity and specificity of the test. The higher the prevalence, the more likely it is that a positive test is predictive of the disease. This measure is referred to as the *predictive value* (PV) of a positive test, or the proportion of true positives (i.e., diseased individuals) among all those who have positive test results.

Disease State

	Disease	No Disease	Predictive Value (PV) of Test
Positive	True Positives (a)	False Positives (b)	PV_{pos} = True Pos/All Positives $\left(\dfrac{a}{a+b}\right)$
Negative	False Negatives (c)	True Negatives (d)	PV_{neg} = True Neg/All Negatives $\left(\dfrac{d}{c+d}\right)$

Figure 9–5 Fourfold table showing true and false positives and negatives and their relationship to predictive values.

Similarly, the predictive value of a negative test is the proportion of nondiseased individuals among all those who have negative test results. These relationships are shown in Figure 9–5. Figure 9–6 shows the relationship between positive and negative predictive value, and prevalence. It is only when prevalence reaches 15 to 20 per cent that a respectable PV is achieved. This means that careful attention must be paid to the group selected for screening.

The following hypothetical data illustrate the calculation of sensitivity, specificity, and predictive value and the relation of these terms to each other. Let us assume that we are dealing with a disease that has a

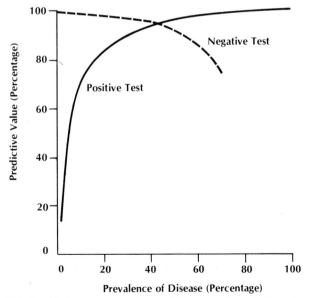

Figure 9–6 Relationship between prevalence of disease and predictive value, with sensitivity and specificity held constant at 95 per cent. (Adapted from Vecchio, 1966.)

prevalence of 2 per cent, that the sensitivity of the test being considered is 90 per cent, and that the specificity of the test is 95 per cent. The population being tested consists of 1000 people. These values can be used to construct a fourfold table. We first use the information on prevalence to separate the population into diseased and nondiseased persons. Since prevalence is 2 per cent, the number of diseased persons is $0.02 \times 1000 = 20$.

		Disease State		
		Disease	No Disease	Total
Test Results	Positive			
	Negative			
	Total	20	980	1000

We next apply the test results for the diseased and nondiseased groups, yielding:

Sensitivity:	$(0.90)(20) = 18$	Specificity:	$(0.95)(980) = 931$
False Negatives:	$20 - 18 = 2$	False Positives:	$980 - 931 = 49$

The data are now displayed in a fourfold table:

		Disease State		
		Disease	No Disease	Total
Test Results	Positive	18	49	67
	Negative	2	931	933
	Total	20	980	1000

$$\text{Predictive value of a positive test:} \quad \frac{18}{18 + 49} = \frac{18}{67} = 27\%$$

$$\text{Predictive value of a negative test:} \quad \frac{931}{933} = 99.8\%$$

Now let us look at what happens with the same sensitivity and specificity at a lower level of prevalence, e.g., 1 per cent. Repeating the computations, we arrive at a predictive value of only 14.5 per cent for a positive test.

Disease State

Test Results		Disease	No Disease	Total
	Positive	9	49.5	58.5
	Negative	1	940.5	941.5
	Total	10	990.0	1000

$$\text{PV of a Positive Test} = \frac{9}{9 + 49.5} = 14.5\%$$

Note also that sensitivity is calculated from the test results of the diseased persons (column I) in Figure 9–4; it is totally independent of the nondiseased group. Similarly, specificity depends only on the test results of the nondiseased (column II). In contrast, predictive value depends on the relation between columns I and II, i.e., on the proportion of diseased individuals in the population, or the prevalence of disease.

It is readily apparent that a high predictive value is desirable. If, for example, only 10 per cent of the persons identified as positive on a screening test are in fact diseased, then 90 per cent of the positive tests will lead to essentially unproductive diagnostic work-ups. Thus, as we have shown, if prevalence of disease is low, even a highly valid test will yield a low predictive value.

Note also that the predictive value of a positive test is of great importance to the practicing physician, who must interpret positive test results and counsel patients about a course of action. Because positive PV depends on the prevalence of disease in the sample tested, this parameter must be considered in determining the next steps in diagnosis.

Reliability (Precision)

A reliable screening test is one that gives consistent results when the test is performed more than once on the same individual under the same conditions. Two major factors affect consistency of results: the *variation inherent in the method* and *observer variation (observer error)*. The variability of a method depends on such factors as the stability of the reagents used and fluctuation in the substance being measured (e.g., in relation to meals, diurnal variation). Observer variation can stem from differences among observers (*interobserver variation*) and also from variation in readings by the same observer on separate occasions (*intraobserver variation*). These variations can usually be reduced by careful standardization of procedures, by an intensive training period for all observers (or interviewers), by periodic checks on their work, and by the use of two or more observers making independent observations.

Yield

The *yield* of a screening program may be defined as the amount of previously unrecognized disease that is diagnosed and brought to treatment as a result of the screening. The following are several factors that affect the yield of a screening program.

Sensitivity of the Test. Obviously, a screening test must detect a sufficient proportion of the cases to be useful. If the test has low sensitivity and therefore identifies only a fraction of the diseased individuals, the yield may be poor, regardless of other factors.

Prevalence of Unrecognized Disease. In the section on predictive value, the importance of prevalence to screening was mentioned. Prevalence level is related to yield of a screening program for other reasons as well. First, the incidence of disease influences yield. In addition, prevalence is also influenced by the duration of the disease and by how recently the population was screened previously. The prevalence of unrecognized disease is at least partially dependent on the level of medical care that has prevailed in a community. When little medical care has been available prior to screening, there may be much undiagnosed and untreated disease, and the yield from initial screening will be high.

Furthermore, from our epidemiologic knowledge, specific groups at high risk of a certain disease can be identified on the basis of age, sex, race, specific occupational exposure, and so on. Screening of such groups will have a higher yield than screening an unselected population. Thus, screening should be aimed at populations with high prevalence. For example, diabetes screening programs are often limited to high-prevalence groups such as persons over the age of 40, the obese, or those with a family history of diabetes.

A problem in screening for disease is that most cases of disease occur in individuals with no known risk factors. For example, in screening for neural tube defects by α-fetoprotein assay, the predictive value of a positive test is very high among high-risk women — i.e., those who have borne a child with a neural tube defect (Allen et al., 1982). However, 90 per cent of neural tube defects occur in women without such a history (Chamberlain, 1978). Thus, screening high-risk women only will cause 90 per cent of the cases to be missed. The dilemma is that, if the general population of pregnant women is screened, the predictive value of a positive test will be low and women with a normal pregnancy but a positive test may undergo abortion unnecessarily.

Multiphasic Screening. An approach that is often cost-effective is *multiphasic screening*, the administration of multiple tests or procedures to detect several pathologic conditions during the same screening visit. Thus, in certain screening programs one finds examination not only for accessible sites of cancer but also for high blood pressure and glaucoma.

When many aspects of health are tested, the probability of finding any positive results is increased. Of course, since each test produces some false positives, the total expense of follow-up increases with the number of tests performed.

Frequency of Screening. It is not possible to generalize about the optimal frequency of screening since (1) each disease has its own natural history, (2) the incidence of disease differs for different groups, and (3) there are also individual differences in risk. One of the benefits of a well-planned, well-executed screening program is the identification of individuals who are at higher risk for a given disease than the demographic group to which they belong. Conditions that increase risk may include previous cancer, family history of cancer or vascular disease, previous medical conditions, specific lifestyle (e.g., smoking or use of alcohol), past exposure to known carcinogens, and so on. With increasing knowledge of the natural history of disease, the benefits from treatment, and the effects of specific risk factors singly and in combination, recommendations for the optimal frequency of screening are subject to repeated revision and refinement. For example, there is currently disagreement about the optimal interval between cervical smear screenings and about whether the interval should be lengthened past one year for many women.

Participation in Screening and Follow-up. Screening will not improve health unless people both participate in the program and act on any problems uncovered. Psychologic and social factors affecting participation in preventive care, usually referred to as "health behavior," are therefore relevant to the success of screening programs. Four factors have been identified that determine the likelihood of participation in screening. First, a threat of disease must be perceived; that is, the disease must be known to the individual. It must also be regarded as a serious threat to health. Further, it must be defined as relevant to the patient; he must feel vulnerable. A feeling of invulnerability will inhibit action. Lastly, there must be a firm belief that action will have meaningful consequences. Fatalism will also inhibit action. In summary, if the disease being studied is perceived as a serious, personal threat, and if action is expected to abort the threat, then participation is likely. If any of these factors is not present, the person is not likely to respond to appeals to participate in the program.

Effective participation in screening by the public involves acceptance of tests and procedures, cooperation in providing needed family and medical history, and compliance with recommendations for further diagnostic tests, treatment procedures, and change in lifestyle to reduce risk. The attitudinal factors just mentioned in relation to acceptance of screening also serve to determine whether a person will follow through on the results of screening. In addition, factors of convenience, expense, and attitudes toward physicians and medical care undoubtedly come into play.

Screening also requires health care providers to be sure to take appropriate action in response to screening results. As the number of tests increases, there is more of a risk that positive test results will be overlooked or charted after the patient's discharge. The process of care must include monitoring of results and appropriate follow-up.

The yield from screening should be monitored periodically so that programs may be revised as needed. For example, for many years mass chest x-rays were a mainstay of tuberculosis case-finding programs. The progressive decrease in yield, coupled with a concern about unnecessary exposure to radiation, resulted in the substitution of routine tuberculin testing of children entering school, with the idea that identification of child reactors would lead to adult source cases. Low reactor rates led shortly to abandonment of this procedure as well. Currently, efforts are being concentrated in high-risk groups and communities.

Screening of all newborns is now routine practice in the United States. While screening programs generally aim for a high yield, programs that detect only a small number of infants with problem conditions may be warranted if serious consequences such as profound mental retardation can be averted through early detection and intervention. Phenylketonuria and hypothyroidism are good examples of such conditions. Of course, conscientious follow-up of infants with positive tests is of critical importance.

Identification of Normal Values and the Relation of Normal Values to Screening

The concept of "normal" and the specifications for separating "positives" from "negatives" deserve some discussion. The term "normal" can refer to the usual, or typical, value of a characteristic for a population group (e.g., average height or weight). It can also be used to describe *functional* status, either present or future. In this sense, any value can be considered normal if no increased risk (i.e., increased probability of disease) has been found to be associated with it. In addition, the term "normal" has a technical, *statistical* meaning, i.e., the normal or Gaussian distribution.

Since the goal of screening is to identify persons who have a disease or are at increased risk for the future, screening is concerned ultimately with a functional definition of normality. However, we must also consider how the statistical use of the term "normal" relates to the goal of screening.

The normal curve refers to a continuous, symmetrical distribution that has certain properties. A major property is that two units of variation (i.e., standard deviation [S.D.] units) above and below the mean correspond to the central 95 per cent of the area under the curve. That is, the central 95 per cent of the cases will be included in the values identified by the mean value ±2 S.D. (Figure 9–7 depicts a normal curve.) By extension, the normal range in laboratory tests or physiologic measures is often defined in terms of the central 95 per cent of values derived from a series of presumably healthy individuals.

This statistical approach to normality is often unsatisfactory for purposes of classification. For one thing, since all the people tested are presumably healthy, we are probably wrong in labelling the 5 per cent with extreme values as "abnormal." In addition, some biochemical measures are not normally distributed (Elveback et al., 1970) and, therefore, items corresponding to the mean ±2 S.D. do not represent the middle 95 per cent of the values. But beyond this, a dichotomous classification of people as "normal" or "abnormal" with respect to a certain value often oversimplifies a complex situation. We know, for example, that even within the central 95 per cent of the total range of blood pressures, there is a gradient such that persons at the upper end are at greater risk of coronary heart disease or stroke than those at the lower end.

In response to problems of this nature, Elveback (1972) has suggested that laboratory data on individuals be presented in terms of a *percentile level* and, furthermore, that this be specific for age and sex. Such specificity is needed because the same level of cholesterol might represent one percentile value for a 60-year-old female, another for a 30-year-old male. The use of age-sex–specific percentiles rather than the 95 per cent central range would emphasize that (1) no assumptions are made that the distribution is normal; (2) the same biochemical value, e.g., 300 mg per 100 ml of cholesterol, could represent a common value for an older woman, but a distinctly unusual one for a young man; and (3) health and disease lie along a continuum and that separation of the two on the basis of a single "cut-off" point may be arbitrary.

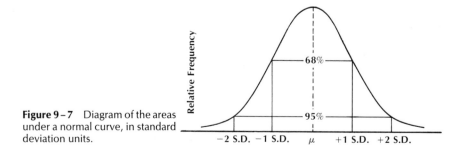

Figure 9–7 Diagram of the areas under a normal curve, in standard deviation units.

The study group from which the values are derived also deserves consideration. Ideally, norms should be based on random samples of defined, healthy populations. With few exceptions, notably the population samples examined in the National Health Survey, random samples have not been used in setting norms for physical measurements (i.e., height, weight, and blood pressure) or laboratory determinations (e.g., serum cholesterol, blood glucose, and serum uric acid). The "normal" ranges for many tests currently used in screening programs have been derived from small numbers of highly selected groups both in and out of hospitals. The development of screening programs for large numbers of healthy persons and the increasing automation of laboratory procedures should make it feasible to retrieve normative data on better samples.

Considerations in Establishing Screening Programs

The requirements for screening have been well summarized by Wilson and Jungner (1968). Following are the major issues they identify:

1. *The condition sought should be an important health problem.* Since screening requires the commitment of large amounts of money, manpower, and other resources, screening should be undertaken only when it has the potential to lead to a significant decrease in rates of disability or death or both.

2. *There should be an accepted treatment for patients with recognized disease.* The goal of screening is to prevent disability or death or both. However, if there is no generally accepted treatment, it is premature to embark on a screening program.

3. *Facilities for diagnosis and treatment should be available.* Many screening programs have had little effect because planning for them did not include adequate and effective mechanisms for follow-up of positives. This has been a major weakness of school health programs in this country.

4. *There should be a recognizable latent or early symptomatic stage.* Because of the dismal prognosis of lung cancer, there has been great interest in the possibility that early detection would improve survival. Earlier studies (Brett, 1969; Boucot and Weiss, 1973) indicated little benefit from screening. A randomized trial testing the efficacy of screening at four-month intervals was begun by the Mayo Clinic in 1971 (Taylor, 1981). Men over 45 years of age known to be heavy smokers were screened by chest x-ray and sputum cytology. Those who were negative on the initial screen were then randomized. The screened group was followed periodically by x-ray and sputum cytology. The other group received only standard advice. Follow-up to date indicates

benefit only for certain subgroups. At this time, it is not possible to reach a final decision about whether it is worthwhile to screen for lung cancer.

5. *There should be a suitable test or examination.*

6. *The test should be acceptable to the population.* Sigmoidoscopy is an effective procedure for detecting presymptomatic colorectal cancer. Unfortunately, people are reluctant to undergo the procedure. This limits the contribution sigmoidoscopy can make to the control of colorectal cancer.

7. *The natural history of the condition, including development from latent to declared disease, should be adequately understood.* This is perhaps the most crucial of all the criteria in determining the feasibility of screening. The point will be illustrated later in the chapter by reference to carcinoma of the cervix.

8. *There should be an agreed-on policy concerning whom to treat as patients.*

9. *The cost of case-finding (including diagnosis and treatment of patients diagnosed) should be economically balanced in relation to possible expenditure on medical care as a whole.* The costs of screening should not be underestimated. Any substantial screening program imposes a heavy load on the medical care system. To the costs of the screening itself must be added the expenses related to medical investigation of the "positives" and long-term follow-up of those diagnosed as having disease. The diseases for which screening is carried out (tuberculosis, diabetes, hypertension, and glaucoma) require sustained supervision. Many patients require drug therapy over a period of years. The expenses and risks secondary to these medications must also be included in the ultimate costs of screening.

A cost-effectiveness analysis should weigh the benefits of early detection (in terms of decreased mortality) against the toll on available resources, the risks, and the inconvenience of screening. Serious risks are often incurred when false positives are subjected to diagnostic work-ups involving invasive procedures.

10. *Case-finding should be a continuing process and not a "once and for all" project.* Some conditions, such as phenylketonuria and certain congenital defects, must be screened for only once, early in life. Others should be monitored repeatedly, but only in young people (e.g., lead poisoning). However, some diseases require repeated screening for many years (e.g., high blood pressure). When repeated screening is necessary, empirical studies are needed to determine the optimal interval between screenings.

One organizational setting for medical care suitable for screening on a large scale is the health maintenance organization (or HMO). The prototype of the HMO may be found in large prepaid group health plans, such as Kaiser-Permanente, HIP in New York City, and Group Health of America in Washington, D.C.

In this type of organization, screening and periodic examination can be incorporated into a comprehensive program of health care for a defined group of people. The large number of persons enrolled in each unit, as well as current technologic advances, makes it economically feasible to perform many tests for a variety of disease conditions. The existence of advanced technology permits diagnostic accuracy to be high. On the other hand, the ease with which multiple tests can be performed may lead to the purposeless ordering of a large number of tests.

Application: Cancer of the Cervix

We will apply the principles of screening to the detection of one specific disease, carcinoma of the cervix. This condition is ideal for illustrating the value of secondary prevention. With today's knowledge, cancer of the cervix cannot be prevented, but its impact can be lessened through early detection and treatment. When we consider Wilson and Jungner's criteria for screening programs, we see that cancer of the cervix basically meets all of the considerations they enumerate.

First, cancer of the cervix is a major health problem. In 1982 in the United States, an estimated total of 55,000 new invasive cases were diagnosed and 10,000 women are estimated to have died from the disease. In addition, there is an accepted treatment, facilities for diagnosis and treatment are generally available, and case-finding is not prohibitively expensive. The screening test is inexpensive, painless, free of risk, and capable of being repeated at intervals. But it is our understanding of the natural history of the disease and the existence of a valid screening test that make it worthwhile to conduct screening programs to detect cancer of the cervix.

Screening for cancer of the cervix originates with Papanicolaou's demonstration in 1943 that cytologic screening of the cervix by examination of exfoliated cells can provide early evidence of malignancy. The usefulness of the test is based on three assumptions: (1) that a high proportion of cancer detected in situ would progress to invasive cancer over time and, conversely, (2) that most cancers remain in situ long enough for screening at reasonable intervals to detect a high proportion of the cancer cases, and (3) that carcinoma in situ is highly curable. All of these assumptions appear to be valid.

Investigations conducted since the Pap test, or cervical smear, was first discovered have led to the concept that there is a continuum in the progression of cancer of the cervix. The first stage, which is thought to last for five to 10 years, is known as dysplasia.

The early changes characteristic of dysplasia are succeeded by changes that are generally labelled carcinoma in situ (CIS). The CIS stage is of variable length and persists for some three to 10 years (Barron et al., 1978). Only at the end of this sequence of changes does invasive cancer appear.°

The concept that the individual phases of cervical cancer are part of one disease process is supported by several lines of evidence:

1. The ages of the different clinical groups are compatible with a progression from preinvasion to invasive disease. The average age at the onset of each stage of the disease is given different values by different authors, but basically there seems to be agreement that the onset of dysplasia occurs before the age of 20; that CIS develops in the late 20s; and that invasive carcinoma of the cervix is first seen in the 30s. Thus, there are a number of years in which histologic changes can be detected by cervical smear and treated, with excellent therapeutic results.

2. CIS has been found at the margins of invasive cancer of the cervix (ICC) (Graham, 1962), and foci of CIS have been demonstrated in earlier biopsies of patients with ICC (Davis, 1967).

3. Follow-up studies have found that 40 to 80 per cent of patients with untreated CIS develop invasive carcinoma (Clemmeson and Poulsen, 1971; Kottmeier, 1961).

However, the situation is more complicated than we have indicated so far. Figure 9–8 presents a model showing the progression of dysplasia. Note that over time, tissue changes move in the direction of increasing abnormality, but that mild changes (mild and perhaps even moderate dysplasia) are reversible. Nasiell and his colleagues (1983) in Stockholm followed 894 women with moderate dysplasia. After an average of six and one-half years of follow-up, 54 per cent of the patients' dysplasia regressed, 30 per cent had progressed, and 16 per cent had not changed. Similar results were obtained in Baltimore (Villa Santa, 1971).

Thus, even though a substantial proportion of dysplasias can regress, the likelihood of progression is high, emphasizing the need for prompt action and continued follow-up. Delay in detection permits the development of invasive disease, which carries with it substantial morbidity and mortality.

The mortality rate from carcinoma of the cervix has been declining

---

° Another system of nomenclature (Nelson et al., 1979) is based on the concept of cervical intraepithelial neoplasia (CIN). Correspondence between CIN and dysplasia is as follows:

    CIN 1 = Mild dysplasia
    CIN 2 = Moderate dysplasia
    CIN 3 = Severe dysplasia and cancer in situ

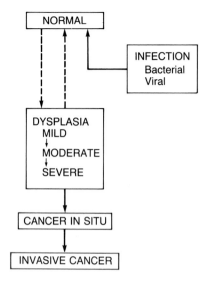

Figure 9-8 Model of the natural history of carcinoma of the cervix.

in the United States for many years—in fact, well before screening programs could have had any impact. Since no controlled evaluation of this procedure was ever done, the contribution of screening to the lowering of the death rate from carcinoma of the cervix can only be estimated. However, there is evidence of the benefits of screening in studies of its effect on incidence and mortality rates from invasive cervical cancer. Several investigators have shown that the incidence rate of ICC among screened women is significantly lower than among unscreened women (MacGregor, 1976; Fidler et al., 1968). Others have reported an inverse relationship between incidence and mortality rates and intensity of screening (Walton Report, 1976).

Figure 9-9 presents data from a cervical smear screening program over a 21-year period and shows the inverse relationship between the incidence of cancer in situ and invasive carcinoma. As more cases of CIS were diagnosed, incidence (and mortality) from ICC fell sharply. The figure also shows that there was relatively little change in the incidence of endometrial cancer during the same period of time.

Efforts are underway to describe the natural history of other cancers, with the aim of identifying a premalignant stage of the tumor during which intervention may be efficacious. Sites that are being studied include the endometrium, breast, bladder, and prostate.

By now, many studies support each other in establishing the place of cervical screening as a major contributor to prevention (Guzick, 1978). Unfortunately, the women at greatest risk of this disease tend to avail

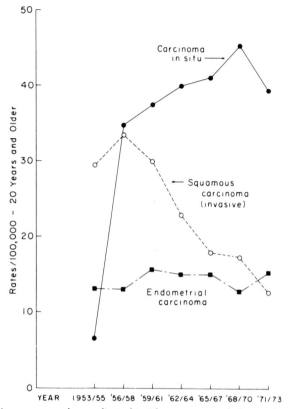

Figure 9-9 Average annual age-adjusted incidence rate trends for carcinoma in situ and invasive squamous carcinoma of the cervix and for invasive endometrial carcinoma for seven time periods, 1953–1973. (From Christopherson, W. M.: Cervical cancer control—A study of morbidity and mortality trends over a twenty-one-year period. Cancer *38*:1360, 1976.)

themselves of cervical cytologic screening less than do others in the population (Kleinman and Kopstein, 1983).

EVALUATION OF SCREENING PROGRAMS

Because of the high costs and risks incurred by screening, the impact of screening must be evaluated (Eddy, 1980). Outcome measures such as physiologic variables associated with disease (e.g., blood cholesterol level), the disease-specific death rate, and the case-fatality rate should be compared between screened and unscreened groups.

Randomized, controlled trials that compare the mortality experience of a group offered screening with a control group (usually observed conventionally) represent the optimal, least biased method of evaluation. For example, the Health Insurance Plan (HIP) of Greater New York initiated a study in 1964 to evaluate the effects of screening for breast cancer on women aged 40 through 65 years (Shapiro, 1977). Sixty-two thousand women were randomly assigned to one of two groups. The study group was offered annual mammograms and physical examinations; the control group was not offered any special screening procedures other than those obtained through their usual source of medical care. Analysis of death rates in the screened and unscreened groups after 10 years showed that, although benefit was noted only in the women aged 50 years and over, the study group had a significantly lower death rate from breast cancer than the control group.

The results of this rigorous trial led to a demonstration project jointly supported by the National Cancer Institute and the American Cancer Society — the Breast Cancer Detection Demonstration Project, or BCDDP. In this project, over a quarter of a million women in 27 centers around the country were enrolled in a program that screened them annually for breast cancer by physical examination and mammography.

Of the 4443 cancers recorded in the project, 80 per cent were detected by the centers; of this number, about a third were either noninfiltrating or less than 1 mm in diameter and over 80 per cent had no lymph node involvement. An additional finding of note was the much greater contribution of mammography than of physical examination to detection. Over 40 per cent of the tumors were detected by mammogram as compared with 8.7 per cent by physical examination. The difference was even greater for "minimal" breast cancers — that is, small and noninfiltrating tumors.

The conclusion of a National Task Force on Breast Cancer Control (American Cancer Society, 1982) was stated as follows:

> Most breast cancers occur in women over the age of 50. In this age group there is definitive proof that screening for breast cancer lowered the death rate by 30 per cent and that mammography and physical examination of the breast accounted for the reduction. It is imperative that screening using both modalities become a routine part of an annual medical examination of women over the age of 50 whenever feasible.

An additional mode of detection depends on a woman's breast self-examination (or BSE) and involves neither exposure to radiation nor cost. Women are encouraged to perform BSE regularly (i.e., monthly, after the menstrual period), because studies such as that by HIP have shown that, since BSE may contribute to early diagnosis, it can also decrease the mortality from breast cancer. However, data on the effectiveness of BSE are not available.

Sources of Bias

Unfortunately, randomized, controlled trials of screening programs are often not carried out. Other approaches to evaluating the effectiveness of screening, which are observational in nature, include comparing the case-fatality ratio of screen-detected versus symptom-diagnosed cases among nonrandomized groups; comparing the incidence rate of advanced disease among screened versus unscreened populations; relating incidence or mortality rates to the intensity of screening; and examining incidence or mortality rates before and after screening in a community.

Such nonrandomized studies are subject to several important sources of bias. The next section discusses biases of particular relevance to the evaluation of screening.

Lead Time Bias. Lead time is defined as the interval between the time a condition is detected through screening and the time it would normally have been detected by the reporting of symptoms or signs.

It is possible that screening, through earlier detection, will advance time of diagnosis without delaying time of death, thereby increasing the diagnosis-to-death interval. Thus, in comparing survival rates between nonrandomized groups, lead time bias may spuriously cause the screened case group to have a higher survival rate than the control group at any particular time after diagnosis. This bias is particularly likely to underlie apparent differences in survival when early detection either has no effect on the course of disease because of lack of an effective therapy or is not sensitive enough to detect the cancer in its earliest stages.

Length Bias. Cases detected through a periodic early detection program tend to have longer preclinical stages than those missed by screening but self-detected between examinations. The preclinical stage is defined as the interval between the time a screening test is capable of detecting disease and the time a patient seeks care as a result of experiencing symptoms. The duration of the preclinical stage is a function of the rate of disease progression and the patient's awareness of symptoms. Since these factors are themselves likely to be associated with a better prognosis, it is possible that screen-detected cases have a better prognosis than symptom-detected cases. This length bias creates an apparent advantage for screen-detected cases that may not exist in reality.

Patient Self-Selection Bias. As in any study that uses volunteers, individuals who choose to participate in early detection programs may differ from those who do not in characteristics that may be related to survival. For example, compared with nonparticipants, participants may generally have higher educational attainment and be more health-conscious, more likely to modify their exposure to risk factors (smoking, diet), more aware of symptoms, and more compliant with prescribed therapy. Any of these characteristics could be independently related to survival.

Screening programs for many conditions, particularly some of our major chronic disease problems, do not fulfill all of the principles set forth by Wilson and Jungner (see p. 228). In Great Britain, great emphasis has been placed on rigorous evaluation of screening. In a group of papers published in *Lancet* in 1974, the benefits from screening for a variety of conditions were examined carefully, and the series concluded with a very cautious statement of the benefits of screening. Among the conditions for which they found evidence of benefit from screening were Rh isoimmunization; detection of phenylketonuria in newborns; carcinoma of the bladder, particularly in exposed industrial groups; and bacteriuria in pregnancy. Multiphasic screening and the use of biochemical profiles were regarded as poor screening tools.

In the United States, screening has been accepted with greater enthusiasm. The American Cancer Society periodically reviews the evidence on the efficiency of screening for cancer and revises its recommendations for the content and periodicity of screening examinations accordingly.

Diseases other than cancer are also subject to detection by screening throughout the life-cycle. Prenatal screening in high-risk groups includes a search for chromosomal abnormalities and measurement of α-fetoprotein (AFP) for detection of neural tube defects. Screening of newborns is carried out for phenylketonuria and other congenital metabolic defects as well as for congenital adrenal hyperplasia, Tay-Sachs disease, and congenital hypothyroidism. In addition, developmental screening, such as the Denver Developmental Screening Test, is started early in the first year of life; in poverty areas, testing is also done at this time for lead poisoning. In later life, screening efforts are directed at hypertension, hyperlipidemia, tuberculosis, and sensory defects.

The special ethical and practical considerations relevant to prescriptive screening of populations have been summarized well in a book of essays, *Screening in Medical Care*, published in Britain for the Nuffield Provincial Hospitals Trust (1968).

. . . although the requirements which should be met by a screening procedure — evidence that it is effective and that it deserves priority over competing medical measures — are not unique to screening, two considerations make them unusually important in this field. First, because investigation is initiated by or on behalf of doctors, there is a presumptive undertaking, not only that the screening method is reliable, but that treatment is possible and will be made available to those who require it. And second, the large scale on which screening should be practiced makes it essential to ensure that it will make better use of limited resources than competing medical measures.

SUMMARY

In this chapter, screening was presented as a form of secondary prevention. High validity, reliability, and yield, as well as feasibility and low cost, were outlined as characteristics desired in screening tests.

Sensitivity and specificity were defined as aspects of validity. We also emphasized the predictive value of tests and the positive relationship between predictive value of a positive test and prevalence of disease. We then went on to discuss the meaning of "normal" values and their relationship to the interpretation of screening tests.

Some of the major problems currently associated with screening were outlined, including cost, lack of public acceptance, and adequate follow-up of positives. These were presented as background for current controversy over the appropriate role for screening in the spectrum of health services. We also noted the expanding potential for screening inherent in large, prepaid groups offering comprehensive care.

Screening for cancer of the cervix was then presented to exemplify a disease that is entirely suitable for screening and meets all of the criteria set forth by Wilson and Jungner as prerequisites for screening programs.

Finally, sources of bias in screening programs were identified. They consist mainly of lead time bias, length bias, and self-selection by patients.

REFERENCES

Allen, L. C., Doran, T. A., Miskin, M., Rudd, N. L., Benzie, R. J., and Sheffield, L. J.: Ultra-sound and amniotic fluid alpha-protein in the prenatal diagnosis of spina bifida. Obstet. Gynecol., 60:169, 1982.

American Cancer Society. CA — A Cancer Journal for Clinicians. 32:226, 1982.

Barron, B. A., Cahill, M. C., and Richart, R. M.: A statistical model of the natural history of cervical neoplastic disease: The duration of carcinoma in situ. Gynecol. Oncol., 6:196, 1978.

Boucot, K. R., Weiss, W.: Is curable lung cancer detected by semiannual screening? J.A.M.A., 224:1361, 1973.

Brett, G. Z.: Earlier diagnosis and survival in lung cancer. Br. Med. J., 4:260, 1969.

Christopherson, W. M.: Cervical cancer control — A study of morbidity and mortality trends over a twenty-one year period. Cancer, 38:1360, 1976.

Clemmesen, J., and Poulson, H.: Report of the Ministry of the Interior, Document 3, Copenhagen, 1971.

Commission on Chronic Illness: Chronic Illness in the United States, Vol. 1. Commonwealth Fund, Harvard University Press, Cambridge, 1957, p. 45.

Davis, H.: Comment on D.U.B. Ashley: the biologic status of carcinoma in situ of the uterine cervix. Obstet. Gynecol. Surv., 22:176, 1967.

Eddy, D. M.: The economics of cancer prevention and detection. Presented at the American Cancer Society National Conference on Cancer Prevention and Detection, Chicago, IL, April 17–19, 1980.

Elveback, L. R.: How high is high? A proposed alternative to the normal range. Mayo Clin. Proc., 47:93, 1972.

Elveback, L. R., Guillier, C. L., et al.: Health, normality and the ghost of Gauss. J.A.M.A., 211:69, 1970.

Fidler, H. K., Boyes, D. A., and Worth, A. J.: Cervical cancer detection in british columbia. J. Obstet. Gynaecol. Br. Commonwealth, 75:392, 1968.

Graham, J. B., Sotto, L. S., Paloncek, F. P.: Carcinoma of the cervix. Philadelphia. W. B. Saunders Co., 1962.

Guzick, D. S.: Efficacy of screening for cervical cancer: a review. Am. J. Public Health, 68:125, 1978.

Hackett, T. P., Cassem, N. H., et al.: Patient delay in cancer. N. Engl. J. Med., 289:14, 1973.

Kleinman, J. C., and Kopstein, A.: Who is being screened for cervical cancer? Am. J. Public Health, 71:73, 1983.

Kottmeier, H. L.: Evolution et traitment des epitheliomas. Rev. Fr. Gynec. Obstet., 56:821, 1961.

Macgregor, J. E.: Evaluation of mass screening programmes for cervical cancer in NE Scotland. Tumori, 62:287, 1976.

Medical Services Administration: Program Regulation Guide–21, Medical Assistance Manual, Part J, 70–20 Implementation. Social and Rehabilitation Service, Dept. of Health, Education, and Welfare, 1972.

Nasiell, K., Nasiell, M., Vaclavinkova, V.: Behavior of moderate cervical dysplasia during long-term follow-up. Obstet. Gynecol. 61:609, 1983.

Nelson, J. H., Averette, H. E., and Richart, R. M.: Detection, diagnostic evaluation and treatment of dysplasia, carcinoma in situ and early invasive cervical carcinoma. Cancer, 29:174–192, 1979.

Papanicolaou, G. N., and Traut, H. F.: Diagnosis of uterine cancer by the vaginal smear. The Commonwealth Fund, New York, 1943.

Screening in Medical Care: Reviewing the Evidence. A Collection of Essays. Nuffield Provincial Hospitals Trust, Oxford University Press, London, 1968.

Shapiro, S.: Evidence on screening for breast cancer from a randomized trial. Cancer, 39:2772, 1977.

Taylor, W. F., Fontana, R. S., Uhlenhopp, M. A., and Davis, C. S.: Some results of screening for early lung cancer. Cancer, 47:1114, 1981.

Thorner, R. M., and Remein, Q. R.: Principles and procedures in the evaluation of screening for diseases. USPHS Pub. No. 846, U.S. Govt. Printing Office, Washington, D.C., 1961.

Vecchio, T. J.: Predictive value of a single diagnostic test in unselected populations. N. Engl. J. Med. 274:1171, 1966.

Villa Santa, U.: Diagnosis and Prognosis of Cervical Dysplasia. Obstet. Gynecol., 38:811, 1971.

The Walton Report: Cervical cancer screening program. Can. Med. Assoc. J., 116:1003–1031, 1976.

Wilson, J. M. G., and Jungner, F.: Principles and practice of screening for disease (Public Health Papers No. 34). WHO, Geneva, 1968.

POPULATION DYNAMICS AND HEALTH

10

Knowledge of the complex interdependence between the demographic° characteristics of a population and its health status and health needs is essential to those responsible for providing health services. We have already discussed the measurement of population through the census (Chap. 4). In this chapter, we will outline the factors that influence size and composition of populations, and then present the current status of world population, with emphasis on the great disparities in population dynamics, economic levels, and health problems in different countries. Finally, we will indicate the major current trends in United States population.

FACTORS IN POPULATION DYNAMICS

Three variables determine the population of any defined area: births (fertility), deaths (mortality), and migration. The balance among these three factors determines whether a population decreases, remains stationary, or increases in number. The relation between births and deaths is referred to as *natural increase*. When the net effect of migration is added to natural increase, this is referred to as *total increase*. Demographers have evolved a number of specific measures of these dynamic factors. Since mortality rates have already been discussed, only fertility and migration will be outlined here.

° The study of population is known as *demography*. Demography has been defined as the statistical study of the characteristics of human populations, especially with reference to size and density, growth, distribution, migration and vital statistics, and the effect of all these on social and economic conditions (Webster's Third New International Dictionary).

Fertility

Many factors influence the fertility of individuals and populations. It is now widely accepted that control of fertility, like the prevention of avoidable deaths, is a public health responsibility. Both lay people and public health professionals have become increasingly concerned about the recent unprecedented growth of population. Uncontrolled fertility influences adversely the economic, physical, and psychologic health of populations and family units, especially those existing at marginal and poverty levels.

For these reasons, measurement of fertility is extremely important. One measure of fertility, the crude birth rate, has already been defined in Chapter 5. This is a very rough indicator of fertility, since everyone in the population—male, female, old, young—contributes equally to the denominator of this rate even though only females of childbearing age are actually at risk of giving birth. The percentage of the population in this category varies with past events and trends. Thus, the crude birth rate can be high either because of a currently high rate of childbearing among women of reproductive age or because women in this age group constitute a high proportion of the population.

A more refined measure of fertility is the *general fertility rate*, whose denominator is restricted to the number of women of childbearing age (i.e., usually 15 to 44 or 15 to 49).

$$\text{General fertility rate} = \frac{\text{number of live births in an area during a year}}{\text{midyear female population aged 15–44 in same area in same year}} \times 1000$$

Other, more specific measures are *age-specific, parity-specific,* and *age–parity-specific birth rates.*

Age-specific birth rate:

$$\text{Birth rate for 15–19 year old females annual} = \frac{\text{number of live births to females aged 15–19 in an area during a year}}{\text{midyear female population aged 15–19 years in same area in same year}} \times 1000$$

Parity-specific birth rate:

$$\begin{array}{c}\text{Parity-specific}\\\text{birth rate}\\\text{(annual)}\end{array} = \dfrac{\begin{array}{c}\text{number of live births of a given}\\\text{birth order occurring in an}\\\text{area during a year}\end{array}}{\begin{array}{c}\text{midyear female population of}\\\text{appropriate parity group in same}\\\text{area in same year}\end{array}} \times 1000$$

These rates are called *period* measures of fertility, because they refer to births in a population over a specified period of calendar time, usually a year. Another way of looking at fertility describes the fertility of a cohort (i.e., *cohort fertility*) of women up to a certain age or over their total reproductive life. A commonly used cohort measure of fertility is the *completed fertility rate* (also called the final birth rate or completed birth rate). This is defined as the number of children ever born per 1000 women (or married women) by the end of the childbearing period (i.e., age 44 or 49).

Closely related to the completed fertility rate is the total fertility rate (TFR), an additional and useful measure of fertility. This summarizes fertility level in a single figure. It is calculated as follows:

$$\text{TFR} = 5 \times \frac{f(15-19) + f(20-24) \ldots . f(45-49)}{1000}$$

Five is used as a multiplier because each age group consists of people from a five-year age-span. Thus, the birth data from the seven five-year age groups (e.g., 15–19, 20–24, and so on), are combined to obtain an expected number of births for the entire group of women of reproductive age. This yields an index that is simple to interpret. For example, an African country might have a TRF of 7. This would mean that if the current age-specific fertility rates were maintained, a group of women surviving to age 50 would have an average completed fertility of seven live births per woman. By contrast, the TRFs for Canada and the United States in a recent year were about 2, indicating an average completed fertility rate of two live births per woman.

The relation between period and cohort measures of fertility is complex. For example, economic recession or war, which can create short-term decline in period fertility, usually does not affect final cohort fertility. Poor economic conditions in one year may cause a couple not to have a child in that year but may not affect the couple's ultimate number of children. Lowering of the average age at which childbearing begins will create a temporary rise in period fertility, which may or may not result in an increase in cohort fertility.

Migration

Migration is defined as a change in residence in which a recognized boundary of some type is crossed. Migration does not affect world population. However, international and internal (intranational) migration can be important sources of change within a particular area. For example, in the United States the proportion of whites who were foreign-born reached a peak around the turn of the century; the census of 1910 indicates that almost one of every five whites in the country was foreign-born (see Table 10–3). This vast influx not only contributed a cheap source of labor and increased the total size of the population but also, as implied by the concept of the "melting pot," enriched and diversified the cultural heritage of the country.

Other recent changes have consisted of new patterns of immigration. As Figure 10–1 shows, the greatest peak of immigration to this country came in the years between 1890 and 1920. More recently, immigration has been largely from Central America, the Caribbean, and Asia. This more recent immigration has greatly increased the percentage of Hispanic people in this country. In 1980, over 14 million people in the United States (i.e., per cent of the population) were Hispanic°. The recent immigration consists of both legal and illegal immigrants, but the exact number of illegal immigrants is unknown.

The Hispanic population in the United States can be expected to increase disproportionately to the current numbers of Hispanic individuals, since their median age is younger than the rest of the United States population (median age of 23 for Hispanics, 25 for blacks, and 31 for whites) and since their fertility rate is high. The Hispanic population is also a disadvantaged group. Their median income in 1980 was only $14,600 as compared with $21,020 for all United States families, and over 20 per cent lived below the poverty level as compared with 10 per cent of all United States families.

Further changes in the technology of agriculture and expanded opportunities for employment in urban areas during World War II led to a mass migration of blacks from rural areas in the South to the northeastern cities. At the same time, new patterns of housing and transportation increased the movement of middle-class whites from inner cities to suburbs. Current trends in internal migration are continued shifts from rural to urban areas, from central cities to suburbs, and from inland to

---

° According to the Census Bureau, Hispanics may be of any race.

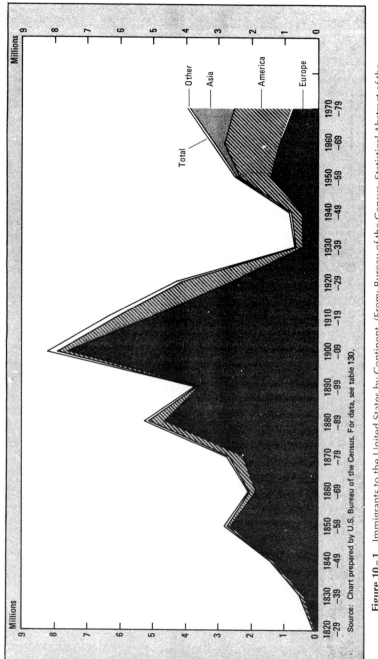

Figure 10–1 Immigrants to the United States by Continent. (From: Bureau of the Census, Statistical Abstract of the United States, 1981.)

Source: Chart prepared by U.S. Bureau of the Census. For data, see table 130.

coastal areas. These changes have had a massive impact on the relative requirements of different areas for facilities and personnel to meet health needs. In many instances, migration has been so great over a short period of time that it has been impossible to maintain an adequate level of services. Adequate social response to such changing needs is immeasurably aided by the use of census data, in conjunction with other kinds of social statistics, to register current population distribution and forecast trends.

Different kinds of population movement within the country compound the problem of satisfactory enumeration. Groups of people without a single, fixed residence include migratory workers, who are mainly but not exclusively engaged in agriculture, and military families. College students tend to have two residences, skid row inhabitants and street people to have none. The Bureau of the Census makes a limited attempt to register internal migration, but it does not request information on all moves made during the ten-year intercensal period. The lack of good information from these migratory groups can be a serious handicap to health planners and other public officials.

UNITED STATES POPULATION PROJECTIONS

One function of the Bureau of the Census is projection of population trends for the future. Figure 10–2 shows projections of United States population growth until the year 2040. The three curves are all based on the same estimates of mortality and migration but differ in assumptions about fertility. Series I, which leads to an estimated population of some 449,000,000 in the year 2040, is based on an assumption of 2.7 births per woman. Series II is based on an assumption of 2.1 births per woman. The current estimate of the number needed for population replacement, Series III, is based on a fertility of 1.7 births per woman and yields a population similar to the total population of the United States today. The estimates of Series II (the medium series) shows a United States population of 306,000,000 people by the year 2025.

Population Pyramids: The Age-Sex Composition of Populations

The effects of the three factors that influence population — births, deaths, and migration — can be shown pictorially by a figure known as a population pyramid. *Population pyramids* present the population of an area or country in terms of its composition by age and sex at a point in time. By convention, males are shown on the left of the pyramid, females on the right, young persons at the bottom, and the elderly at the top. The

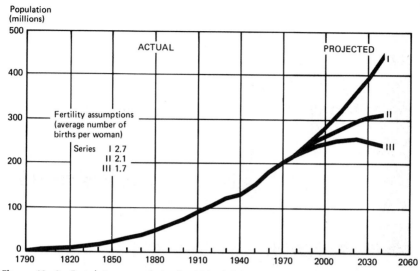

Figure 10-2 Population growth in the United States, 1790-2040, according to three different assumptions about fertility. (From: Bureau of the Census, Social Indicators. 1976, p. 4.)

pyramid consists of a series of bars, each drawn proportionately to represent the percentage contribution of each age-sex group (often in five-year groupings) to the total population; that is, the total area of the bars represents 100 per cent of the population. The shape of the pyramid reflects the major influences on births and deaths, plus any changes due to migration, over the three or four generations preceding the date of the pyramid. The following pyramids (Fig. 10-3) contrast the differences in composition of the United States in 1900 and 1970.

The essentially triangular, broad-based pattern of 1900 reflects high birth rates over a long period of time. Only a small proportion of persons have survived into the older age groups; as a result, the median age is relatively young. In contrast, the pyramid for 1970 has a narrow base and steeper sides. Life expectancy is higher, and therefore, a higher proportion of the population survives into old age, resulting in a higher median age. In other words, in 1900 the United States was a "young" country, whereas in 1970 it was an "old" country. The pyramid for 1900 is typical of developing countries; that for 1970 is typical of economically developed areas.

Irregularities in the shape of a pyramid reflect prior events in the history of a country. Severe famines affect age distribution by taking a disproportionately high toll of infants, young children, and the aged. Wars not only reduce the number of young males but also affect patterns of conception by delaying or reducing births. In Figure 10-3, for

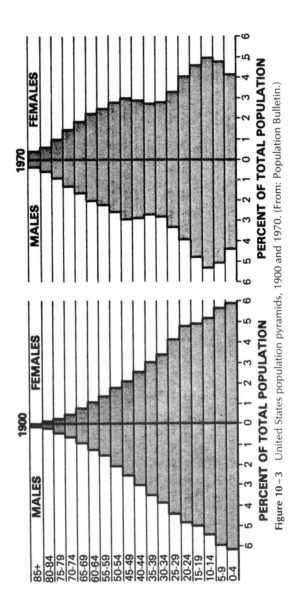

Figure 10 – 3   United States population pyramids, 1900 and 1970. (From: Population Bulletin.)

example, the slight bulge for ages 10 to 14 in 1970 suggests that the number of births was higher during 1945 to 1949 (post–World War II baby boom) than it was during 1950 to 1954.

Dependency Ratio. Another important concept is that of the *dependency ratio*. The dependency ratio describes the relation between the potentially self-supporting portion of the population and the dependent portions at the extremes of age.

$$\text{Dependency ratio} = \frac{\text{population} < \text{age 20} + \text{population} \geq \text{age 65}}{\text{population ages 20–64}} \times 100$$

The period of economic self-sufficiency is defined variously as starting at age 15, 18, or 20. The upper limit of the working population is usually set at 64, but is sometimes defined as 59. To illustrate the dependency ratio, we will assume age 15 to be the lower limit and age 65 to be the upper limit for the self-supporting population. The proportion of dependent persons was about the same in both years (Fig. 10–3), but in the earlier year 31.5 per cent were under age 15 and 4.5 per cent were age 65 or over. In 1970, 27.6 per cent were under 15 and 10 per cent were 65 or over. Clearly, the older portion of the population will require an increasing allotment of resources.

WORLD POPULATION

Concern about the size of world population goes back at least to Thomas Malthus (1766–1834), the English clergyman who warned of the dire effects of uncontrolled population growth. Malthus proposed that production of food can only increase arithmetically, whereas population increases geometrically. Malthus' analysis understated the potential for technical advances in agriculture, but his basic view of the imbalance between resources and population is nevertheless correct. His concern with the harmful effects of unchecked fertility is echoed by many modern scientists with more accurate insights into the mathematical aspects of demography and the processes of economic development.

Data about the past numbers of people on the planet are fragmentary, but available evidence indicates an exponentially increasing rate of population growth (Dorn, 1962). Figure 10–4, which is based on United Nations projections prepared in the 1950s, has been widely reproduced as an estimate of past, current, and future population figures. In considering the figures, it is well to note that no accurate information is available on the current population of many countries, and that the projections for the future are based on a number of

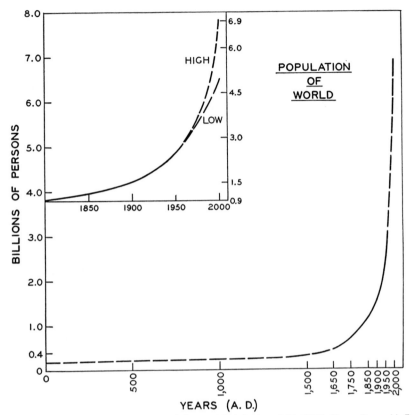

Figure 10–4 Estimated population of the world, A.D. 1 to A.D. 2000. (From Dorn, H. F.: World population growth: An international dilemma. Science, *135*:283, 1962.)

assumptions, such as the idea that food supply will be adequate to permit continued rapid growth of population.

One country for which population data recently became available is China, which conducted its first population census in 1982. This census showed a population of more than one billion people, making China the most populous country in the world. The birth rate in China was estimated to be 13.5 per 1000 in 1982. The Chinese government has set as a goal reduction of the birth rate 9.5 per 1000 for the rest of the century, so that by the year 2000 the population will not exceed 1.2 billion. To accomplish this, the government is adopting a policy of promoting one-child families and encouraging birth control and sterilization. In certain places, sanctions (e.g., reduction in income) have been applied to those exceeding the stipulated one-child family size. The social changes resulting from this new policy will affect Chinese life and family structure profoundly.

TABLE 10–1 Estimated World Population and Doubling Time in Different Eras°

Year (A.D.)	Population in Billions	Number of Years to Double
1	0.25	1650
1650	0.5	200
1850	1.1	80
1930	2.0	45
1975	4.0	35
2010	8.0†	?

° From Dorn, H. F.: World population growth: An international dilemma. Science, 135:283, 1962. Copyright 1962 by the American Association for the Advancement of Science.
† Projection based on United Nations estimates.

It is estimated that there are about four billion people on the earth today. This number is greater than it has ever been. Estimates of the length of time that man has been on the earth vary widely. Nevertheless, there is general agreement that the numbers of people on earth increased very slowly in the early millennia; by the start of the Christian era there were perhaps one-quarter of a billion people on earth. It took

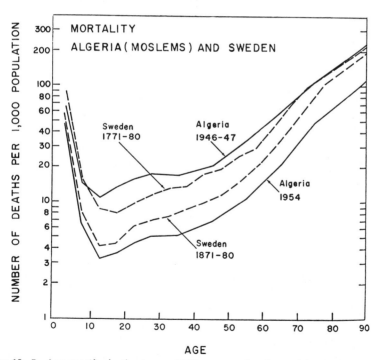

Figure 10–5 Age-specific death rates per 1000 per year, Sweden and the Moslem population of Algeria, various time periods from 1771–1954 (semi-logarithmic scale). (From Dorn, H. F.: World population growth: An international dilemma. Science, 135:283, 1962.)

approximately 1650 years for this number to double, but the rate of growth has continued to accelerate so that the next doubling, i.e., to one billion, took about 200 years, the next 80, and the next only 45 years. It is projected that the next doubling will take 35 years, so that by the year 2010 there will be eight billion people on earth. These figures are summarized in Table 10–1.

The major factor in the recent increase in world population has been a decline in death rates, especially in childhood. As a consequence, more people live into the reproductive ages. Local increases in fertility have not been of sufficient magnitude to account for the rapid rise in population.

The rapidity with which change in death rates can occur is demonstrated in Figure 10–5. Age-specific death rates are shown for Sweden and the Moslems in Algeria, each at two different time periods. Note that between 1946 to 1947 and 1954, the decrease in the death rate for the Moslems in Algeria was greater than that which occurred in Sweden over the 100-year period between 1771 to 1780 and 1871 to 1880.

THE STAGES IN DEMOGRAPHIC DEVELOPMENT

The explosive increase in the number of people in the world in the recent past has resulted from the complex series of developments accompanying the industrial revolution and the worldwide spread of advanced technology

Demographic transition is a term used to describe the major demographic trends of the past two centuries. As we have seen in Figure 10–2, the rate of growth in population since 1790 exceeds anything previously known on this earth. The change in population basically consists of a shift from an equilibrium condition of high birth and death rates characteristic of agrarian societies to a newer equilibrium in which both birth and death rates are at much lower levels. The period of

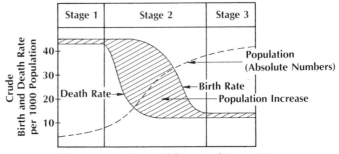

Figure 10–6 Stages of demographic transition.

transition, at least in Western Europe, was initiated by a drop in death rates that was followed some years later by a fall in birth rates. The intermediate period was one of rapid population growth, as illustrated in Figure 10–6, a schematized illustration of the demographic transition.

Figure 10–7 shows the demographic shift that occurred in England and the United States. In 1750, both crude birth and death rates were high in England. The crude death rate began to fall toward the end of the seventeenth century, but it was only about 100 years later that the birth rate fell similarly.

In the United States, the pattern was different. The crude death rate (extrapolated for the country from Massachusetts, the only source of data before 1900) fell throughout the nineteenth century. The crude birth rate, which had been extremely high in the early part of the nineteenth century, dropped from 1800 on, but it was only after 1900 that crude birth rates below 25 were observed.

The demographic changes that we have traced in the United States and England are in accord with our knowledge of different societies. We know that agrarian civilizations are characterized by stable or slowly growing populations. Agricultural existence favors large families: children are needed to work the soil; sons are desired to inherit the farm; and the tradition-bound lifestyle militates against such innovations as the adoption of new techniques for family planning. However, high birth rates are balanced by high death rates from disease, famine, and war (stage 1).

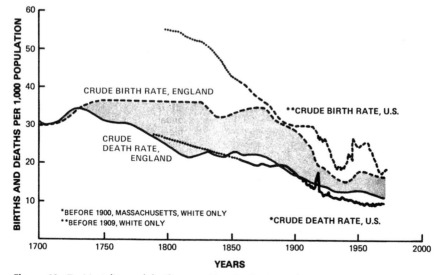

Figure 10–7 Mortality and fertility transition in the United States and England. (From: Population Bulletin.)

Advances in sanitation and improved availability and quality of food, water, and shelter lead to a fall in death rate and an increase in life expectancy. This has usually occurred without an immediate change in birth rate; however, the improved conditions of life may favor an increase in fertility. During this period (stage 2), a marked excess of births over deaths develops, leading to a rapid expansion in population.

After a time, birth rates tend to fall, largely as a reflection of industrialization and consequent urbanization. With industrialization, people tend to migrate from rural to urban areas. Urban living not only breaks the traditional patterns but also creates incentives for having small families. Living quarters are cramped. Children begin to represent a financial liability rather than an asset. There is a greater need for cash, since food and clothing can no longer be produced at home. For these reasons, husbands and wives are impelled to seek work outside the home for wages. There is a greater geographic proximity to health care services and to the availability of information about family planning. These various factors increase the likelihood that contraceptive practices will be adopted. In some places, abortion has also been included in the measures available for the control of fertility.

The end-stage (stage 3) of this demographic transition is a situation in which birth and death rates are again essentially in balance but at a lower level (e.g., about 10 to 15 per 1000 population) as compared with those of the primitive first stage, when both rates were in the vicinity of 35 to 45 per 1000.

The form of demographic transition exhibited by England and the United States is not duplicated exactly elsewhere, owing to a variety of factors. Several local variants shown in Figure 10–8 are referred to as the "accelerated," "delayed," and "western" models. As compared with the "western" model, the first two models are characterized by (1) later onset of demographic change, (2) a rapid drop in the death rate, and (3) an accelerated rate of population growth.

Population Momentum

The extent to which past trends in population will be reflected into the future is of great importance. Consider a country with high birth rates: Even if this country's population would reduce its fertility rate abruptly to replacement levels, the population would continue to grow for many years because it would contain so many young people who would still have to pass through the childbearing years. This population momentum is very significant for developing countries that have been undergoing rapid growth in the recent past.

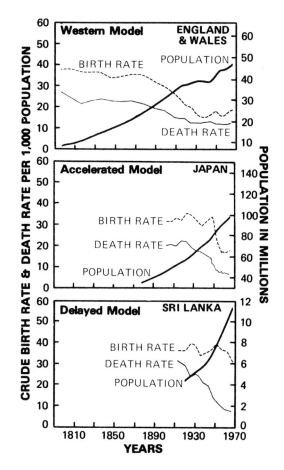

Figure 10-8 Western, accelerated and delayed epidemiologic transition patterns. (From: Omran, A.R.: The epidemiologic transition: A theory of the epidemiology of population change. Milbank Memorial Fund Quarterly 49:515, 1971.)

Consequences of Demographic Status

There are epidemiologic consequences of demographic status. For example, the diseases characteristic of the pretransition period are largely epidemics of infectious disease — typhoid, tuberculosis, cholera, plague, diphtheria, and so on. All of these are superimposed on a high endemic death rate caused by a variety of less dramatic illnesses, such as respiratory and gastrointestinal infections. A clear illustration of this is seen in the graph of deaths over time in New York City (Fig. 10-9). Sharp peaks of mortality and a high base rate of deaths is apparent. Omran (1971) has referred to this as the "Age of Pestilence and Famine." As various environmental controls were introduced (e.g., purification of water, pasteurization of milk, improved personal hygiene and

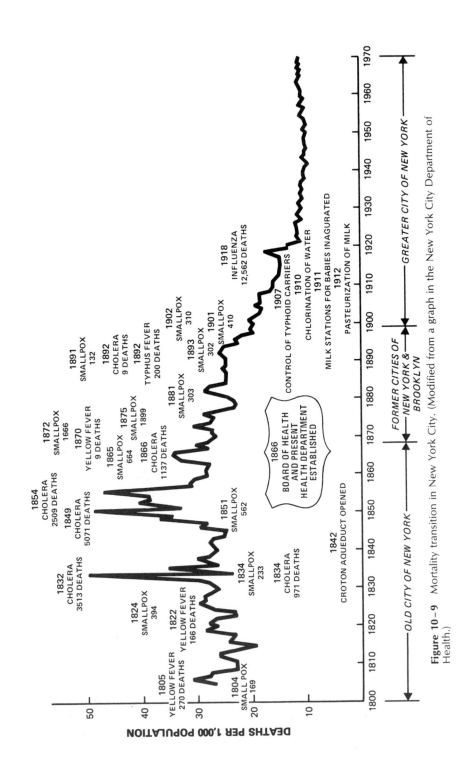

Figure 10–9 Mortality transition in New York City. (Modified from a graph in the New York City Department of Health.)

nutrition), there was a shift into the "Age of Receding Epidemics." This, in turn, gave way to what we know of disease patterns today. We are now in an "Era of Degenerative and Man-made Diseases." These latter diseases have their greatest impact on older people, whereas the diseases of the pretransitional era affected mainly children and young adults.

Comparison of Countries at Different Stages of Transition

To sharpen our understanding of the profound differences between countries at different stages in the demographic transition, it might be useful (Table 10–2) to compare the developed countries (industrialized, stage 3) with those that are essentially agrarian (stage 1) or only partly through the process of demographic change ("developing," stage 2).

As we look at the features of the developing countries, we see a constellation of forces that operate to maintain a static level of economic development and create a cycle of poverty and ill health. Solutions to the total complex of problems presented by developing countries cannot be

TABLE 10–2 Comparison of Some Major Demographic and Economic Characteristics of Developing and Developed Countries

Characteristic	Developing	Developed
Birth rate	High (e.g., 35–50 per 1000)	Low (e.g., under 20 per 1000)
Infant mortality rate	High (e.g., 50–180 per 1000 live births)	Low (e.g., 10–18 per 1000 live births)
Crude death rate	High° (e.g., 25 per 1000)	Low (e.g., 10 per 1000)
Life expectancy	Low (e.g., 45–65 years)	High (e.g., 65–78 years)
Average age of population	Young	Old
Percentage under 15	High (35–45 per cent)	Low (20–25 per cent)
Percentage 65 and over	Low (e.g., 3 per cent)	High (e.g., 13 per cent)
Literacy	Low	High
Per capita income	Low (e.g., $150 per year)	High (e.g., $7300 per year)
Percentage of males engaged in agriculture	High (e.g., 80 per cent)	Low (e.g., ≤ 5 per cent)
Productivity of land	Low	High
Food-to-population ratio	Low	High
Animal protein in diet	Low	High
Disease due to poor environmental conditions	Common	Rare but increasing with industrialization
Physician-to-population ratio	Low (e.g., 1 : 10,000– 15,000)	High (e.g., 1 : 800)
Accumulation of capital	Little or none	Great

° Crude death rate may be low because of the young age of the population even with high age-specific death rates.

simple, nor can "health" problems be resolved solely through provision for health needs alone, since these are woven so firmly into the total fabric of life.

Whatever the optimal combination or sequence of interventions, it is clear that decreased fertility is an essential component in economic advance. In a number of countries, herculean efforts at economic development have been negated by an ever-increasing number of people to be fed, housed, clothed, educated, and given medical care. The problem of population in technically developed nations is somewhat less acute but nonetheless real.

Governments throughout the world vary in their population policies, which may be divided into three categories: antinatalist, pronatalist, and neutral. Most Western countries, such as the United States and the United Kingdom, are basically neutral, although some of their tax policies are favorable to large families. The antinatal policy is typical of such countries as mainland China and India. But the approaches of these two countries differ greatly: the stern, restrictive measures employed in China contrast with the relatively ineffectual attempts used in India to persuade the population to limit family size.

Pronatalism was characteristic of Nazi Germany and Fascist Italy, and France was conspicuously pronatalist for many years. In 1939, the French government introduced the Code de la Famille, which encouraged larger families through subsidies, a policy that persisted until recently.

Despite local variations, on a worldwide basis it is generally agreed that the potential threat lies in over-, not underpopulation, and efforts should be directed toward the control of fertility, not its encouragement.

TRENDS IN UNITED STATES POPULATION

In the final section of this chapter, we would like to point out the major current trends in population in this country (Fig. 10–10, Table 10–3), with particular focus on their relevance to health and social needs.

The *net growth rate* of a population reflects the net difference between additions to the population through births and immigration and losses from deaths and emigration. Thus, the net growth rate for the United States in 1979 was 9.7 per 1000 population, or approximately 1 per cent. Its components were:

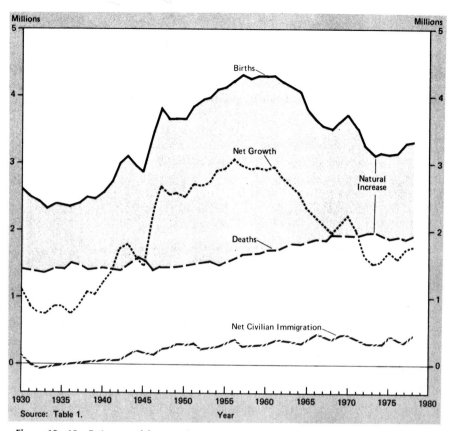

Figure 10–10 Estimates of the population of the United States and components of change: 1940–1978. (From Series P-25, No. 802, Bureau of the Census, May 1979.)

$$\text{Net growth rate}^\circ = \text{Birth rate} - \text{Death rate} + \text{Net immigration rate}$$
$$8.2 \qquad = \qquad 14.8 \quad - \quad 8.7 \quad + \qquad 2.1$$

Figure 10–10 shows yearly rates of net growth of population and its components over a 50-year period. The outstanding feature evident is the abrupt rise in net growth rate in the late 1940s followed by a decline after the peak period (1947 to 1960). Crude death rate and net immigration increased slightly over the entire interval, but the major influence on growth rate has been fluctuation in births — the birth rate has been declining since 1957. The increase in age of the population over this time undoubtedly accounts for most or all of the rise in the crude death rate.

The striking increase in the size of the United States population

---

° Rates can be added or subtracted directly only if they are based on the same common denominator.

from 1790 to 1980 is evident in Table 10–3. Other features of population change also indicated in the table include the following:

Variation in Rate of Increase. In general, the rate of increase has declined. Until 1860, the population increased by more than 30 per cent each decade (i.e., 3 per cent per year). Between 1860 and 1910, the rate of increase each decade dropped to between 20 and 30 per cent. Since 1910, it has consistently been below 20 per cent. The lowest rate, 7.2 per cent, was recorded in 1940 as an aftermath of the depression.

Changes in Proportion of Nonwhites. Until 1920, there was a constant decline in the proportion of nonwhites in the population (from 19 to 10 per cent), partially owing to the heavy immigration of whites.

TABLE 10–3 Summary of United States Population Growth and Change, 1770–1980 °

Census Year	Total Population	Percentage Increase in Previous Decade	Percentage Nonwhite	Percentage White Foreign-born	Percentage Urban-C†
1770-A†	2,205,000	37.0	D†	D†	D†
1780-A	2,781,000	26.1	D	D	D
1790	3,929,214	41.3	19.3	D	5.1
1800	5,308,483	35.1	18.9	D	6.1
1810	7,239,881	36.4	19.0	D	7.3
1820	9,638,453	33.1	18.4	D	7.2
1830	12,866,020	33.5	18.1	D	8.7
1840	17,069,453	32.7	16.8	D	10.8
1850	23,191,876	35.9	15.7	11.6	15.3
1860	31,443,321	35.6	14.4	15.2	19.8
1870	39,818,449	26.6	12.9	16.4	25.7
1880	50,155,783	26.0	13.5	15.1	28.2
1890	62,947,714	25.5	12.5	16.6	35.1
1900	75,994,575	20.7	12.1	15.3	40.0
1910	91,972,266	21.0	11.1	19.5	45.7
1920	105,710,620	14.9	10.3	16.9	51.2
1930	122,775,046	16.1	10.2	14.5	56.2
1940	131,669,275	7.2	10.2	9.7	56.5
1950	150,216,110	14.1	10.5	7.5	64.2
1960-B†	179,323,175	19.4	11.4	5.9	69.9
1970-E†	203,211,926	13.3	12.6	4.9	73.5
1980	226,505,000	16.4	16.9	6.2‡	73.7

° From U.S. Decenniel Censuses. Bureau of the Census, U.S. Govt. Printing Office, Washington, D.C., selected years.

† A, Estimated; B, includes Alaska and Hawaii; C, definitions of "urban" have changed many times, and generally reflect contemporary political, social, and economic developments; D, data not available; E, preliminary.

‡ 6.2% of population is foreign-born, but for 1980 this is based not just on whites but on the entire population.

Since 1940, the proportion of nonwhites has increased from 10.2 to 16.9 per cent, because of immigration, higher birth rates, and greater proportionate gains in life expectancy among nonwhites.

Changes in Proportion of White Foreign-born Population. The variations in the proportion of the white population born abroad was discussed earlier in the chapter (see section on migration, p 242).

Steady Increase in Urbanization. Whereas in 1790 only one out of 20 persons were city-dwellers, today three out of four people live in urban areas. The typically small size of apartments and homes in urban areas tends to reduce the size of households. Three-generation households have become less common. The difficulty of absorbing persons other than members of the nuclear family has led to a need for nursing homes and similar facilities for elderly and chronically ill persons.

Other trends in population that are apparent from neither Figure 10–10 nor Table 10–3 include the following:

Movement from Cities to Suburbs. A migration of population from city to suburb was a major feature of the 1980 census. In that year, city residents were outnumbered by suburbanites in a ratio of three to two. Extensive movements of population within a country create problems for public health workers. Not only is there difficulty in planning health facilities for a shifting population, but there is also a problem with the scattering of health records and lack of continuity for individuals.

Increase in Proportion of Women. The male-to-female ratio, which was 104 in 1920, has dropped continuously since then and was 94.5 in 1980. This decrease has been caused primarily by the proportionately greater increase in life expectancy for females than for males, and possibly also to changes in patterns of immigration.

Industrialization. Closely tied to the urbanization noted previously is industrialization. Over the years, there has been a progressive decrease in the proportion of people engaged in farming and an increase in those working in industry and service occupations. In 1980, the proportion of the working population engaged in agriculture, forestry, and fisheries reached an all-time low of 3 per cent. Within industry, automation and changes in the relative importance of capital-intensive and labor-intensive industrial processes have led to a massive shift away from production toward service and white-collar activities. The change from the relative self-sufficiency characteristic of farm life to specialization and dependence on monetary earnings has resulted in a greater need for old-age, unemployment, and disability benefits.

Increase in Literacy and Level of Education. The increased level of education in the population over the past decades, along with advances in medical science, has generated a rising level of expectation for medical services. The concept of medical care as a right rather than a privilege has increasingly permeated social thinking.

Increase in the Proportion of Women in the Labor Force. This is one of the more important trends of our times. For instance, whereas women comprised 28 per cent of the labor force in 1950, this proportion had risen to 45 per cent by 1980. This is due only partly to a decrease in the proportion of older men who work.

Changes in the Composition of Households. Husband-wife households, with or without children, used to be the "normal" social arrangement, but this is no longer the case. Many different types of households are seen today, including the following:

1. Households with persons of the opposite sex living together (cohabitation)

2. Other arrangements made by adults of the same or opposite sex

3. Single-person households; this is seen increasingly among persons of all ages but particularly with elderly people. In 1975, almost 10 per cent of all women over 65 were living alone.

4. Families with female heads-of-household. In 1979, no husband was present in 31.9 per cent of households. This was particularly true in black families. In 1975, 35 per cent of black family units were headed by females, as compared to 10.5 per cent of white family units.

Current Economic Status

Until recently, the majority of Americans have been more prosperous than any other people in the history of the human race. This condition no longer prevails. When individuals become unemployed, many lose not only their incomes but also their health insurance benefits. The combination of loss of benefits for individuals and the withdrawal of government supports for health care and nutritional supplements is creating a large number of people who qualify neither for preventive nor for curative services. The fact that there is no universal United States health insurance means that health services will be available primarily only to those who can afford to pay for them, with the exception of the most impoverished individuals, who qualify for such programs as Medicaid. The impact of this situation on health may be profound and disastrous.

Implications for Health

Each of the trends and population features just outlined has important consequences for health and needs for health services. For example, the high proportion of working mothers requires that there be adequate arrangements for child care and for health supervision to accommodate the working mothers' schedules. This is particularly true in view of the current high rate of divorce and separation. In 1980, one-fourth of all children under the age of 18 were living with either no parent or only one parent. An attempt is being made to meet these needs through the development of day care centers.

Our high rates of utilization of resources create, and urbanization and associated industrialization intensify, environmental problems of all kinds, such as water and air pollution, solid waste disposal, and noise "pollution." In addition, shifts in population have left the inner cities with a concentration of problems at the interface of medical and social pathology: alcoholism, delinquency, drug abuse, suicide, venereal disease, tuberculosis, and mental illness. These problems are compounded by the loss of revenue-producing industries and the flight of middle-class householders from the cities.

The population problems facing the United States are well expressed in the following quotation from the Presidential Commision on Population Growth and the American Future (1972):

Demographic events have the quality of persisting over time, for example, the baby boom generation born after World War II is still working its way through the age structure, with many repercussions. . . . Because the lead time is decades in length, it is necessary to face the issue now and come to deliberate and informed decisions about population problems. . . . The major contribution to growth now comes from the advantaged majority in our society. Because of their smaller number, our "have-not" groups—our racial and ethnic minorities—do not bear the primary responsibility for population growth, and inducing them to limit the number of children they have would not in itself stabilize our population. However, there are strong connections between high fertility and the economic and social problems that affect the 13 per cent of our people who are poor. Therefore, we recognize that unless we address our racism and poverty we will not be able to resolve the question of population growth for our racial and ethnic minorities. As deprived groups are brought into the educational, occupational, and residential mainstream, their fertility will probably decline to the level of the people already there.

SUMMARY

Births, deaths, and migration are the three variables that determine the size and composition of the population of any defined area. The operation of these factors over several decades is mirrored in population pyramids that depict percentage distribution of the population by age and sex at a point in time. Developing countries with high birth and death rates have a triangularly shaped pyramid, whereas countries with low birth and death rates have pyramids of a more rectangular shape. Past levels of fertility and mortality determine the dependency ratio, a measure of the relative proportions of economically productive and unproductive persons (i.e., those at the extremes of life) in the population.

In this chapter, a historic account of trends in world population led to a series of projections for the future. The demographic transition was identified as the changes in birth and death rates that have typically accompanied the shift from agrarian to industrialized societies. The rapid population growth characteristic of countries in the process of transition was noted. The economic status and health needs of developed and developing countries were contrasted.

Lastly, we focussed on trends in United States population. Excerpts of the report of the Presidential Commission on Population Growth and the American Future were cited in support of the need for stabilization of the United States population.

REFERENCES

Dorn, H. F.: World population growth: An international dilemma. Science, *135*:283, 1962.

Omran, A. R.: The epidemiologic transition. A theory of the epidemiology of population change. Milbank Mem. Fund Q., *49*:509, 1971.

Omran, A. R.: Epidemiologic transition in the United States. The health factor in population change. Pop. Bull. *32*, No. 2, 1980 (updated reprint).

Population and the American Future. Final Report, Commission on Population Growth and the American Future. U.S. Govt. Printing Office, Washington, D.C., 1972.

General Reference

Ewbank, D., and Wray, J. D.: Population and public health. In Last, J. M. (Ed.): Maxcy-Rosenau: Public Health and Preventive Medicine, 11th Ed. Appleton-Century-Crofts, New York, 1980.

EPIDEMIOLOGIC ASPECTS OF INFECTIOUS DISEASE[*]

11

Despite the great scientific advances that have reduced morbidity and mortality from infectious diseases over the past decades, these conditions continue to account for a major proportion of acute illness, even in technically advanced countries. Current estimates put the toll from infectious disease in the United States at 145 million school-loss days and 130 million days lost from work, in addition to 140,000 deaths annually.

In this chapter, we will discuss various aspects of infectious disease, beginning with variations in the severity of illness, which includes inapparent infection, and progressing to host-parasite interactions, methods of transmission, person-to-person spread of disease, types of epidemics, and the investigation of an epidemic.

VARIATIONS IN SEVERITY OF ILLNESS

Infectious processes can result in a wide variety of clinical effects, ranging from inapparent infection to severe clinical illness or death.

Recovery may be either complete or associated with mild or severe sequelae. Some infections that are usually inapparent may nonetheless be considered severe because they have a high case fatality rate (CFR) or a high rate of severe clinical manifestations in those who are clinically ill. For example, St. Louis encephalitis in an urban setting has a ratio of

---

[*] With the assistance of C. Stephen Bowen, M.D.

clinical to inapparent infections of approximately 1 to 200, but the CFR among the clinically ill, especially those over age 60, may be as high as 15 to 20 per cent.

The CFR is defined as the number of deaths from a particular disease divided by the number of clinically apparent cases of that disease:

$$CFR = \frac{\text{Number of deaths from a disease}}{\text{Number of clinical cases of that disease}}$$

The CFR for a disease must be distinguished from the mortality rate caused by that disease, which, it may be recalled, is defined as follows:

$$\text{Mortality rate} = \frac{\text{Number of deaths from a disease}}{\text{Population at risk of acquiring a disease}}$$

A disease is considered severe if the case fatality rate is high or if a substantial proportion of the surviving patients are left with sequelae. In addition to the effect of a disease on individuals, the severity of a disease may also be considered from the point of view of its public health impact (i.e., impact on the entire population). Diseases of low incidence and high CFR (e.g., rabies) may be severe for individuals, but a disease of high incidence and lesser severity (e.g., influenza) may be a much more serious problem from a public health standpoint because it causes a great deal of excess mortality in the population as a whole. Excess mortality is mortality above expected levels for the season and geographic area in question in nonepidemic years.

The following discussion will focus on characteristic or modal severity of diseases, as shown in Figure 11–1. The first bar chart (Class A) describes infections of which a high proportion are inapparent, i.e., the infection does not become manifest at any stage. These infections have a low pathogenicity (see further on); only a small fraction are clinically evident, an even smaller proportion severe or fatal. This type of infection has been likened to an iceberg, whose visible tip represents only a small fraction of the whole. For example, the number of people with positive tuberculin tests (an indication of infection with tubercle bacilli at some time in the past) far exceeds the number who develop clinical tuberculosis. Other examples would be infections with St. Louis encephalitis virus, with polio virus or hepatitis A virus in early childhood, and with the meningococcus. Only a small fraction of the total number of Class A infections can be identified without special diagnostic tests.

The second horizontal bar (Class B) represents infections in which the inapparent component is relatively small. Most of the cases are

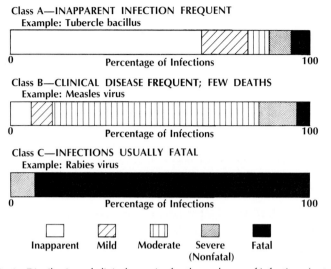

Figure 11-1 Distribution of clinical severity for three classes of infections (not drawn to scale).

clinically apparent and readily diagnosable (i.e., they appear to be "classic" cases); only a small fraction are severe or fatal. Examples would include measles and chickenpox.

The last bar (Class C) portrays infections in which the outcome is typically severe or fatal illness. Rabies is an outstanding example, since virtually 100 per cent of infections with rabies virus end in death. Other very severe but not uniformly fatal diseases include primary amoebic meningoencephalitis, the African hemorrhagic fevers caused by Marburg and Ebola viruses, and infections from agents such as Lassa fever virus and Machupo virus.

In contrast to overt disease, which can sometimes be detected by clinical evaluation alone, inapparent infection cannot be diagnosed without such procedures as tuberculin tests or throat cultures for diphtheria organisms. The number of human infections with rabies virus may be adequately estimated by clinical examination, but infections with polio virus or meningococci will largely go undetected. For accurate estimates of the extent of inapparent infection in a population, epidemiologic surveys may be needed in which apparently well persons are tested for direct or indirect evidence of the presence of specific organisms. Such information on inapparent infection is important for practical reasons as well as for academic curiosity. Laboratory evaluation may also be essential for treatment of many common clinical syndromes (e.g., meningitis, urethritis, vulvovaginitis, and so on) as well as for epidemiologic investigation.

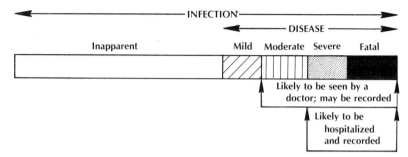

Figure 11-2 The relation of severity of illness to disease statistics.

Inapparent Infection and Control of Disease. Procedures for control must be directed toward all infections capable of being transmitted to others. Since many inapparent infections can be transmitted and can produce disease in others, it is insufficient to direct procedures solely to clinically apparent cases. Before inapparent infection was well understood, control measures were directed mainly toward persons known to be ill. Emphasis was placed on isolation of patients, disinfection of their belongings and excreta, and quarantine of exposed persons (e.g., household contacts) who might be incubating disease. While isolation is still an essential part of control procedures for some diseases, the focus on isolation and disinfection has been replaced by a more general concern with the spread of organisms through a community. The current focus on discovery and treatment of asymptomatic carriers of gonorrhea illustrates the importance of detecting inapparent infection for control of disease. In fact, efforts at control may include deliberate spread of inapparent infections, such as the administration of live, attenuated oral polio vaccine.

Inapparent Infection and Disease Statistics. The impact of inapparent infection on disease statistics is shown in Figure 11-2 for Class A infections. Only the small fraction of infections that cause obvious disease or severe symptoms will come to medical attention; an even smaller fraction will find their way into hospital records. Therefore, statistics on infections with this kind of gradient are likely to be inaccurate. The number of infections diagnosed and reported will be understated, i.e., it will be lower than the true number of infections, while the severity of the disease will be overstated. Thus, when the discrepancy between "infection" and "disease" is large, it is particularly important to know the criteria used for diagnosis. Many more infections will be recorded if those detected by laboratory methods or skin tests are included than if only clinically diagnosed cases are tabulated.

COMPONENTS OF THE INFECTIOUS DISEASE PROCESS

Infectious Agents

A wide variety of infectious agents, from the simplest viral particles to complex multicellular organisms, can produce disease in man. No discussion of infectious disease would be complete without specification of infectious agents as essential links in the chain of events resulting in infection in man. A detailed or comprehensive account of the various agents is beyond the scope of this text. However, an introduction to some basic concepts of agent factors and host-agent interactions is essential to an understanding of the biology and epidemiology of infectious diseases.

Intrinsic Properties of Infectious Agents

Many characteristics of infectious agents are agent-determined or intrinsic to the agent itself and do not depend on any interaction with a host. Among these are morphology, size, chemical character, antigenic make-up, growth requirements (temperature, nutrients, and so on), ability to survive outside a host in a variety of vehicles (e.g., water, milk, soil), viability under different conditions of temperature and humidity, spectrum of hosts (animals and arthropods), ability to produce toxins, ability to become resistant to antibiotics or other chemicals, and (for bacteria) ability to acquire new genetic information from plasmids or other subviral particles. All infectious agents vary considerably in these intrinsic characteristics. Understanding a particular intrinsic property may be essential to understanding an agent's epidemiology, including its mode of transmission. In addition, strains or isolates of a particular agent from different outbreaks or different geographic areas at different times may vary significantly in some of the properties just given.

Host-Parasite (Infectious Agent) Interactions

Many properties that are ascribed to infectious agents are not actually intrinsic to the agent but are dependent on the interaction between the agent (parasite) and the host. Included in this category are infectivity, pathogenicity, virulence, and immunogenicity. Environmental conditions, dose, and route of infection can, of course, change these properties of infectious agents. The same pathogen obtained from different sources may, as noted, differ in these four properties. Host factors such as age, race, and nutritional status may also dramatically change an agent's ability to infect, produce mild or severe illness, or immunize a host or population of hosts.

Infectivity is defined as the ability of an agent to invade and multiply (produce infection) in a host. Experimentally, infectivity may be thought of as the minimum number of particles or agents required to establish infection in 50 per cent of a group of hosts of the same species (ID_{50}). This number varies, of course, with the agent, route of administration of the agent (in some cases), source of the agent, and with many host factors such as age or race. An example of an infection of high infectivity would be measles; one of low infectivity would be leprosy.

Infectivity in humans can often only be inferred, because ethical considerations prohibit experimental infection. Some of the techniques for evaluating infectivity are studies of the ease or speed with which an agent spreads in a population, the proportion of close contacts (such as household contacts) who become infected (secondary attack rate), and serosurveys after epidemics to determine the proportion of persons recently infected.

Pathogenicity is defined as the ability to produce clinically apparent illness. If a population is studied by laboratory methods during and/or following an outbreak of a particular disease for which reliable, sensitive, and specific laboratory diagnostic methods exist, the pathogenicity or proportion of infections resulting in clinical illness can be determined. As was noted for infectivity, many host and environmental factors as well as the dose, route of entrance of the infection, and source of the infection may alter the pathogenicity of a particular infectious disease or agent. For example, staphylococci are not pathogens when located in the rectum, but the same organism found in the peritoneal cavity or meninges would cause severe illness. Some of the mechanisms by which pathogens produce mild or severe pathogenic effects in a host will be discussed next.

Virulence can be defined as the proportion of clinical cases resulting in severe clinical manifestations (including sequelae). The CFR discussed previously is one way of measuring virulence. Virulence may depend on dose, route of infection, and host factors such as age or race. For example, the plague bacillus is more likely to produce severe clinical manifestations if it is inhaled into the lungs than if injected into an extremity by a flea, and infection with the rickettsia responsible for Rocky Mountain spotted fever leads to more severe disease when transmitted by aerosolization than when spread by tick bites. Likewise, infections with bacteria such as *Neisseria meningitidis* or *Hemophilus influenzae* will be much more severe if they enter the brain through a fracture in the cribriform plate than if they simply enter through the nasopharynx. Severe clinical illness is more likely in adults than in young children in the case of poliomyelitis, whereas children are more susceptible than adults to clinically severe infections from the viruses of California or Western equine encephalitis.

Immunogenicity can be defined as the infection's ability to produce specific immunity. Depending on the type of pathogen, this may be primarily humoral immunity, cellular immunity, or a mixture of both. Immunogenicity can be affected by host factors such as age, nutrition, dose, and virulence of infection. Agents that replicate in local areas such as the respiratory tract (rhinoviruses), genital tract (gonococci), or gastrointestinal mucosa may produce only local, and not systemic, immune responses. Agents also differ in their intrinsic ability to induce an effective, lasting immune response. For example, the agent of measles produces lifelong immunity, whereas gonococci have no such ability and it is therefore possible to have multiple attacks of gonorrhea.

Pathogenetic Mechanisms

The pathogenetic effects produced by infectious agents may result from a variety of mechanisms. Among these mechanisms are (1) direct tissue invasion, (2) production of a toxin, (3) immunologic enhancement or allergic reaction leading to damage to the host, (4) persistent or latent infection, (5) enhancement of host susceptibility to drugs of otherwise minimal toxicity, and (6) immune suppression. More than one mechanism may be involved simultaneously, or different mechanisms may lead to illnesses with clinically different characteristics as a result of infection by the same pathogen.

A large number of pathogens produce disease by direct invasion of tissue. Included are many parasitic diseases, such as amoebiasis, giardiasis, and many nematodes, trematodes, and cestodes; bacterial meningitides, urinary tract infection, pharyngitis or otitis, and skin abscesses; and viral infections such as upper respiratory and gastrointestinal viruses, and encephalitis (rabies, arbovirus encephalitides).

Some diseases result primarily from toxin production. Among these are tetanus, diphtheria, and infections by enterotoxigenic *Escherichia coli*. In addition to direct invasion of tissue, infection by *Staphylococcus aureus* may result in illness by toxin production as occurs in toxic shock syndrome or staphylococcal food poisoning.

An unusual environment for replication, such as high-absorbency tampons for staphylococci or intradermal replication of tetanus bacteria as a result of "popping" among drug abusers, may promote unusually severe diseases caused by toxin-producing agents.

In many diseases, immunologic mechanisms including allergy form part of the pathogenetic processes. Among the many diseases that are thought to have significant immunologic components are tuberculosis, post-streptococcal glomerulonephritis, dengue hemorrhagic fever, and alveolar hypersensitivity syndromes produced by fungi encountered during occupational exposure to hay, sugar cane fibers, wood dust, mushroom compost, cheese mold, or malt dust.

Persistent or chronic bacterial infection and latent viral infection are important pathogenetic mechanisms in the production of a variety of diseases. Bacteria may persist asymptomatically or after clinical infection in the pharynx (*Hemophilus influenzae, Neisseria meningitidis,* streptococci, and so on), in the gallbladder *(Salmonella typhi),* in the gastrointestinal system (many species of salmonellae), or in the urinary tract *(E. coli, Serratia, Pseudomonas,* and so on). In these instances, whole bacteria are produced by the infected area and can be cultured. In the case of persistent viral infections (herpes I and II, varicella zoster, cytomegalovirus, hepatitis B, measles virus in subacute sclerosing panencephalitis, Epstein-Barr virus in Burkitt's lymphoma), the viral nucleic acids persist in the cell, but cellular mechanisms prevent completion of the viral replication cycle and no complete virus is expressed. When some stress, hormonal, or environmental factor alters the host-cell regulatory mechanisms, then production of complete viruses occurs and may result in clinical disease.

An infectious agent may produce severe disease by sensitizing the host to otherwise relatively nontoxic drugs. Such is thought to be a possible pathogenetic mechanism in Reye's syndrome, in which infection by such viral agents as varicella and influenza B viruses may result in severe disease (encephalopathy) when the patient is treated with medication containing salicylates.

In recent years, a new condition, acquired immune deficiency syndrome (AIDS), has been recognized. This disease has a case fatality rate estimated to be as high as 70 per cent. In this condition, a variety of opportunistic organisms, including *Pneumocystis carinii,* atypical *Mycoplasma* species, *Toxoplasma gondii,* and cytomegalovirus infection, and a malignancy, Kaposi's sarcoma, have been found. AIDS is associated with a suppression or alteration of cellular immune mechanisms resulting in altered helper/suppressor T-cell ratios and anergy in response to common skin-test antigens. Attempts are being made to isolate and identify the etiologic agent(s) that can produce the immune suppression leading to the later malignant and infectious manifestations.

Table 11–1 shows some of the pathogenetic mechanisms responsible for several common diseases.

Reservoirs

Reservoirs may be defined as the living organisms or inanimate matter (such as soil) in which an infectious agent normally lives and multiplies. Thus, the reservoirs of infection consist of human beings,

TABLE 11-1 Spectrum of Pathogenetic Host-Parasite Interactions °

Disease	Invasion of Tissues	Toxin Production	Hyper- sensitivity
Botulism	0	++++	0
Tetanus	+	++++	0
Diphtheria	++	++++	0
Staphylococcosis	+++	++	±
Pneumococcosis	++++	0	0
Streptococcosis	+++	++	++
Tuberculosis	+++	0	++++

° Adapted from Hoeprich, P. D. (Ed.): Infectious Diseases: A Guide to the Understanding and Management of Infectious Processes. Harper and Row, New York, 1972.

animals, and environmental sources. The concept of the reservoir is central in infectious disease because the reservoir is an essential component of the cycle by which an infectious agent maintains and perpetuates itself. The specific reservoir for an agent is thus intimately related to the life-cycle of that agent in nature.

In the simplest cycle, the reservoir is the human, and the cycle may be diagrammed as follows:

$$Human \rightarrow Human \rightarrow Human$$

This type of cycle is characteristic of many of the common infectious diseases to which humans are subject: most of the viral and bacterial respiratory diseases, most staphylococcal and streptococcal infections, diphtheria, venereal diseases, the childhood exanthemata, mumps, typhoid fever, amoebiasis, and many others.

In addition to the diseases that are acquired from other human beings, we are also subject to some diseases that are acquired from other species, such as bovine tuberculosis (from cows), brucellosis (from cows, pigs, and goats), anthrax (from sheep), leptospirosis (from rodents), and rabies (from dogs, bats, foxes, and other wild animals). These diseases are known as *zoonoses*, infections transmissible under natural conditions from vertebrate animals to man. In these diseases the human is not an essential part (usual reservoir) of the life-cycle of the agent. Thus:

$$Animal \rightarrow Animal \rightarrow Animal$$
$$\searrow$$
$$Human$$

Certain other infectious diseases are characterized by more complex cycles. Features may include multiple reservoirs and different developmental stages of the agent. The cycle may involve an alternation of widely divergent host species. More complex cycles are illustrated by echinococcosis, tapeworm infestations, schistosomiasis, malaria, and vectorborne viral infections.

Humans as Reservoirs: Cases and Carriers. The section on pathogenicity and virulence was concerned primarily with characteristics of the agent. In this section, the focus will be on humans as reservoirs of infection.

Infection is said to have occurred if an infectious agent has entered and established itself in a host. A range of reactions to this occurrence is possible. At a minimal level, the agent may be present on the surface of the body and propagate at a rate sufficient to maintain its numbers without producing identifiable evidence of any reaction in the host. This phenomenon, which is referred to as *colonization,* is exemplified by the presence of *Staphylococcus aureus* on the nasal mucosa.*

At the next level is *inapparent infection* (covert or subclinical infection). In this type of relationship, the organisms not only multiply in the host, but also cause a measurable reaction that, however, is not clinically detectable. When infection leads to clinical (overt) disease with symptoms, physical findings, or both, *infectious disease* is said to exist. Thus, infection encompasses (1) colonization, (2) inapparent infection, and (3) infectious disease. This range of interactions between host and parasite is indicated by the Venn Diagram in Figure 11–3.

---

* A related term is *contamination.* This refers to the presence on the surface of the body or on inanimate objects (fomites) of an infectious agent that can serve as a source of infection.

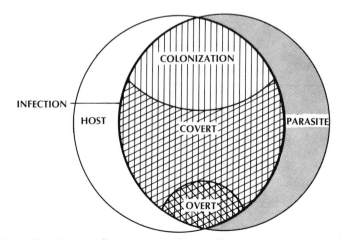

Figure 11–3 Venn Diagram illustrating several types of host-parasite interaction. (Adapted from Hoeprich, P.D. (ed.): Infectious Diseases: A Guide to the Understanding and Management of Infectious Processes. Harper and Row, New York, 1972, p. 40.)

All infected persons, including those with colonization only, are potential sources of infection to others. A *carrier* is an infected person who does not have apparent clinical disease, but is, nevertheless, a potential source of infection to others. The term "carrier" includes persons whose infection remains inapparent (asymptomatic) throughout, as well as those for whom the carrier state precedes or follows manifest disease (incubatory and convalescent carriers, respectively). When the carrier state persists for a long period of time, the person is referred to as a chronic carrier. Some examples of infectious agents that give rise to each of these types of carriers follow:

Type of Carrier	Examples
Inapparent throughout	Polio virus, meningococcus, hepatitis viruses
Incubatory carrier	Viruses of chickenpox, measles, and hepatitis
Convalescent carrier	C. diphtheriae, hepatitis B virus, and Salmonella species
Chronic carrier	S. typhosa, hepatitis B virus

A person with an inapparent infection is not necessarily a carrier. For example, most persons with positive tuberculin tests do not actively disseminate tubercle bacilli and, therefore, are not labelled carriers, even though they probably harbor tubercle bacilli.

MECHANISMS OF TRANSMISSION OF INFECTION

A central aspect of the spread of infectious disease is *transmission of infection,* or the various mechanisms by which agents reach and infect the human host. This involves escape of the agent from a source or reservoir, conveyance to a susceptible host, and entry into that host. Transmission may be direct or indirect as shown in the following scheme:

Classification of the Mechanisms of Transmission

Direct transmission	Indirect transmission
	Vehicleborne
	Vectorborne
	Airborne (droplet nuclei and dust)

Direct transmission consists of essentially immediate transfer of an infectious agent from an infected host or reservoir to an appropriate portal of entry. Note that this can involve not only direct contact, such as kissing and sexual intercourse, but also spray by *droplets* through sneezing and coughing onto the mucous membranes of others. Such droplet spread is classified as direct transmission because it occurs over short distances—the droplets travel only a few feet before falling to the ground. Direct transmission also includes exposure of susceptible tissues to fungal agents, bacterial spores, or other parasites (e.g., hookworm) lying in the soil or vegetation.

A special category of direct transmission is that of sexually transmitted diseases (STDs). In addition to the traditional venereal diseases (syphilis, gonorrhea, lymphogranuloma venereum, chancroid, and granuloma inguinale), other STDs have now been recognized, including infections caused by *Chlamydia trachomatis, Trichomonas vaginalis*, and herpes simplex types I and II. In addition, sexual practices such as orogenital contact and anal intercourse, when combined with promiscuity, have contributed to the increased sexual transmission of hepatitis B, herpes simplex type II, giardiasis, amoebiasis, salmonellosis, and shigellosis. Acquired immune deficiency syndrome (AIDS) may fall into this category as well. Some groups of homosexual males have been shown to be at especially high risk for these diseases.

A major risk factor for AIDS among male homosexuals is frequent sexual contact with different partners. However, the disease is not confined to this group; heterosexual males, women, and children are also affected. Additional risk factors include intravenous drug use and blood transfusions, Haitian ancestry, and possibly inhalation of amyl nitrate. Affected children tend to have parents with the aforementioned risk factors.

To date there is no satisfactory treatment or program of prevention for AIDS. So far, there have been programs to persuade people to reduce the number of sexual partners, to warn against intravenous drug use, to discourage homosexuals from handling food in the service of the public and from donating blood, and to encourage frequent screening to detect disease.

Indirect transmission may be vehicleborne, vectorborne, or airborne. *Vehicleborne* transmission is indirect contact through inanimate objects (fomites), such as bedding, toys, or surgical instruments, as well as contaminated food, water, and intravenously administered fluids. The agent may or may not multiply or develop in or on the vehicle before it is introduced into the human.

In *vectorborne* transmission, the infectious agent is conveyed by an arthropod to a susceptible host. The arthropod may merely carry the agent mechanically, by soiling its feet or proboscis, in which case multiplication of the agent in the vector does not occur. The vector may also be truly biological if the agent multiplies in the arthropod before it is transmitted. In this case, there is an incubation period in the arthropod, known as the extrinsic incubation period, before the arthropod can become infective.

Finally, indirect transmission may be *airborne*. Two types of particles are implicated in this kind of spread — dusts and droplet nuclei. *Dusts* are particles of varying size that result from resuspension of particles that have settled on floors or bedding as well as particles blown from the soil by the wind. Coccidioidomycosis (San Joaquin Valley fever, page 137) is an example of a disease spread through airborne transmission of fungal spores.

Droplet nuclei are very tiny particles that represent the dried residue of droplets. They may be formed in several ways. One is from the evaporation of droplets that have been coughed or sneezed into the air. Droplet nuclei are also formed from aerosolization of infective materials in the course of laboratory procedures and of processes for rendering animals in slaughterhouses. Because of their small size, these droplet nuclei can remain suspended in the air for long periods of time and are also capable of being inhaled and carried into the alveoli.

Figure 11–4 shows the relationship between particle size and

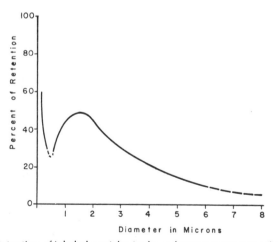

Figure 11–4 Retention of inhaled particles in the pulmonary spaces in relation to particle size. (From Langmuir, A. D.: Contact and airborne infection. *In* Sartwell, P. E. (ed.): Maxcy-Rosenau Preventive Medicine and Public Health, 10th ed. Appleton-Century-Crofts, New York, 1973.)

retention within the alveolar spaces. Most particles over 5 microns in diameter do not reach the lungs, because they are removed in the upper respiratory passages. As particle size decreases, more of the inhaled particles penetrate into the lungs and are retained there. When particles 1 to 2 microns in diameter are inhaled, approximately half are deposited in the lungs.

Airborne infection is important in a number of diseases. For example, coughing by a person with an open cavitary, tuberculous lesion can result in the formation of droplets that travel only a few feet and then either fall to the ground or are inhaled (direct contact). Because of their large size, these droplets, if inhaled, are promptly removed from the upper airways. However, as described earlier, some droplets form droplet nuclei that can be inhaled directly into the alveoli. Airborne spread from droplet nuclei is now considered to be the major mode of transmission of tuberculosis from person to person.

With a few exceptions, general acceptance of the importance of airborne spread has developed only recently. Interest in airborne disease has been stimulated since World War II by research on the pulmonary effects of particle size (see earlier), by experimental studies largely related to biological warfare, and by investigations of epidemics that could only be attributed to airborne transmission. Among these have been outbreaks of Q fever, histoplasmosis, tuberculosis, and legionnaires' disease. For example, in one outbreak of Q fever in the San Francisco Bay region, 75 cases of the disease occurred in an area approximately one-half to one mile wide and seven miles long, downwind of a rendering plant that processed sheep and goats. In addition, among laboratory personnel, there have been outbreaks of Q fever, brucellosis, and psittacosis that have clearly been airborne in origin. An important finding of these studies on airborne spread has been that with this mechanism very small numbers of organisms can induce infection.

The distinction between direct and indirect spread of respiratory secretions has been emphasized because of its importance to the control of disease. When disease is spread by direct transmission, control depends on the proper handling of the source case. Reliance must be placed on treatment of the patient and on proper handling of secretions. Airborne spread of infection poses essentially an engineering problem. Measures such as adequate ventilation and proper air hygiene are needed to reduce the incidence of infection. For a historic perspective on airborne infection and on the controversies over the years between proponents of contact and airborne spread in respiratory diseases, the reader is referred to Langmuir (1980) and Riley (1980).

SOME ASPECTS OF PERSON-TO-PERSON SPREAD OF DISEASE

Three important aspects of person-to-person spread of disease are generation time, herd immunity, and secondary attack rates.

Generation Time

With person-to-person spread, the interval between cases is determined by the *generation time,* the period between the receipt of infection by a host and maximal communicability of that host (Sartwell, 1973). In general, the generation time is roughly equivalent to the *incubation period,* the time interval between the receipt of infection and the onset of illness. However, the two terms are not identical. The time of maximal communicability may precede or follow the end of the incubation period. In mumps, for example, communicability appears to reach its height about 48 hours before the onset of swelling in the salivary glands. A further difference is that the term "incubation period" can only be applied to infections that result in manifest disease, whereas "generation time" refers to transmissions of infection, whether apparent or inapparent. Since infectious agents can be spread by persons with inapparent infection as well as clinically manifest cases, the concept of generation time is essential in studies of the dynamics of transmission of infection.

Herd Immunity

Herd immunity, the term used to express the immunity of a group or community, has been defined by Fox (1970) as the "resistance of a group to invasion and spread of an infectious agent, based on the immunity of a high proportion of individual members of the group." We can illustrate this concept through an oversimplified diagram.

Figure 11–5 depicts two groups of people **before** and **after** an epidemic. Each group consists of Mr. Jones and two office mates, X and Y, with whom he has close contacts. Both co-workers also have close association with three other individuals. The two groups are the same except that in group A all individuals are susceptible to the illness, whereas in group B coworker X is immune. Let us assume that during the course of the epidemic Mr. Jones becomes ill, that the disease is highly contagious, and also that Mr. Jones' contacts have no other exposures.

Note that in group A in which everyone is susceptible, all come down with the illness. In group B only the contacts of Y become ill.

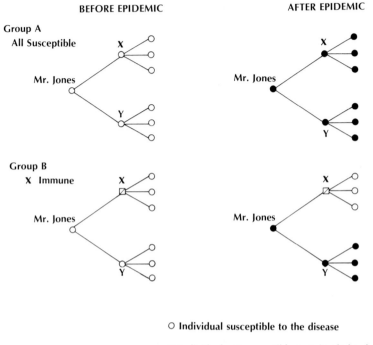

Figure 11-5 Schematic illustration of herd immunity.

○ Individual susceptible to the disease

▨ Individual not susceptible (previously has had the disease or has been immunized against it)

● Susceptible individual who develops the disease

Because of X's immunity, he does not transmit the infection from Mr. Jones to his three contacts. Thus, in group A, Mr. Jones' illness led to eight other cases of disease. In group B, his illness resulted in only four cases of disease even though only one of the other four people was immune. By his immunity, X protected three other people against the disease.

Herd immunity is believed to be an important factor underlying the dynamics of propagated epidemics and the periodicity of diseases such as chickenpox and measles (prior to widespread use of vaccine). During the course of an epidemic a number of susceptible people come down with the disease, thus providing multiple sources of infection to others. However, since the disease victims develop immunity, as the epidemic progresses the proportion of nonsusceptibles in the population increases and the likelihood of effective contact between patients with the disease and remaining susceptibles declines. With the birth of additional babies or immigration of nonimmunized persons into the community, the number of susceptibles gradually increases enough to support a new wave of transmission.

This view of the dynamics of periodicity in measles was applied by Hedrich (1933). On the basis of reported cases, births, and deaths in children under age 15, he estimated the relationship between number of susceptibles and monthly attack rates from measles over a 30-year period in Baltimore (Fig. 11 – 6). Note that the proportion of susceptibles ranged from 30 to 50 per cent and that a build-up in the estimated proportion of susceptibles preceded the peaks in case rates.

Another important consequence of herd immunity is that, in general, it is not necessary to achieve 100 per cent immunity in a population in order to halt an epidemic or control a disease. Just how far short of 100 per cent is safe is, of course, a crucial question. No definite answers can be given here, although, for example, it has been customary to cite 70 per cent for diphtheria. However, studies of several outbreaks of diphtheria, including one involving 196 persons in San Antonio, Texas, in 1970 (Marcuse and Grand, 1973), suggest that in densely settled areas immunization of the total population may be needed to prevent the occurrence of clinical diphtheria. Since immunized persons can harbor diphtheria organisms, they are a potential source of infection to the nonimmune portion of the population. Recent studies to evaluate the success of rubella immunization campaigns have shown that herd immunity does not operate well in prevention of rubella. Outbreaks have occurred even in populations in which 85 to 90 per cent have presumably been immune owing to natural infection or vaccination.

Another problem has been that an apparently satisfactory overall

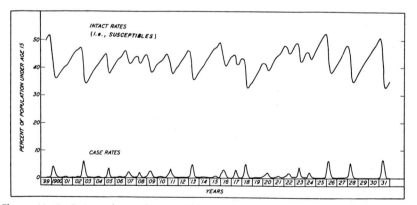

Figure 11–6 Estimated complete monthly attack rates from measles, and intact rates (proportions not previously attacked) for the population under age 15, Old Baltimore, Md., July, 1899–December, 1931. (From Hedrich, A. W.: Monthly estimates of the child population "susceptible" to measles, 1900–1931, Baltimore, Md. Am. J. Hyg. *17*:626, 1933.)

level of immunity of a population may obscure the existence of pockets of unimmunized persons. In this country, small outbreaks of poliomyelitis and diphtheria have occurred among such population subgroups. For example, in the 1970 outbreak of diphtheria in San Antonio, the 5- to 14-year-olds had higher case rates than the 1- to 4-year-olds, a reflection of the fact that a smaller proportion of the older children had been fully immunized. It has recently been recognized that for some highly contagious diseases, such as measles, transmission may occur among susceptibles if the organism is introduced into even a well-immunized community.

Two situations are particularly conducive to the development of large-scale propagated epidemics. (1) A large epidemic can result from the introduction of infectious agents into populations that have never been exposed to the agent previously or from which the agent has been absent for many years (so-called virgin populations, see page 27). (2) Epidemics also occur following the introduction of a large number of susceptible persons into a closed community, such as a barracks, where crowded living arrangements and intimate contact facilitate the spread of infection. Examples of this are outbreaks of meningococcal infections and of adenovirus types 4 and 7 among young military recruits, with those from isolated rural areas particularly affected.

Secondary Attack Rates

An important aspect of propagated spread is the concept of the family, household, or other closed group (e.g., barracks) as an epidemiologic unit within which infections tend to disseminate. The case that brings a household or other group to the attention of public health personnel is called the *index case.*° Spread of disease within a group is measured through the *secondary attack rate.* This is defined as the number of cases of a disease developing during a stated time period among those members of a closed group who are at risk:

$$\text{Secondary attack rate} = \frac{\text{number of new cases in group minus initial case(s)}}{\text{number of susceptible persons in group minus initial case(s)}} \quad \text{during specified time period}$$

The index case is excluded from both numerator and denominator as are *co-primaries,* cases that are related to the index case so closely in time that they are considered to belong to the same generation of cases.

° Investigation may reveal cases that antedate the index case. That is, the index case is not necessarily the first case in a family or group.

Because members of a household have intimate contact with each other, much can be learned from intrahousehold spread. The value of the secondary attack rate is illustrated by the following study (Ward et al., 1979). To determine the risk of illness from *H. influenzae* among household contacts of patients with this infection, the Centers for Disease Control (CDC) undertook a nationwide investigation of 1147 families containing an index case of *H. influenzae* meningitis. Over the next 18 months, the occurrence of *H. influenzae* in the families was monitored. It was found that within 30 days of the onset in the index case, the risk of infection was almost 600 times higher within the household than in the general population. Thus, the household is seen to be a meaningful unit in which to study the transmission of disease. Studies of intrafamilial spread also provide information on the type of family member to introduce the disease into the household. For respiratory infections, this is primarily the young school child.

TYPES OF EPIDEMICS: COMMON SOURCE VERSUS PROPAGATED

We are now ready to apply the information about transmission of infectious agents to community patterns of disease occurrence. These mechanisms of spread account for the usual level of morbidity (endemic disease) as well as levels above those expected (i.e., epidemics). Two principal types of epidemics can be distinguished: (1) common source, and (2) propagated, or progressive. In general, these can be differentiated primarily by plotting the distribution of cases by time of onset (i.e., by determining the *epidemic curve*).

Common source epidemics are outbreaks caused by exposure of a group of persons to a common, noxious influence. When the exposure is brief and essentially simultaneous (a *point*, or *point source*, epidemic), the resultant cases all develop within one incubation period. In a common source epidemic, the epidemic curve follows a log-normal distribution. That is, if the cumulative proportion of cases are plotted by the log-time of onset, a straight line results. The median incubation period can be determined easily by reading off the time at which 50 percent of the cases have occurred on the resulting graph. Knowledge of the median incubation period may help to identify the etiologic agent, since agents have characteristic incubation periods.

Figure 11 – 7 shows the times of onset of illness during an outbreak of food intoxication at a military base. The rapid rise and fall of the epidemic curve is compatible with a point, or point source, epidemic.

If the vehicle or source of the epidemic (food, water, air) remains

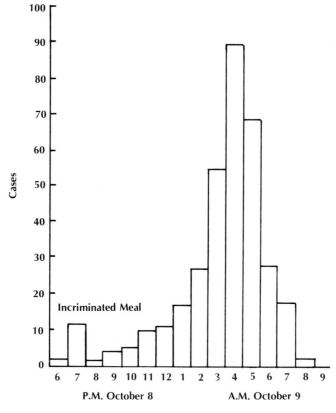

Figure 11-7 Food intoxication at a military base in Texas, October 8-9, 1968. (From Morbidity and Mortality Weekly Report, CDC, U.S. Public Health Service, *18*:20, 1969.)

contaminated, the situation is more complex. Because the epidemic curve results from multiple exposures at different times and because incubation periods are variable, there will be a less distinct peak and the outbreak will be of longer duration.

A probable common source epidemic of major proportions came to light in Philadelphia in the summer of 1976, following an American Legion convention. The investigation of this outbreak led to the discovery of a previously unknown pathogen, *Legionella pneumophila*, and revealed that the disease was not, in fact, new but that the organism had caused several previous outbreaks. Since the large Philadelphia outbreak of 1976 (with 221 cases and 34 deaths), several additional outbreaks have been identified.

There are two types of disease caused by this organism. One kind, known as legionnaires' disease, which results in epidemic illness, is a multisystem disease, with pneumonia and a high case fatality rate. The other type, which is less severe, is known as "Pontiac fever" because Pontiac, Michigan, was the site of an outbreak of this nonfatal and nonpneumonic form of the disease in 1968. There is now considerable evidence that the organism is widespread.

Several features of the epidemic form of the disease have been identified. The disease occurs seasonally, mainly in the summer. The incubation period is between two and 10 days, with a median of five days. There is a distinct male preponderance, with two to three times as many cases in males as in females. Several risk factors for the disease (i.e., cigarette smoking, ingestion of alcohol) may contribute to this male predilection. Another important risk factor is the presence of underlying disease, such as renal failure, malignancy, or immunosuppressed state. Serosurveys in different areas have yielded different estimates of the prevalence of prior infection; these have varied from 1 to 25 per cent of the population.

Several investigations of the mode of transmission have indicated the importance of environmental factors. Transmission of the epidemic form of the disease appears to be mainly airborne. Several outbreaks have been traced to storage towers and to cooling or air-conditioning systems. In addition, several outbreaks have been traced to persistence of the organism in shower facilities or in institutional water systems.

Point source epidemics can also arise from common exposure to noninfectious agents, such as chemical poisons and polluted air. Figure 11 – 8 shows the relationship between atmospheric pollution and deaths in London for the period that included the great fog of December 1952. The figure also shows that shortly after the fog there was an epidemic of influenza, which also caused an excess number of deaths in comparison with the corresponding week of the previous year. This type of epidemic (propagated) will be discussed next.

Propagated or progressive epidemics result from transmission, either direct or indirect, of an infectious agent from one susceptible host to another. This can occur through direct person-to-person transmission or it can involve more complex cycles in which the agent must pass through a vector to be transmitted from one human host to another, as in yellow fever and malaria. Figure 11 – 9A depicts the distribution of onsets of hepatitis A in an institution for the mentally retarded during an epidemic. Even though the incubation period of hepatitis A can be long, it does not generally exceed 50 days. Therefore, it is apparent that the epidemic extended over a number of incubation periods. The probable path of transmission among patient-employees, contacts, and ward groups is shown schematically in Figure 11 – 9B.

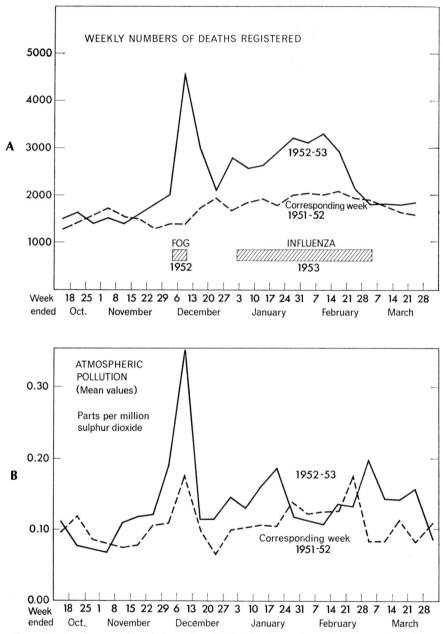

Figure 11–8 The great fog of December, 1952. Weekly numbers of deaths registered in Greater London (A) in relation to levels of air pollution, indicated by SO$_2$ (B). All causes of death; all ages, both sexes. Comparison of 1952 with ordinary year, 1951. Effects of the 1953 influenza epidemic are also shown. (From Morris, J. N.: Uses of epidemiology. Rep. Public Health Med. Subj. (Lond.), 95:200, 1954; with permission of the Controller of Her Majesty's Stationery Office.)

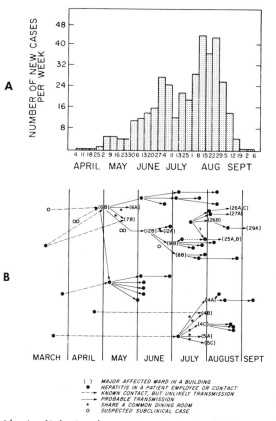

Figure 11–9 Epidemic of infectious hepatitis in an institution for the mentally retarded. *A*, Weekly clinical case rate. *B*, Schematic representation of possible hepatitis transmission. (From Matthew, E. B., Dietzman, D. E., et al.: A major epidemic of infectious hepatitis in an institution for the mentally retarded. Am. J. Epidemiol., *98*:199, 1973.)

The upward trend at the onset of a propagated epidemic reflects an increasing number of cases in each successive time period. As a consequence, the increased probability that a susceptible will have contact with one or more cases more than offsets the decline in the number of susceptibles. However, eventually the number of susceptibles falls below a critical level and the number of cases declines.

It is clear from comparison of the point source epidemics (i.e., food intoxication and the London fog in Figures 11–7 and 11–8) with the propagated spread of influenza and hepatitis (shown in Figures 11–8 and 11–9) that the two types of epidemics show different temporal curves. Typically, the curve of onsets for a common vehicle epidemic shows a rapid rise and fall within one incubation period, whereas new cases in a propagated epidemic continue to develop beyond one incubation period. Sometimes it is possible to identify "generations" of cases. However, the variability in incubation periods often obscures such patterns.

In addition to the first two types, there is a third type of epidemic, which is the result of vectorborne disease. This type of epidemic usually has a small geographic area as a "common source" but may have a zoonotic, human, or mixed cycle as the source of the pathogen to the vector. Most vectorborne epidemics have multiple cycles of transmission between vector and host before enough human cases are recognized to define an epidemic.

It may be difficult to identify the nature of an epidemic from the shape of the epidemic curve alone. The typical point source curve may be affected by the development of secondary cases, by the continued contamination of the source, or by a long and variable incubation period. Conversely, propagated spread of a disease like influenza, which has a short incubation period and is highly infectious, can create a rapidly rising and rapidly falling epidemic curve similar to that of a point source epidemic. However, geographic distribution can help to differentiate the two types of epidemics; propagated epidemics tend to show geographic spread with successive generations of cases.

The origins of an epidemic can be primarily behavioral rather than infectious or chemical. Like infectious agents, ideas and behavioral patterns can be transmitted from person to person. The communicable nature of behavior has been noted over the centuries, from the dancing manias of the Middle Ages to recent outbreaks of hysteria. Drug abuse is one of the most serious behavioral phenomena of our times and can lead to spread of infectious diseases in previously unknown ways. For example, hepatitis B and malaria have been spread by paraphernalia used for the intake of drugs. The development of cases is dependent not only on person-to-person transmission but also on group reinforcement. The rituals associated with the act of injecting the drug, or smoking the cigarette, are as important as physiologic effects in the early stages of initiation. The person-to-person spread of intravenous heroin use to boys in one town from other boys who had acquired the habit elsewhere is shown vividly in Figure 11–10.

The chain of events in a common vehicle epidemic is relatively simple to conceptualize. Following a common exposure, a proportion (not necessarily all) of those exposed develop an illness; the times of onset vary over the range of the incubation period for that condition. The forces determining the extent and course of a propagated epidemic are more complex. The rate of transmission of infection from one person to another depends upon a number of factors, especially the proportions of susceptible and immune persons in the population. A historic review

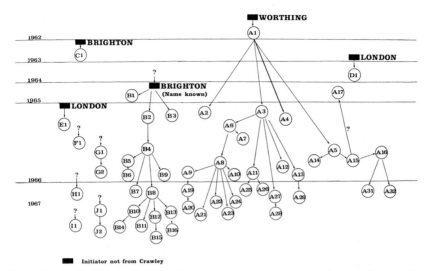

Figure 11–10 Pathways of spread of intravenous heroin use in Crawley New Town, 1967. (From de Alarcon, R.: The spread of heroin abuse in a community. Bull. Narc., *31:17*, 1969.)

of attempts to develop mathematical models of the course of propagated epidemics may be found in Serfling (1952).

OUTLINE OF THE INVESTIGATION OF AN EPIDEMIC

The investigation of an epidemic is an exciting exercise in medical detection. However, successful investigations require painstaking accumulation of information in the field ("shoeleather" epidemiology), and careful analysis of data, as well as flashes of insight. Therefore, we will present a systematic outline of the essential steps in the investigation of an outbreak even though some may seem self-evident. These steps are not necessarily accomplished in the order given and, in fact, the investigator usually sets in motion the activities needed for answering several questions simultaneously. However, *verification of the diagnosis* and *establishment of the existence of an epidemic* always deserve early attention when report of an apparent outbreak is received.

Preliminary Analysis

Verify the Diagnosis. Do clinical and laboratory studies to confirm the diagnosis.

Always consider whether initial reports are correct. For example, an outbreak of jaundice initially diagnosed as "leptospirosis" (a spirochetal disease usually transmitted by water contaminated by the urine of infected animals) was found to be infectious hepatitis. The confirming tests indicated that one laboratory reagent was faulty. Investigation of a purported epidemic of "gonorrhea" among the girls in a grade school revealed a "phantom epidemic" based on rumors (Mausner and Gezon, 1967).

It is necessary to establish criteria for labelling persons as "cases." Depending on the type of problem being investigated, the classification will be based on symptoms, laboratory results, or both.

Verify the Existence of an Epidemic. Attempt to compare the current incidence with past levels of the disease to determine whether an excessive number of cases have occurred.

Describe the Epidemic with Respect to Time, Place, Person. Plot the cases by time of onset (epidemic curve).

Plot the cases by location (spot map).

Calculate rates of illness in population at risk, by age, sex, occupation, exposure to specific foods, and other relevant attributes. The identification of "relevant" attributes may be a crucial step in the solution of the problem. For example, in the winter of 1960 to 1961 the New Jersey State Health Department became aware that an unexpectedly large proportion of the cases of hepatitis reported to them were occurring in adult males. This intelligence led eventually to identification of contaminated clams taken from Raritan Bay as the vehicle of spread for these cases (Dougherty and Altman, 1962).

Formulate and Test Hypotheses. Identify type of epidemic — common source versus propagated.

Using the previously given descriptive characteristics to define the population that has been at highest risk of acquiring the disease, consider the possible source or sources from which disease may have been contracted. Compare ill population (cases) with well population (controls) with regard to exposure to the postulated source. Calculate relative risk for exposed and nonexposed persons. Carry out statistical tests to determine probable source. When appropriate, attempt to confirm epidemiologic findings by laboratory tests (samples of blood or feces, samples of suspect food, and so on).

Possible Further Investigation and Analysis

Search for Additional Cases. Locate unrecognized or unreported cases by:

1. Canvass of physicians or hospitals or both in the area to determine if they have seen other patients who might have the disease under investigation.

2. Intensive investigation of asymptomatic persons or those with mild illness who may be contacts of cases. For example, in an investigation of an outbreak of hepatitis one might do liver function tests (e.g., serum transaminase levels) to search for cases of anicteric hepatitis (i.e., nonjaundiced), which ordinarily would not come to diagnosis.

Analyze the Data. Assemble the results. Interpret findings.

Make a Decision About the Hypotheses Considered. By the conclusion of the investigation all of the known facts should be consistent with one, and only one, hypothesis.

Intervention and Follow-up. As called for by the specific circumstances.

Report of the Investigation

At the termination of an investigation a report is usually prepared and submitted to the appropriate agency (or agencies). The report generally includes discussion of factors leading to the epidemic, evaluation of measures used for control, and recommendations for prevention of similar episodes in the future.

Example: Investigation of a Foodborne Outbreak

Outbreaks of foodborne disease provide good examples of the application of epidemiology to the solution of public health problems. We will consider data from an outbreak that occurred in Oswego County, New York, in 1940 (Gross, 1976). Over a period of a few hours, 46 people became ill with gastrointestinal symptoms. Inquiry revealed that all had attended a church supper the previous evening. The physician in charge of investigating the outbreak set out to obtain a history from the 75 people who had attended the supper (attack rate of 61 per cent). Table 11–2 presents a partial example of a line listing of persons who attended the dinner, along with an indication of which foods each person had eaten and whether the individual had become ill or had remained well.

The next step in analysis of the problem is to construct an attack rate table, which further subdivides ill and well people according to their intake of specific foods (Table 11–3). Comparison of attack rates by ingestion of specific foods shows that only for vanilla ice cream was the attack rate substantially greater among those who ate the item than among those who did not. (Any differences that appear to be of interest can be analyzed by the χ^2 test for statistically significant differences.)

If more than one food appears to be suspicious, one can develop a cross-reference table parallel to the analysis of matched pairs (see p. 291). For example, in this problem one may wish to examine the joint effect of eating chocolate ice cream or vanilla ice cream or both. Table 11–4 shows how this problem may be set up. Note that those who ate chocolate ice cream had a different risk, depending on whether they also ate vanilla ice cream (78.6 per cent attack rate) or did not eat vanilla ice cream (15.8 per cent attack rate). The two groups that ate vanilla ice cream had almost identical attack rates — 78.6 and 80.0 per cent — regardless of whether they also ate chocolate ice cream. An analysis of this type confirms the etiological role of one or more foods in causing the outbreak. Once the source has been identified (contaminated food or infected food handler), appropriate control measures may be possible.

Many infectious diseases that are problems in other countries are of little concern in the United States. These differences are related partly

TABLE 11–2 Selected Characteristics of 8 Persons Attending the Church Supper on April 18, 1940, in Oswego County, New York

Identity Number	Age	Sex	Time of Eating Church Supper	Date of Onset: April	Date of Onset: Time	Baked Ham	Spinach	Mashed Potatoes	Cabbage Salad	Jello	Rolls	Brown Bread	Milk	Coffee	Water	Cakes	Ice Cream: Vanilla	Ice Cream: Chocolate	Fruit Salad
1	11	M	Unknown	WELL														X	
2	52	F	8:00 pm	19	12:30 am	X	X	X			X			X			X		
3	65	M	6:30 pm	19	12:30 am	X	X	X	X					X			X	X	
4	59	F	6:30 pm	19	12:30 am	X	X							X		X	X	X	
5	13	F	Unknown	WELL														X	
6	63	F	7:30 pm	18	10:30 pm	X	X		X	X					X		X		
7	70	M	7:30 pm	18	10:30 pm	X	X	X		X	X	X		X	X		X		
8	40	F	7:30 pm	19	2:00 am												X	X	

From: Centers for Disease Control. An Outbreak of Gastrointestinal Illness Following A Church Supper. Atlanta, July 1976.

TABLE 11-3 Food-specific Attack Rates Among Persons Attending a Church Supper, Oswego County, New York

Food or Beverage	Group A— Persons who ate specified food				Group B— Persons who did not eat specified food			
	Ill	Not Ill	Total	Attack Rate (Per cent)	Ill	Not Ill	Total	Attack Rate (Per cent)
Baked ham	29	17	46	63.0	17	12	29	58.6
Spinach	26	17	43	60.5	20	12	32	62.5
Mashed potato°	23	14	37	62.2	23	14	37	62.2
Cabbage salad	18	10	28	64.3	28	19	47	59.6
Jello	16	7	23	69.6	30	22	52	57.7
Rolls	21	16	37	56.8	25	13	38	65.8
Ice cream (van.)	43	11	54	79.6	3	18	21	14.3
Ice cream (choc.)°	25	22	47	53.2	20	7	27	74.1
Fruit salad	4	2	6	66.7	42	27	69	60.9

° One history indefinite as to consumption of mashed potato (#19), another as to chocolate ice cream (#44); both omitted from the tabulation.

From Centers for Disease Control: An Outbreak of Gastrointestinal Illness Following a Church Supper. Atlanta, July 1976.

to geography, but primarily to differences in levels of environmental hygiene and medical technology. A tropical climate can support parasites and vectorborne organisms not seen in more temperate areas. Enteric infections are a major problem in tropical areas, probably in great measure because of inadequate hygienic practices and sanitary protection. On the other hand, large numbers of legal and illegal immigrants have entered the country within the past decade. Many of them

TABLE 11-4 Cross-Reference Table

		Ate Chocolate Ice Cream	Did Not Eat Chocolate Ice Cream	Total
Ate vanilla ice cream	Ill/Total	22/28	20/25	43°/54
	Per cent ill	78.6	80.0	79.6
Did not eat vanilla ice cream	Ill/Total	3/19	0/2	3/21
	Per cent ill	15.8	0.0	14.3
Total	Ill/Total	25/47	20/27	46/75
	Per cent ill	53.2	74.1	61.3

° Case #44 ate vanilla ice cream but gave a questionable history of consumption of chocolate ice cream.

From Centers for Disease Control: An Outbreak of Gastrointestinal Illness Following a Church Supper. Atlanta, July 1976.

have substantial health problems, and this is increasing the need for health services.

In the United States, the sharp decline in infectious diseases has necessitated ongoing evaluation and restructuring of control programs. Traditional aspects of control have been supplemented by programs based on surveillance. Eradication has also been proposed as a realistic goal for several conditions. We will discuss some specific control measures first and then comment briefly on surveillance and eradication.

Specific Control Measures

These may be grouped as measures directed against the reservoir of the organism, those designed to interrupt transmission of infection, and those that reduce the susceptibility of the host.

Measures Directed Against the Reservoir. The nature of the reservoir is of paramount importance in determining the appropriate methods of control and their likelihood of success. If the reservoir of infection is in domestic animals, the problems can be approached through immunization, testing of herds, and destruction of infected animals. These procedures have been applied very successfully to brucellosis and bovine tuberculosis.

This approach is less applicable to wild animals, although experimental studies of methods of control are being conducted. Infection of wild animals with plague and rabies continues to pose a threat to domestic animals and human beings. Although for the last decade there has been an average of only one or two cases of human rabies each year, a large number of persons receive postexposure prophylaxis annually.

When humans are the reservoir, eradication of an infected host is not a viable option. However, in some circumstances it may be possible to remove the focus of infection (e.g., cholecystectomy in a chronic typhoid carrier). Related control measures include isolation of infected persons, treatment to render them noninfectious, and disinfection of contaminated objects.

Isolation is the separation of infected persons from those not infected for the period of communicability. While isolation is still an essential element in the control of certain diseases, there is decreasing reliance on this measure. It is futile to impose isolation if there is a large component of inapparent infection or if maximal infectivity precedes overt illness.

A control procedure closely related to isolation is quarantine. Classically, *quarantine* is the limitation of freedom of movement of apparently well persons or animals who have been exposed to a case of infectious disease. Quarantine is imposed for the duration of the usual maximal incubation period of the disease. Currently in the United

States, even for the three[*] diseases that are quarantinable by international agreement (cholera, plague, and yellow fever), quarantine has been replaced by active *surveillance of individuals*. In such surveillance, close supervision is maintained over possible contacts of ill persons to detect infection or illness promptly; their freedom of movement is not restricted. For example, travellers from countries where there have been cases of a disease of serious concern may be required to remain in touch with their local health officer during the incubation period of the disease. Quarantine of animals is still important in the control of zoonoses. It is used, for example, to control hog cholera and swine influenza. An outbreak of Venezuelan equine encephalitis in Texas in 1971 led to restriction of the movement of equine animals (horses and mules) (Zehmer et al., 1974).

Measures that Interrupt the Transmission of Organisms. Environmental measures to prevent transmission of disease by ingestion of contaminated vehicles include purification of water, pasteurization of milk, and inspection and other procedures designed to ensure a safe food supply. These public health measures, along with improvements in housing, nutrition, and other social conditions, are largely responsible for the great reduction in sickness and death due to infectious disease in developed countries during this century.

Attempts to reduce transmission of respiratory infection in classrooms in the 1930s by chemical disinfection of air and use of ultraviolet light gave generally disappointing results (Riley, 1980). Work on ventilation patterns, including unidirectional ("laminar") airflow to reduce the transmission of organisms in hospitals, is still in the process of evaluation (Schimpff, 1980; Pizzo, 1981).

Success in interrupting transmission of diseases whose cycles involve arthropods or alternative hosts or both has been variable. Schistosomiasis, a parasitic disease whose cycle includes snails, has no public health significance in the United States; it causes considerable debilitation and economic loss in other parts of the world. Unfortunately, in certain places irrigation to increase food production has also increased the prevalence of schistosomiasis. The construction of the Aswan High Dam in Egypt has provided a notable example of this particular dilemma. Other unsolved problems include the arthropodborne viral encephalitides, such as eastern and western equine encephalitis, and various rickettsial diseases.

Measures that Reduce Host Susceptibility. Active immunization against diphtheria, tetanus, and pertussis (DTP) has been a mainstay of public health practice for many decades. In the mid-1950s vaccine

---

[*] Smallpox has been included in the list of quarantinable diseases, but is now considered eradicated worldwide.

against poliomyelitis became available. More recently, vaccines against measles, mumps, and rubella have been added to the armamentarium and have been incorporated into routine pediatric practice. The immunization schedule recommended by the American Academy of Pediatrics (1982) is shown in Table 11–5. Other vaccines with more limited application include those against typhoid, typhus, and cholera for persons travelling abroad and immunizations against anthrax and rabies for persons occupationally exposed. Routine smallpox vaccination is no longer recommended.

Annual nationwide immunization surveys provide an estimate of the overall level of immunization in the country and among subgroups of the population. Table 11–6 shows that levels of immunization against poliomyelitis, measles, diphtheria, tetanus, and pertussis are lower among preschool children from central cities than among all children of the same ages from the remainder of the standard metropolitan statistical area (SMSA). In addition, the table shows that immunization levels for DTP and polio were lower in 1978 than they were a decade earlier. The failure to achieve immunization of the total population of young children has persisted over a number of years despite clinics where immunization is provided without cost. Laws in some states that require proof of

TABLE 11–5 Recommended Schedule for Active Immunization of Normal Infants and Children

Recommended Age	Vaccine(s)	Comments
2 mo	DTP,[1] OPV[2]	Can be initiated earlier in areas of high endemicity
4 mo	DTP, OPV	2-mo interval desired for OPV to avoid interference
6 mo	DTP (OPV)	OPV optional for areas where polio might be imported (e.g., some areas of Southwest United States)
12 mo	Tuberculin Test[3]	May be given simultaneously with MMR at 15 mo (see text)
15 mo	Measles, Mumps, Rubella (MMR)[4]	MMR preferred
18 mo	DTP, OPV	Consider as part of primary series — DTP essential
4-6 yr[5]	DTP, OPV	
14-16 yr	Td[6]	Repeat every 10 years for lifetime

[1] DTP—Diphtheria and tetanus toxoids with pertussis vaccine.
[2] OPV—Oral, attenuated polio virus vaccine contains polio virus types 1, 2, and 3.
[3] Tuberculin test—Mantoux (intradermal PPD) preferred. Frequency of tests depends on local epidemiology.
[4] MMR—Live measles, mumps, and rubella viruses in a combined vaccine.
[5] Up to the seventh birthday.
[6] Td—Adult tetanus toxoid (full dose) and diphtheria toxoid (reduced dose) in combination.
From Report of the Commission on Infectious Diseases, American Academy of Pediatrics, Evanston, Illinois, 1982.

TABLE 11-6 Percentage of Population Age 1-4 Years With History of Receiving Specified Vaccines by Standard Metropolitan Statistical Area (SMSA), for Central Cities and Remaining SMSA, United States, 1969 (or 1970) and 1978 °

	Year	SMSA Central Cities (%)	Component Area Remaining SMSA (%)
Rubella	1970	38.3	39.2
	1978	58.5	64.3
Measles	1969	57.3	66.6
	1978	60.0	66.1
DTP (3 + doses)	1969	73.8	87.6
	1978	60.3	71.6
Polio (3 + doses)	1969	62.4	72.5
	1978	55.4	64.0

° From United States Immunization Survey — 1978. U.S. Dept. of Health, Education, and Welfare, U.S. Govt. Printing Office, Washington, D.C., 1979.

immunization at time of school entry are helpful but do not ensure that children will receive immunizations early enough to provide protection when it is needed most.

The prophylactic measures discussed so far are examples of *active immunization* in which either the altered organism or its product induces the host to produce antibodies. Protective antibodies produced by another host can also be introduced into a susceptible person, a procedure known as *passive immunization.* Passive immunization plays a role, albeit a somewhat lesser one than active immunization, in infectious disease control. The transfer of maternal antibodies to the fetus through the placenta is a form of passive immunization. Other examples of passive immunization include administration of immune serum globulin (ISG) for the prophylaxis of measles and infectious hepatitis (hepatitis A) and of tetanus antitoxin for unimmunized persons who receive penetrating wounds. (The latter should never be necessary, as active immunization against tetanus is far preferable.) Other substances available for passive immunization include antitoxin against *Clostridium botulinum* and antiserum against rabies following animal bites. Another prophylactic measure is the use of antibiotics for known contacts of cases — for example, in tuberculosis, gonorrhea, and syphilis.

Surveillance

Data on past occurrence of an infectious disease in a geographic area of concern may be generated by a system of surveillance in that area. This is essential to the recognition of the existence of disease outbreak and to any understanding of its epidemiology. The area of concern may be a nursing home, ward of a hospital, school, city, county, state or country—any defined locale for which demographic data are known and in which data are systematically collected and summarized. *Surveillance of infectious diseases* is defined as the regular collection, summarization, and analysis of data on newly diagnosed cases of any infectious disease for the purpose of identifying high-risk groups in the population, understanding the mode(s) of transmission of the disease, and reducing or eliminating its transmission. Each case should be reported promptly; information about the patient should include diagnosis, date of onset of symptoms, and critical demographic variables such as name, age, sex, address of residence, telephone number, and his or her source of referral (e.g., physician, clinic, emergency room, hospital, nursing home, school nurse). Regular analyses of such data for a variety of diseases can lead to recognition of seasonal and long-term trends; geographic areas of elevated or decreased transmission; high-risk groups categorized by age, sex, race, or religious or socioeconomic background; and occupational diseases.

There are two general categories of surveillance: active and passive. *Passive surveillance* refers to data generated without solicitation, intervention, or contact by the health agency carrying out the surveillance. All states and many city health departments have laws requiring the reporting of a large number of infectious (and some noninfectious) diseases. Forms are provided for returning by mail to the health department. A few states have instituted telephone reporting systems. Laboratory diagnosis is encouraged but not required for most diseases. These data provide the basic information necessary for studying infectious diseases in specific areas, and they form the basis for recognition of problems requiring further investigation.

Active surveillance is the collection of data (usually on a specific disease) for a relatively limited period of time by regular outreach on the part of health department personnel. By arrangement, designated medical personnel are called at regular intervals (e.g., twice a week, weekly, monthly) to collect information on presence or absence of new cases of a particular disease and to record demographic data, date of onset, and other information relevant to that particular disease, such as travel, personal habits, occupation, food consumption, and so on. Negative information is also recorded.

This mode of data collection may be undertaken when a new disease is discovered, when a new mode of transmission is being investigated, when a high-risk season or year is recognized, and when a disease appears in a new geographic area or is found to affect a new subgroup of the population. It may be done when a previously eradicated disease, a particularly severe disease, or a disease of previously low incidence suddenly reappears or occurs at a high level of incidence.

Surveillance in Hospitals: Nosocomial Infection

A special setting in which environmental factors may contribute significantly to the risk of acquiring an infectious disease and in which specialized techniques of surveillance, data analysis, and disease control may be required is the modern hospital. Many factors combine to make this setting a particularly fertile one for transmission of infectious diseases. First, of course, people who are sick may bring pathogens with them to the hospital. Once in the hospital, the patient receives care from many individuals, any one of whom may be the vehicle for transporting pathogens among patients or from staff to patients. Patients may be particularly susceptible because of their own preexisting disease (e.g., premature infants), their treatment (e.g., immunosuppression, chemotherapy, radiation therapy, transplantation, hemodialysis, surgery), and their exposure to blood products, intravenous fluids, needles, catheters, and so on. Despite disinfection of instruments or parts of instruments (e.g., respirators, mist tents, and equipment for urinary or reproductive tract visualization), the repeated use of such instruments may lead to nosocomial infections. In addition, hospitals are places in which virulent organisms may develop and prosper. Widespread antibiotic use leads to passage of resistance in genetic materials, such as plasmids, and specialized machines that recirculate body fluids create an unusually favorable environment for pathogens. Examples include pseudomonas in respiratory equipment and hepatitis B in dialysis units. Contaminated ventilation or water systems may spread agents such as that of legionnaires' disease to susceptible hosts.

Because the hospital environment is such a fertile setting for transmission of infectious diseases, an epidemiologic subspecialty has developed to provide effective surveillance and control of nosocomial infections in hospitals. Most hospitals now have full- or part-time infection control practitioners (ICPs) and many have hospital epidemiologists as well. These may be physicians, nurses, or graduates of epidemiology training programs. Regular surveillance may be performed on laboratory records, and rates of infection by ward, service, or surgical procedure can be calculated. These activities—plus regular analysis of a statistically valid sample of charts and active surveillance by ICPs or hospital epidemiologists of known high-risk areas in the hospital—may lead to early recognition, investigation, and control of outbreaks in the hospital setting.

Eradication of Disease

The concept of eradication of disease, i.e., total elimination of a disease worldwide, was considered visionary only a few decades ago, but has now been accomplished for one disease, smallpox.

The decision to make an all-out effort to eradicate smallpox was taken by the World Health Organization in the mid-1960s. Factors leading to this decision included the continued danger of importations from endemic to disease-free areas, the complications from vaccination, and the key fact that man is the only known reservoir. Since then, progress was steady, and on January 1, 1982, the World Health Assembly removed smallpox from the list of diseases subject to reporting. This represented a tremendous triumph in the application of epidemiologic principles to the solution of worldwide problems in health.

The elimination of measles in the United States will not lag far behind the conquest of smallpox. The incidence of measles has declined steadily since 1950 (Fig. 11–11). The rate of progress was so striking that in 1978 the Secretary of Health, Education, and Welfare announced the goal of eliminating indigenous cases of measles from the United States by October 1982. That date is now past and the goal has so far not been entirely met, but progress toward it has been striking, as can be seen from Table 11–7. It is clear that the number of cases now is only a fraction of what it had been and that transmission has been interrupted in much of the country. Only about 5 per cent of all counties have had recent transmission of measles virus. These results can be attributed to

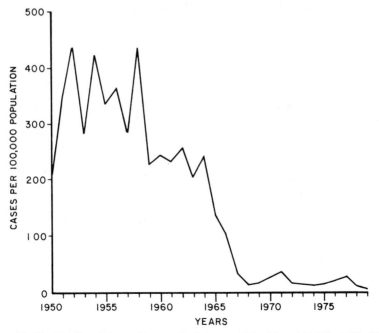

Figure 11–11 Measles: Reported case rates by year, United States, 1950–1979. (From Morbidity and Mortality Weekly Report, CDC, U.S. Public Health Service, 1979, pg. 49.)

TABLE 11-7 Number of Measles Cases Reported, Weeks 1-37, 1977-1982 — United States

Year (Weeks 1-37)	No. of cases	Change from previous year (%)	Percentage of counties
1977	53,023		45.5
1978	22,904	-56.8	31.1
1979	12,135	-47.0	28.3
1980	12,843	+5.8	22.8
1981	2,668	-79.2	10.1
1982	1,230	-53.9	5.0

From: Centers for Disease Control. Morbidity and Mortality Weekly Report. Vol. 31, No. 38, p. 518, October 1, 1982.

an effective vaccine, to high levels of immunity in the population, and to the use of school systems to enforce immunization, a strong surveillance network, and aggressive responses to any outbreaks of disease. This policy will have to be continued in order to achieve a definitive victory over measles in this country.

Measles is a serious illness in any country, but in underdeveloped countries it is a particular threat. It has been estimated that approximately 900,000 deaths from measles occur each year in developing nations. It is a leading cause of death in these nations. On the basis of a number of factors, including the success of smallpox eradication, the heat-stability of current measles vaccines, and the experience gained from control efforts in the United States and Africa, officials of the CDC have proposed the desirability and feasibility of a program for the global eradication of measles (Hopkins et al., 1982).

Malaria has been eradicated from large areas of the world, largely owing to spraying of dwellings with insecticides, effective surveillance, and treatment of parasitemic individuals. In several areas, however, advanced control efforts have met with setbacks because of the emergence of insecticide-resistant strains of Anopheles mosquitoes and of drug-resistant Plasmodium. Once importation occurs, the potential exists in the United States for the spread of malaria by indigenous vectors and by parenteral transmission through shared needles and syringes.

The prospect of eradication of diseases such as rabies, plague, and other zoonoses that involve an extensive reservoir among nondomestic animals appears a more remote possibility.

SUMMARY

This chapter focussed on the epidemiology and control of infectious disease. We first discussed variations in the spectrum of disease and, in particular, the implications of inapparent infection for the control of disease and the collection of statistics. We then discussed important characteristics of infectious agents and host-agent interactions, specifically infectivity, pathogenicity, virulence, and immunogenicity. Among the pathogenetic mechanisms discussed were direct invasion of tissues, toxin production, allergic and immunologic reactions, and prolonged persistence of infection.

Mechanisms of spread of infection were discussed next and were classified as direct or indirect. Direct spread occurs through direct contact and respiratory droplets. Mechanisms of indirect transmission include fomites and other vehicles, arthropod vectors, and airborne spread through dusts and droplet nuclei. The importance of airborne droplet nuclei in the spread of tuberculosis and certain other diseases has received increasing acceptance in recent years.

The difference between epidemics spread by a common vehicle (common source) and propagated spread (person-to-person) was discussed. Generation time, herd immunity, and infection of members of a closed group by an index case (secondary attack) are features of propagated spread.

A formal outline for the investigation of an epidemic was presented next. Verification that an epidemic exists, confirmation of diagnosis, and orientation by time, place, and person were emphasized.

The chapter ended with a section on the control of disease. Specific control measures were classified as those designed to eliminate the organism, those that interrupt the transmission of infection, and those that reduce susceptibility of the host. The newer concepts of surveillance of disease and eradication were discussed with respect to current levels of infectious disease in the United States and to conditions affecting control of disease worldwide.

REFERENCES

Alexander, J. W.: Nosocomial Infections. Current Problems in Surgery. Yearbook Medical Publishers, Inc., Chicago, 1973.

American Academy of Pediatrics: Report of the Committee on Infectious Diseases. Evanston, IL, 1982.

American Hospital Association: Proceedings of the International Conference on Nosocomial Infections, 1970, Center for Disease Control. Waverly Press, Inc., Baltimore, 1971.

Benenson, A. S. (Ed.): Control of Communicable Diseases in Man, 11th Ed. Amer. Public Health Assn., New York, 1970.

Broome, C. V., and Fraser, D. W.: Epidemiologic Aspects of Legionnellosis. Epidemiol. Rev., 1:1–16, 1979.

Dougherty, W.J., Altman, R.: Viral hepatitis in New Jersey. Am. J. Med., 32:704, 1962.

Fox, J. P., Hall, C. E., et al.: Epidemiology: Man and Disease. Macmillan Publishing Co., Inc., New York, 1970.

Gross, H.: Oswego County Revisited. Pub. Hlth. Rep., *91*:168, 1976.

Hedrich, A. W.: Monthly estimates of the child population "susceptible" to measles, 1900–1931, Baltimore, Md. Am. J. Hygiene, *17*:626, 1933.

Hopkins, D. R., Hinman, A. R., Koplan, J. P., and Lane, J. M.: The case for global measles eradication. Lancet, *1*:1396, 1982.

Langmuir, A. D.: Air-borne infection. *In* Sartwell, P. E. (Ed.): Maxcy-Rosenau Preventive Medicine and Public Health, 9th Ed. Appleton-Century-Crofts, New York, 1965.

Langmuir, A. D.: Changing concepts of airborne infection of acute contagious diseases: A reconsideration of classic epidemiologic theories. N.Y. Acad. Sci., *353*:35, 1980.

Marcuse, E. K., and Grand, M. G.: Epidemiology of diphtheria in San Antonio, Texas, 1970. J.A.M.A., *224*:305, 1973.

Mausner, J. S., and Gezon, H. M.: Report on a phantom epidemic of gonorrhea. Am. J. Epidemiol., *85*:320, 1967.

Pizzo, P.: Value of protective isolation in preventing nosocomial infections in high risk patients. Am. J. Med., *70*:631, 1981.

Riley, R. L.: Airborne contagion. Historical background. Ann. N.Y. Acad. Sci., *353*:3, 1980.

Sartwell, P. E.: Infectious Disease Epidemiology. *In* Sartwell, P. E. (Ed.): Maxcy-Rosenau Preventive Medicine and Public Health, 10th Ed. Appleton-Century-Crofts, New York, 1973.

Schimpff, S.: Infection prevention during profound granulocytopenia. New approaches to alimentary canal microbial suppression. Ann. Int. Med., *93*:358, 1980.

Serfling, R. E. Historical review of epidemic theory. Hum. Biol., *24*:145, 1952.

Ward, J. I., Fraser, D. W., Baraff, L. J., and Plikaytis, B. D.: *Haemophilus influenzae* meningitis. A national study of secondary spread in household contacts. N. Engl. J. Med., *301*:122, 1979.

Zehmer, R. B., Dean, P. B., Sudia, W. D., Calisher, C. H., Sather, G. E., Parker, R. L.: Venezuelan equine encephalitis epidemic, Texas-1971. Health Serv. Repts., *89*:278, 1974.

OCCUPATIONAL EPIDEMIOLOGY

12

PETER GANN

Occupational epidemiology is the study of health effects of factors to which people are exposed in the workplace environment. These factors may be chemical, physical (such as heat, noise, radiation, or mechanical energy), or biological. Exposures that tend to occur either through individual behavior or cultural habits, such as smoking, drug use, and diet, are generally beyond the scope of occupational epidemiology except as secondary or modifying variables.

The purpose of this chapter is to illustrate how the epidemiologic techniques discussed in the book are applied to the study of occupational and environmental illness. Unique problems in applying these techniques to occupational illness will be discussed, and the important social policy considerations relating to the use of these study results will then be explored. No attempt can be made to cover the entire factual content of the field, which includes a seemingly infinite variety of exposures and illnesses.

Emphasis will be on occupational rather than environmental studies, because they are more numerous and because their findings can often be extrapolated to the environmental situation. Certain infectious diseases — for example, brucellosis in sheep handlers or hepatitis B in renal dialysis technicians — are clearly work-related, but techniques for their investigation and prevention belong to the general field of infectious disease epidemiology and are covered elsewhere.

Health problems arising from the nature of an individual's occupation are certainly at least as old as the pyramids. The kind of occupational illness and the health hazards encountered at any place or time are directly related to the means of economic activity that prevail and the type of technology available. The worker dyeing cloth in a nonindustrialized part of the world today may be exposed to hazards that have not been seen for centuries in more industrialized areas. The introduction of powerful machinery created the physical force required to liberate the toxic potential of such naturally occurring substances as coal dust, asbestos, and uranium. For instance, the modern-day quarry worker cutting silica rock with a pneumatic drill is at higher risk for silicosis than the worker who cut the same rock with a pick years ago.

Changes in such historic economic forces have led to the recent increased attention to occupational and environmental illness. The development of the internal combustion engine and subsequent growth in the importance of petroleum opened what some have called "the petrochemical era." Sudden bursts in the discovery and use of petroleum-based chemicals occurred, particularly during the two world wars. Today more than four million chemicals have been identified, and over 60,000 are commonly used in industry. Approximately 700 new chemicals are introduced every year. A rapidly increasing proportion of the materials we use for furniture, clothing, and building construction are derived from synthetic organic chemicals. Biologist Barry Commoner has emphasized that most of these chemicals have never been encountered by the living organisms that have evolved over millions of years. According to the National Occupational Health Survey conducted from 1972 to 1974, 58 per cent of urban workers in the United States are exposed to potentially hazardous chemicals on the job.

The rapid growth in the use of potentially hazardous materials has been accompanied by numerous observations of serious health effects in humans as a result of community or occupational exposure. Examples include the Minamata Bay disaster in Japan, where 1200 cases of neurologic disease and severe birth defects occurred among people eating fish contaminated with methyl mercury (Kurland, 1960). In another episode, workers at plastic manufacturing plants who handled the gas vinyl chloride were discovered in 1974 to be developing an unusual cancer, hepatic angiosarcoma (Waxweiler, 1976). At about the same time, infertility and extreme decrease in spermatogenesis were discovered in workers in a California plant producing dibromochloropropane (Whorton, 1977).

It is important to note that these and other chemical-related epidemics were first discovered by clinicians or by the victims themselves. Epidemiologic studies were used to confirm and extend the basic findings. This points to an important interaction between clinical observation and epidemiology in the environmental/occupational area. When the disease in question is rare in the general population, discovery of its occupational or environmental origins can usually be made by clinical observation. However, when the disease is more common, such as lung cancer or chronic nephritis, epidemiologic study is often needed to distinguish chemical or physical exposures from other causes.

At present, there have been some basic advances in improving work environments and avoiding dangerously uncontrolled industrial plant emissions. For example, the epidemics of severe, often fatal bronchitis associated with polluted atmospheric inversions are no longer found in the industrialized world, as they were in London and the Donora Valley, Pennsylvania, in the early 1950s. Epidemiologists' main concerns have shifted from acute health effects to those of a more insidious or subtle nature; this is according to the power of the epidemiologic approach in resolving complex exposure-disease associations. Epidemiologists now working in this field are focussing on three such complex areas: carcinogenesis, chronic diseases (particularly involving the respiratory, neurologic, and cardiovascular systems), and reproduction.

The systematic application of epidemiologic techniques to the study of occupational and environmental disease has only recently begun to evolve. Early works, such as Sartwell and Seltser's mortality study of radiologists (see Chap. 6) or Selikoff's study of asbestos insulation workers in the 1960s (Selikoff, 1968), were of great interest not only because of their findings but also because they demonstrated that the workplace, an organized context of exposure with its own record-keeping systems, was a fertile area for epidemiologic study. In occupational medicine, the emphasis had previously been on recognizing, treating, and preventing acute illnesses and injuries arising from the work process; studies of populations were not needed to establish, for instance, that working with carbon tetrachloride can lead to a severe form of hepatitis. The past 20 years has shown a shift of emphasis from acute to chronic illness, as new methods for statistics and design became available in the general area of chronic-disease epidemiology. Occupational epidemiology may be considered a branch of chronic-disease epidemiology; in both, the attempt is usually made to explore the association between an exposure with an imprecise but prolonged duration and a disease with a delayed and obscure onset.

Most studies in occupational epidemiology are analytic rather than descriptive. Once a disease is recognized as being occupational in origin, it may be described with respect to person, place, and time. However, the primary goal in occupational epidemiology is the identification or confirmation of new occupational diseases and the study of dose-response characteristics in order to prevent illness. The various types of study in occupational epidemiology are discussed subsequently.

ECOLOGICAL STUDIES

Ecological studies provide a crude way of exploring associations between occupation or environment and disease. More precisely, these studies are considered to be "hypothesis-generating" rather than "hypothesis-testing" in nature. In ecological studies, the group—rather than the individual—is the unit of comparison. Disease rates in various groups, usually defined as groups living within specific geographic areas, are compared. The variation in rates from one area to another may be explained by correlations between these rates and factors distinct to certain areas. In another type of ecological study, time trends are compared; changes in exposure among various groups may be correlated with observed changes in disease rates. An example would be the comparison of the trend in saccharin usage to the trend in bladder cancer rates in the United States.

The former (geographic) type of study is more often encountered in occupational epidemiology. As an example, the National Cancer Institute (NCI) published maps showing the age-adjusted mortality rates for cancer in the United States by county for the period 1950 to 1969 (Mason, 1975). Figure 12 – 1 shows the age-adjusted mortality rate map for cancers of the trachea, bronchus, and lung in white males. Clustering of high-rate counties in the Northeast and Southeast and on the Gulf coasts is evident. An ecological study correlating these county rates with industry concentration data revealed that lung cancer mortality was elevated in counties with paper, chemical petroleum, and transportation industries (Blot and Fraumeni, 1976). This study in turn hypothesized that lung cancer in certain coastal areas was associated with the ship-building industry. A case-control study of lung cancer in coastal Georgia (Blot et al., 1978) was a logical next step and confirmed the association between shipbuilding and lung cancer, possibly as a result of asbestos exposure.

Several major reservations exist regarding the use of ecological studies in occupational epidemiology. In some instances, as the example shows, they may provide a reasonable and inexpensive means for generating hypotheses. On the other hand, these studies are subject to the "ecological fallacy" (Morgenstern, 1983) that states that conclusions regarding individual risk (e.g., the risk of lung cancer) on the basis of group risk must be made cautiously, because data on individual behavior that may influence risk have not been collected. One does not know which in the county are currently in the process of developing lung cancer. For example, the correlation between lung cancer and certain industries could be explained by a higher prevalence of cigarette smoking among individuals in the counties with those industries. It is impossible to refute this explanation without data on prevalence of smoking with respect to county, which are not available.

Another problem with ecological studies lies in the difficulty of selecting groups of proper size. Groups that are too small will have too few cases and unstable rates for the disease in question or will be affected by migration. Groups that are too large may have such a small proportion of the population with a particular exposure that the effect of

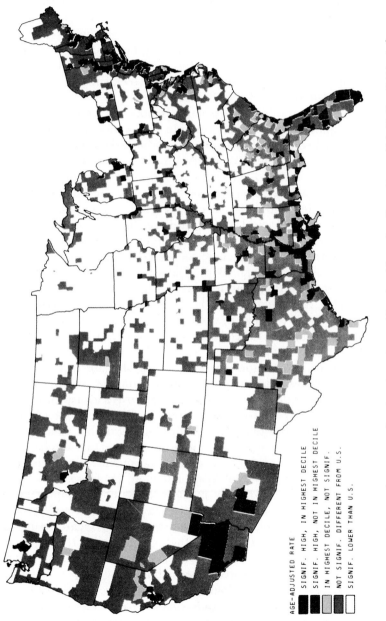

AGE-ADJUSTED RATE

SIGNIF. HIGH, IN HIGHEST DECILE

SIGNIF. HIGH, NOT IN HIGHEST DECILE

IN HIGHEST DECILE, NOT SIGNIF.

NOT SIGNIF. DIFFERENT FROM U.S.

SIGNIF. LOWER THAN U.S.

Figure 12–1 Map for cancers of trachea, bronchus and lung in white males. (From Mason, T. J., McKay, F. W., et al.: Atlas of cancer mortality for United States counties: 1950–1980. U.S. Government Printing Office, DHEW Publ. (NIH) 75-780, Washington, D.C., 1975.)

that exposure on disease rates for the group is diluted. Looked at another way, small increases in disease rates for a county may be the result of an enormously increased relative risk for a small segment of the population of that county.

CROSS-SECTIONAL STUDIES

In the cross-sectional study, observations of a group are made during a cross-sectional slice in time, usually employing clinical tests, interviews, and measures of exposure. Data collection is therefore basically handled in the same way as a screening or periodic health study. All current workers, or all living retirees, might be included. Sometimes repeated cross-sectional observations may be combined to compare trends between exposed and nonexposed groups. For example, in a study of pulmonary function in Boston firefighters (Musk et al., 1977), a drop in certain indices over a two-year interval was found, compared with the expected loss over the same interval in the general population.

The cross-sectional study is especially suited for inquiry into subtle, perhaps even subclinical health effects for which records are unlikely to exist. Since these are essentially prevalence studies, the relationship between the health effects and time cannot be readily explored. The prevalence of the health effect is compared among subgroups with varying exposures, ages, personal habits, or medical histories.

With a cross-sectional design, the principal weakness lies in the possible relationship between a worker's having the health problem and the likelihood of his or her appearing in the study group. Since workers who become ill may stay home from work, quit, or retire early, at any one time the current workers are probably relatively healthy. (The "healthy worker effect" will be discussed later in more detail in the context of the cohort study.) The exclusion of some affected workers will obviously minimize an association or decrease the chances of its being detected. Conversely, if presence of the health effects or correlates of exposure make an individual more likely to volunteer for study, an overestimate of the association may occur.

A special type of cross-sectional study is involved when an acute epidemic of illness occurs in the workplace. In that case, the techniques employed resemble those used in classic infectious or foodborne outbreak investigations: cases are defined, epidemic curves are plotted, and cases are compared with noncases for various potential risk factors.

CASE-CONTROL STUDIES

Case-control studies, which were fully discussed in Chapter 7, play an important role in the study of occupational disease. Although the cohort method is more often used when a specific exposure is of interest, the case-control method may be preferred if either of the following exist:

1. One disease of interest that is relatively rare and would require a large cohort for follow-up

2. Several occupations or substances that may be associated with the disease of interest.

The latter situation implies that many different jobs involve handling the same materials and that diseases often have multiple causes. For example, a study of sinonasal cancer may disclose that the condition is associated with nickel, isopropyl, oil, and wood dust exposure. Many occupational cohorts can contribute to the sum total of cases and controls with each of these exposures (Rousch, 1980). In addition to providing an opportunity to test many potential etiologic hypotheses, the rich variety of data collected on the individual case or control allows the influence of various modifiers of the exposure-disease relationship to be studied. A simple example of this in occupational disease is the enhanced risk of lung cancer among asbestos workers who also smoke. This modifying, or synergistic, effect (i.e., the combined risk is greater than that expected by adding the independent risks) would be difficult to determine in anything but a case-control study.

Recently developed techniques for multivariate analysis have added to the strength of the case-control method, providing an effective means for evaluating confounding and interaction of variables, as well as allowing for more flexibility in study designs (Schlesselman, 1982).

Jobs held in the past are often of greater relevance than a worker's current occupation, particularly if the disease under study has a delayed onset following exposure (as is the case for occupationally related cancer). Furthermore, the development of an occupational disease may itself lead to a change in work because of physical disability. The emphasis in case-control studies, then, must be on an overview of the individual's entire work history.

Several sources of data may be used by the epidemiologist to obtain these histories. The most commonly used is the personal interview, in which cases and controls relate details of their past work. If a case or a control has died by the time of the interview, as is often true for rapidly fatal illnesses, the individual's next of kin may provide the needed information. The reliability of data on work history gathered from next of kin has not yet been fully studied, but there are some indications that it is reasonably accurate for broadly defined job categories (Rogot and Reid, 1975).

Existing record systems may also be used as a source of occupational data for case-control studies. Death certificates usually contain information on the decedent's usual occupation and the industry that employed him. These data, most often recorded by the funeral director, can provide for a rapid, inexpensive study, since both cause of death and occupation are contained in the same document. However, the completeness and accuracy of occupational data on death certificates is strongly suspect and therefore should only be used in studies of an exploratory nature or in surveillance systems. When compared with data obtained from cohort records or interviews, death certificates appear to reflect the true usual lifetime occupation about 70 to 75 per cent of the time (Wegman and Peters, 1978). This degree of accuracy is even lower for women and nonwhites (Steenland and Beaumont, personal communication).

Other sources have been or could be used as sources of occupational data for case-control studies. For example, commercial city directories, available for 1200 municipalities, list the occupations and employers of individual residents annually (Rousch et al., 1980). Several major health maintenance organizations and hospitals record occupation, and some companies and unions have record systems large enough to construct series of cases and controls from a wide variety of occupations. Some population-based cancer incidence registries also collect and code the usual occupation of cancer cases. Two very complete systems containing occupational data, private medical insurance programs, and federal tax returns, are not yet available for epidemiologic studies. When completeness, accuracy, and the handling of confounding variables are all considered, the interview remains the preferable means of collecting these data.

A study on bladder cancer and occupation done in the Boston area (Cole et al., 1972) serves as a useful illustration of the case-control method. An attempt was made to identify all newly diagnosed cases of lower urinary tract cancer in the defined geographic area during an 18-month period. Following the selection of controls from residence lists in the area, interviews were conducted in order to obtain information on occupational history as well as other factors. For each job held longer than 6 months, the following data were obtained: name, address, and nature of the employer's industry, job title, time interval on the job, specific duties performed, and history of exposure to chemical or physical hazards. Both job titles and nature of industry were used to construct a reduced list of basic exposure and industry categories. Table 12–1 shows the relative risks for persons employed at any time in the 13 exposure categories in this study. Relative risks were controlled for age

TABLE 12-1 Relative Risks of Lower Urinary Tract Cancer Among Men Ever Employed in Various Industry Categories

Industry Categories	Relative Risk°	95% Confidence Limits
Suspect		
Dyestuffs	2.33	0.66–8.24
Rubber, rubber products	1.63	1.04–2.56
Leather, leather products	2.25	1.46–3.46
Printing	1.30	0.68–2.49
Paint	1.19	0.69–2.05
Petroleum products	1.18	0.82–1.69
Other organic chemicals	1.44	0.74–2.80
Other chemicals	0.99	0.54–1.81
All suspect categories	1.54	1.19–1.98
Nonsuspect		
Fumes, dust, dirt, smoke	1.00	
Manufacturing, nonspecific	1.00	
Ranching, farming	1.00	
Service	1.00	
Office	1.00	

° Relative to a risk of 1.00 for men never employed in a suspect industry, controlled for age and smoking.

Adapted from Cole, P., Hoover, R., and Friedell, G. H.: Occupation and cancer of the lower urinary tract. Cancer 29:1250, 1972.

and smoking, the two important confounding variables. The data confirmed previous reports of an association between bladder cancer and work in the rubber and leather industries. Analysis of exposure subcategories allowed further delineation of excess risk; for instance, among those employed at any time in the leather industry, most of the excess cases occurred among those who had worked in finishing leather, which involves cutting, assembling, and buffing leather pieces.

Case-control studies of occupation must be evaluated in light of the vulnerable areas common to all studies of this type, such as recall bias and biased selection of cases or controls. An additional problem is that for the null hypothesis to be accepted (that is, for there to be no association between disease and occupation), cases and controls must have had equal opportunity to have experienced occupations and exposures. If, because of the nature of the disease among cases, this is not true, false estimates of the association may result. A simple example can be seen in a study of occupation and chronic lung disease in which cases may have less opportunity for exposure, owing to their illness. The opposite effect may occur if the cases have a disease that does not lead to prolonged restriction of participation in the workforce but a sizable proportion of controls (particularly if they are hospital controls) have such diseases.

The usefulness of the case-control approach in studying occupational factors in disease is limited primarily by the difficulty in determining the precise nature and extent of past exposures on the basis of an interview. This tends to lead to the use of broadly defined job or industry categories, such as "usual employment in the leather industry," which dilute the true risk by including individuals with widely disparate histories of exposure to specific chemicals. On the other hand, if exposures are defined too narrowly, the prevalence of certain exposed groups in the study may be too low, and the case-control comparison will be based on numbers that are too small for interpretation. This can be seen for some groups in the bladder cancer study. The statistical power of an occupational study is greatly enhanced when subjects can be grouped according to an exposure they actually have in common rather than by job title and industry, which are poor indicators of exposure. For instance, grouping textile finishers with morticians may at first appear incongruous but in fact makes sense if maximum power in exploring the effects of formaldehyde exposure is to be achieved.

The problem of identifying which subjects in the study were actually exposed to a particular substance and which were not is being addressed in two different ways. First, Canadian researchers are conducting studies on cancer and occupation using chemist-engineers to interview the study subjects. More precise past chemical exposures are thus determined on a case-by-case basis through informed probing of the subjects (Siematycki et al., 1981). Second, a number of researchers are working on data linkage systems that tie together various industry-specific job titles for which exposure to a particular substance is presumed to exist a priori (Hoar, 1981). The exposure-linkage systems consist of thousands of pairs linking a specific job and a chemical or physical agent (Table 12–2). An indication of the intensity of exposure (heavy, moderate, or light) may also be used. Table 12–2 shows the agents linked to the job of carpenter in the construction industry. A list of job titles and industries linked to a particular agent could also be generated. It is important to note that these linkages are only inferred; exposure may not occur for some individuals, and some exposures may be missed. A reanalysis of the data from the previously mentioned bladder cancer study was performed using a linkage system that combined various job titles with similar patterns of exposure regardless of industry category. The result was a higher relative risk (RR = 3.1) for persons with jobs that had heavy presumptive exposure to aromatic amines, compared with the relative risk obtained for the rubber and dye industries in general. Aromatic amines are used in these two industries and are known to cause bladder cancer.

It appears that both approaches to the problem of assembling more accurate occupational exposure data in case-control studies are promising. However, the use of this study design to discover new risks is

TABLE 12-2 Agents Linked to Employment as a Carpenter in the Construction Industry

Agent	Degree of Exposure
Azo compounds	Moderate
Creosote	Moderate
Aromatic hydrocarbons	
Coal, tar and pitch	Moderate
Petroleum, coal tar, and pitch	Moderate
Aliphatic compounds	
Water-insoluble carbon polymers	Light
Polysiloxanes	Light
Metals	
Chromium	Heavy
Minerals	
Asbestos	Moderate
Physical agents	
Wood dust	Heavy
UV radiation	Moderate

From Hoar, S. K.: Epidemiology and occupational classification systems. *In* Peto, R., and Schneiderman, M. (Eds.): Banbury Report 9: Quantification of Occupational Cancer. Cold Spring Harbor Laboratory, 1981.

sometimes limited to hypothesis-generation, and confirmation by cohort studies will often be necessary. In most instances, case-control studies will not permit identification of specific worksites at which preventive actions can be directed. An exception to this may occur if a study covers a narrow geographic area where large numbers of cases are likely to have worked in a small number of plants (Axelson, 1979).

COHORT STUDIES

Cohort studies are particularly useful and effective in occupational epidemiology. The various types of cohort studies have been discussed in Chapter 7. Although true prospective studies on work cohorts can be conducted, the historic prospective cohort method is far more commonly used. Records maintained by employers or labor unions permit the epidemiologist to identify readily a cohort to be traced for a variety of health outcomes. Occupational cohort studies are usually mortality studies, since records of cause of death are generally more accessible and less biased than cause of illness records. Furthermore, the emphasis is often on cancer mortality, since cancer of most sites is usually ultimately fatal and diagnosis is more accurate for neoplastic disease than, for instance, for cardiovascular disease.

The central and unique element of occupational cohort studies is the individual work history. This history, which can be reconstructed to one degree or another through existing records, provides the exposure data for the hypothesized disease–exposure associations. Various problems in utilizing work histories will be discussed later.

The historic cohort method is a relatively new tool. Its beginnings trace back to studies by Wade Hampton Frost in the 1930s on the follow-up of families in contact with pulmonary tuberculosis cases (Frost, 1933). The method has undergone rapid refinement over the past 15 years, primarily because of its usefulness in occupational epidemiology.

The basic design of the historic prospective cohort study was presented earlier in this text. The general sequence of steps in conducting such a study on an occupational group are presented here:

1. *Setting up hypotheses.* Hypotheses in occupational cohort studies often arise from concern over the health effects of exposure to a particular substance. For instance, when the results of animal studies on the carcinogenicity of formaldehyde became known, researchers began to look for groups of workers with a history of exposure to formaldehyde. As a result, large ongoing studies of textile workers, formaldehyde producers, and embalmers were initiated. Sometimes the hypothesis derives from concern about a whole industry or process rather than a specific substance. The rubber industry — tire-building in particular — was studied because of its associated exposure to multiple carcinogens (Monson and Fine, 1978). These industry-based studies can result in confirming hypotheses linking a process to a disease without identifying any specific etiologic exposures. For instance, shoemaking has been associated with nasal cancer, but the actual carcinogen is unknown (Acheson, 1976).

2. *Defining the cohort.* Records from employer personnel departments, union seniority lists, or benefits programs are the usual sources for establishing the cohort. These records should reveal who worked where and when in the workplace under study. Ideally, epidemiologists prefer to define the cohort as broadly as possible, to include all individuals who worked at the site 1 day or more from a point in the distant past until the present. If record sources are limited, the cohort may be defined as all persons at work on a given day or year in the past. This is a "prevalence" type of cohort and, although easier to assemble, it may be biased owing to an overrepresentation of long-term workers.

In Figure 12–2, A is a prevalence cohort, whereas B, C, and D represent incidence cohorts, and entry and follow-up overlap in cohorts C and D. Very short-term workers or workers with only recent exposure may later be dropped from the cohort. This type of incidence cohort, in which members are entering and leaving the cohort at different times, is linked with the person-years at risk, or modified life table, technique. This technique maximizes the population available for study and hence

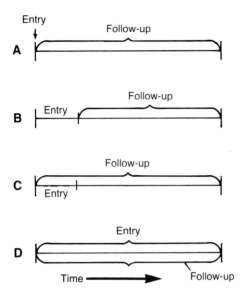

Figure 12-2 Relation between entry and follow-up periods in cohort studies.

the statistical power. Figure 12-2 illustrates four possible ways of defining cohorts in terms of entry and follow-up periods.

Verification of a cohort by external sources is recommended. Union seniority lists and employer records may be checked against each other. An alternative method, using periodic reports by employers that give individual names and social security numbers to the Social Security Administration, has also been used (Enterline and Marsh, 1982). Workers who leave employment (other than by death) are more difficult to follow up in a cohort study. In the past, some studies have eliminated these workers from the cohort and included only people who are active workers in the plant or are listed as retired for disability at the time of death or end of the study period. This exclusion of "terminated" workers can lead to serious biases in assessing mortality, since it may distort the age distribution of the cohort and omit workers who left employment for reasons of poor health.

3. *Follow-up of mortality.* Once the cohort is established, the next step is to determine the vital status of each cohort member at the end of the study period. For many workers, this can be done by checking personnel, union, or benefit plan records. In some cases even telephone books, post offices, obituaries, or notices in company newsletters have been used. Social Security, a nearly universal benefit plan for working people since 1935, has also proved helpful. This system can inform the researcher of an individual's vital status and, if the individual has died, of the date and place of death. State or local governments will locate these certificates if a name and approximate date of death are supplied. Cause

of death is then coded, usually according to the International Classification of Disease (ICD). If the study period encompasses several revisions of the ICD, as is often true, the revisions may have to be merged into a single coding scheme for the study.

Follow-up in an occupational cohort mortality study must be nearly complete, at least over 90 per cent. Cohort members who are lost to follow-up present a problem, since their elusiveness may be associated with mortality rates different from the general population. Women are more likely to be lost to follow-up than are men, partly resulting from marital name-changing. Because of the potential for bias, the best approach to handling workers who have been lost to follow-up is to assume that they are alive at the end of the study period. This ensures that if bias occurs, it tends to reduce the relative risks observed.

The creation of a National Death Index in the United States, which began collecting data in 1979, will greatly facilitate the follow-up of cohorts in future studies. This index uses name and birthdate to locate individual death certificates of United States residents.

4. *Exposure data.* Cohorts are very seldom homogenous with respect to the exposure of interest. There are numerous ways to divide the cohort into exposure level groups, in order to search for dose-response relationships or to identify high-risk jobs within the workplace. Work histories, including date of hire and calendar period in each job title or work area, must be abstracted from available records. The simplest surrogate for dose is duration of exposure, in years. Job titles and work areas must each be weighed in terms of historic exposures. This can be extremely complex; a single shipyard may have 20,000 job titles in its personnel files. One way to rate jobs for exposure is to use a panel of industrial hygienists, engineers, physicians, and workers to place each job, in part by subjective impression, into an exposure category (Gamble and Spirtas, 1976). Changes in exposure over time in a particular job must also be considered. If the investigator is fortunate, past air-sampling data from various jobs within the workplace may be available. These data, if complete enough, may allow calculation of each individual worker's total cumulative exposure. In a study of chrysotile asbestos miners in Quebec, a cumulative dust exposure, expressed as million particles per cubic foot years (mpcf·y), was calculated on the basis of average dust concentrations in each job and the worker's years in these jobs. Figure 12–3 shows the dose-response relationships between this measure and lung cancer risk in this study (McDonald et al., 1980). In very rare instances, biologic monitoring data—that which is collected on the actual concentration of toxins absorbed into the body (e.g., blood lead levels)—may also be available.

There are several models that can be used in creating an index to represent a worker's lifetime exposure to a potentially toxic agent. Since

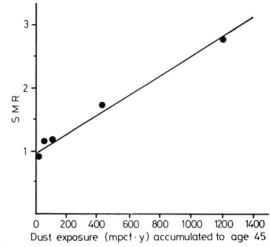

Figure 12 - 3 The relationship of lung cancer, SMR to cumulative asbestos dust exposure in Quebec miners. (From McDonald, J. C., Liddell, F. D. K. et al.: Dust exposure and mortality in chrysotile mining, 1910 – 1975. Br. J. Ind. Med., *37:* 11, 1980.)

the decision of which is best may depend on the biologic half-life and tendency of the chemical to accumulate in the body, a cumulative-dose model, as just presented, may be ideal. For other toxins, which have a hit-and-run effect, peak or highest exposure may be relevant. In general, exposure classification models that utilize less than the whole work history, such as "last job held" or "job held longest" are suspect, since early exposure is often more significant and workers who gain seniority or become ill usually try to leave heavily exposed jobs. On the other hand, attempts to utilize every detail of the work history may either make study costs prohibitive or reduce group sizes to the point of statistical instability, while adding little to the overall precision of the study.

   5. *Analysis.* The modified life table method, which allows persons to enter and exit the cohort at different times during the study period and therefore maximizes the population at risk, is the most commonly used method for analysis of occupational cohort studies. A matrix consisting of age and calendar year cells or strata is created, as in Figure 12 – 4. Once a worker becomes eligible and enters the cohort, he or she begins contributing person-years at risk to various strata. In the example given, it can be seen that persons move diagonally through the matrix. The expected number of deaths in each stratum is calculated by applying a comparison population death rate to the sum of the person-years in the stratum. (The assumptions behind use of a person-time technique are

			Age, Yrs			
	30–34	35–39	40–44	45–49	50–54	Total
1950–54	(1) 3 yrs					3 p-yrs
1955–59		(1) 5 yrs				5 p-yrs
1960–64		(2) 2 yrs	(1) 5 yrs			7 p-yrs
1965–69			(2) 3 yrs †	(1) 5 yrs		8 p-yrs
1970–74					(1) 5 yrs*	5 p-yrs
Total	3 p-yrs	7 p-yrs	8 p-yrs	5 p-yrs	5 p-yrs	28 p-yrs

(left axis label: Calendar Period)

Figure 12 – 4 Contribution of two individual workers to a person-years matrix.

discussed in Chapter 3.) This application of a larger comparison population rate to the age distribution of the study population is a form of indirect adjustment (see Chap. 13), and leads to the Standardized Mortality (or Morbidity) Ratio (SMR) as the measure of outcome. The overall summary SMR can be expressed as follows:

$$\text{SMR} = \frac{\text{Observed deaths in the study population}}{\text{Expected deaths in the study population}} \times 100$$

The expected number of deaths in the denominator is the sum of the expected deaths from each age/time stratum. Cause-specific SMRs are also calculated the same way, from observed and expected deaths from a specific cause. The age/time matrix of person-years at risk may be further divided or stratified by race, sex, and work history or exposure categories, yielding SMRs specific for these variables. The result, for instance, may be a lung cancer SMR for nonwhite females over age 45 with a minimum of 10 years in a high-exposure job, which incorporates a comparison with nonexposed, nonwhite females in the same age category. The flexibility of the method is obvious.

The SMR, although widely used in occupational studies as a measure of relative risk, has a number of limitations. For example, it is usually used as a summary statistic adjusted for the age distribution of the cohort. The problem this may create in masking risks occurring only within age-specific groups has been mentioned earlier (Chap. 3). Occasionally, a study may include many young workers who are not yet at full risk for the development of an occupational disease, or it may include many older workers for whom the risk of that disease may have begun to decline. In addition, since the SMR is derived by indirect age adjustment, SMRs calculated for two or more separate cohorts cannot be directly compared, even though the same standard population rates may have been used to determine expected deaths.

Before completing the discussion of problems with methodology, an illustration of the use of SMRs in occupational cohort studies will be presented.

Arsenic and Respiratory Cancer

In order to study the carcinogenic potential of arsenic trioxide in humans, Lee and Fraumeni gathered a cohort of 8047 white male smelter workers. Workers were eligible if they worked for at least 12 months prior to 31 December 1956. The follow-up period was from 1938 through 1963. Vital status was determined for 90.4 per cent of the cohort. Persons lost to follow-up were considered to be at risk until the year they were last known to be alive. Mortality rates for the general population of the states in which the smelters existed were used to compute expected deaths. Exposure was handled by grouping the smelter workers by length of employment, as shown in Table 12–3.

Sampling measurements for arsenic were also used to rate each work area from 1 to 10 with respect to arsenic exposure. This scale was then divided into heavy-, medium-, and light-exposure work areas. Table 12–4 shows the SMRs stratified by these exposure categories.

Cohort studies may also be used to localize a high-risk group within a workforce with varied job activities. In a well-known example, Lloyd and co-workers found that the elevated risk of lung cancer in coke plant workers was attributable to a very high risk among nonwhite steelworkers who worked atop the coke ovens (Lloyd, 1971).

Several major issues regarding the use of the historic prospective cohort study in occupational epidemiology are under debate. Selection

TABLE 12-3 SMRs for Various Causes Among Smelterers with Arsenic Exposure

	Respiratory Cancer			Heart Disease		
Length of Employment	*Observed*	*Expected*	*SMR*	*Observed*	*Expected*	*SMR*
>15 years, completed before 1938	61	13.0	469°	280	258.3	108
>15 years, completed between 1938–1963	37	10.0	370°	138	115.0	120†
10–14 years	10	4.3	233†	68	51.9	131†
5–9 years	15	5.6	268°	87	60.4	144°
1–4 years	24	11.8	203°	152	128.4	118†

° Significant at 1% level
† Significant at 5% level

TABLE 12-4   Respiratory Cancer SMR by Length of Employment and
Maximum Level of Arsenic Exposure

Length of Employment	Maximum Exposure		
	Heavy	*Medium*	*Light*
>15 years, completed before 1938	800°	667°	250°
>15 years, completed 1938-1963	667°	545°	310°
<15 years	444°	263°	214°
All lengths above combined	667†	478†	239°

° Significant at 1% level
† Significant at 5% level

of the comparison or standard population to compute expected deaths is one such issue. National mortality rates are readily available but do not necessarily agree with the local rates in the area where the cohort actually lives. For example, a particular county may have an elevated rate for mortality from pancreatic cancer. The county rate may prove to be more acceptable for computing expected deaths in a study of pancreatic cancer in a cohort of workers in that county; national rates may yield falsely elevated SMRs. On the other hand, if the comparison population is too local, the mortality rates for specific causes or age-groups may be unstable or, even worse, heavily influenced by the very cohort under study. Internal comparisons, in which the standard population is an entire heterogeneous cohort, can be used to investigate mortality in a subset of the cohort, as illustrated by Lloyd's study.

The use of mortality rates from a large working population for computing SMRs has the major advantage of minimizing what is known as the "healthy worker effect," mentioned earlier. This advantage may be so important that data bases consisting of mortality rates from mixed groups of workers may eventually become available to epidemiologists. Mortality figures from standard general populations include individuals who are too sick to work. The very fact of employment implies a certain level of health. Occupational cohorts, therefore, usually have SMRs below 100, in comparison with general populations, when no excess risk is present. Selection for healthy workers operates both at the time of hiring and throughout the duration of work, since some workers will leave employment as a result of ill health, perhaps related to their job. Theoretically, these workers may move on to less hazardous jobs, creating an "unhealthy worker effect" on mortality in these jobs.

The magnitude of the healthy worker effect can be influenced by several factors: the particular disease under consideration, the length of follow-up, age, and race. Table 12-5 presents data from a study of vinyl

TABLE 12–5 SMRs by Cause and Length of Time Since Entering Vinyl Chloride Industry

Cause of Death	Length of Time Since Entering Industry				
	0–4 yrs	5–9 yrs	10–14 yrs	15+ yrs	Total
All causes	37.4	62.9	75.1	94.2	75.4
All cancers	44.5	70.6	94.0	111.8	90.7
Circulatory disease	21.5	70.3	84.7	90.7	76.9
Respiratory disease	20.9	38.8	31.3	93.0	62.6

chloride–exposed workers in Great Britain that illustrate some of these concepts (Fox and Collier, 1976).

For each cause of death, the healthy worker effect diminishes with increasing time in the industry or follow-up, which is logical, since the workers observed for longer periods are farther from the health-selecting event of hiring. The healthy worker effect on cancer SMRs is less than that for circulatory or respiratory disease. This is because most fatal circulatory or respiratory illnesses are chronic conditions whose symptoms or disabilities appear long before death, allowing selection out of the workplace to occur; in contrast, cancer is unlikely to influence employment until much later in its course. In comparing different age groups while keeping length of follow-up constant, it can also be observed that older workers show a larger healthy worker effect than do younger ones; older people able to enter the workforce are far healthier than their overall age counterparts. Similarly, nonwhites show a consistently greater healthy worker effect than do whites at all ages, owing to the presence of more nonwhite individuals who are poor, unemployed, or too ill to work (McMichael, 1976).

Occupational cohort studies must also cope with the phenomenon of latency (alluded to earlier), the delay between onset of exposure and appearance of the related disease. Mesotheliomas associated with asbestos exposure may not appear for an average of 30 years after initial exposure; bladder cancers may not appear for a mean of 20 years following exposure to aromatic amines. If too many early years after initial exposure are mistakenly included as person-years at risk, the disease association will be diluted. Although the precise date at which risk begins can never be known, many epidemiologists routinely require that a subject begin contributing person-years at risk (and observed death or morbidity) only after 5 or 10 years from initial exposure have elapsed.

Only very rarely does an occupation involve a single potentially hazardous exposure. The problem of multiple exposures demands that the epidemiologist be sensitive to many factors in the work environment simultaneously that may explain risk. In a related sense, occupational disease may be multifactorial; that is, it may have two or more etiologic factors, each of which is necessary but insufficient for explaining the risks observed. This type of problem is discussed in Chapter 7 as a problem generic to the investigation of chronic diseases. For example, in the smelter study on arsenic, exposure levels to sulfur dioxide, silica, lead, and ferromanganese were also determined. It was found that sulfur dioxide exposure also was related to an increased risk of lung cancer, and the independent or joint effects of arsenic and sulfur dioxide could not be clearly identified.

The inability to examine many variables related to disease outcome is a basic weakness of the historic prospective cohort method. Modifying variables may be found inside or outside the work environment and may interact negatively or positively with the exposure-disease association. An important example of this is the relationship between cigarette smoking, occupational exposure, and lung cancer risk. Smoking data on individuals in a historic study are very rarely available, so whether the workers in the study smoked more or less than the comparison population may be only speculated on. There is a relationship between socio-economic status and smoking habit (Covey and Wynder, 1981). Once again, if internal comparison or external worker populations are used for computation of expected death rates, the problem of a lack of smoking data in a cohort study may be partially negated.

Alternatives to the SMR

Sometimes past records on a cohort are inadequate to determine work histories and years at risk. Notices of death or death certificates themselves are all that may be available, perhaps collected as part of a benefit program for long-term workers. In this case, the investigator must abandon the SMR and rely on the proportionate mortality (or morbidity) ratio (PMR), which has been presented in a different form in Chapter 5. In occupational studies, the PMR is expressed as observed/expected deaths from a specific cause in an occupational cohort times 100.

$$PMR = \frac{\text{Observed deaths from a specific cause}}{\text{Expected deaths from the same cause}} \times 100$$

The numerator, deaths observed in the cohort or a subgroup of the cohort, is identical to the numerator of the SMR. The expected deaths, however, are computed by applying the proportion of total deaths due to a particular cause in the comparison or general population to the total deaths in the study population. Consider the following example, shown in Table 12–6:

TABLE 12-6 Hypothetical Example of a PMR Calculation

Age	(1) Total Deaths Observed	(2) Deaths Observed Due to Lung Cancer	(3) Lung Cancer Death Proportion General Pop.	(4) = (1) × (3) Expected Lung Cancer Deaths
30–39	2	0	0.02	0.04
40–49	8	3	0.03	0.24
50–59	10	4	0.06	0.60
60–69	20	6	0.10	2.00
		Σ Observed = 13		Σ Expected = 2.88

$$\text{PMR} = \frac{13}{2.88} \times 100 = 451$$

Like SMRs, PMRs are also often used as a standardized summary statistic; expected deaths from various age at death and calendar period strata are summed. Deaths among the cohort may also be stratified by work area, job title, duration of exposure, or latency, to yield PMRs specific for these variables. The chief problem with PMRs is that the PMR for one cause is not independent of the PMR for other causes. If the total number of deaths in the cohort is unusual, the proportion due to the particular cause of interest may be distorted. In an extreme example, if the total number of deaths in each age group is doubled as a result of a large number of accidental deaths, the lung cancer PMR will be halved. PMRs also do not work well for common causes of death, for which small increases in risk easily affect the total number of deaths. Nevertheless, under the conditions existing in many occupational cohort studies, the PMR provides a reasonably accurate substitute for the SMR. In another analysis of the data from the coke workers mentioned earlier, SMR and PMR values based on internal comparison to all steelworkers in the study and comparison to county death statistics were calculated. See Table 12–7 (Redmond and Breslin, 1975).

In this table, the SMRs and PMRs are in the same direction relative to 100, and for whites, whose rates are more stable owing to larger numbers, the internal comparison yields a closer approximation of PMR to SMR, since the overall mortality of the study population (coke plant) and comparison population (all steelworkers studied) are more nearly equal.

In some instances, the epidemiologist may be interested in studying only one or two diseases within a cohort. Furthermore, it may be too expensive to assemble work histories on everyone in the workplace. A "nested" case-control or case-control-within-a-cohort study may then be the method of choice. Cases consist of all workers, or a representative sample, within a cohort who have developed a particular disease of

TABLE 12-7 Comparison of SMR and PMR for Selected Causes of Death Among Coke Plant Workers Using Total Steelworker and County Populations as Comparison Groups

	White				NonWhite			
	Total Steelworker Population		County Population		Total Steelworker Population		County Population	
Cause	SMR	PMR	SMR	PMR	SMR	PMR	SMR	PMR
Lung cancer	68	71	71	86	322	254	322	380
Genitourinary cancer	203	193	137	175	148	119	151	177
Cardiovascular/ renal	95	94	72	93	98	79	63	74

interest. Controls may be randomly selected workers from the same cohort who developed other diseases or remained healthy. Work histories from the cases and controls are abstracted and the analysis proceeds as in any case-control study. It can be assumed that the prevalence of a particular exposure among the total study population is fairly high, compared with cases and controls from the general population, so that the statistical power of the nested study is likely to be enhanced. This method is already being used to explore elevated SMRs in workplaces in which the cause is unclear and multiple exposures occur. Detailed and expanded exposure histories on a small number of workers can help distinguish among potential causal agents.

EPIDEMIOLOGIC SURVEILLANCE FOR OCCUPATIONAL DISEASE

When data on cases of actual or potential occupational disease are routinely collected, the opportunity to use these data for surveillance of a population exists. The most universal data base for this purpose is death certificates, which contain the decedent's usual occupation and employer and which allow the calculation of PMR for specific occupational groups. These certificates have been used notably in Washington State to scan occupations for excess mortality from a variety of causes (Milham, 1976). Unfortunately, only a handful of states code and store occupational data from vital statistics. In the United Kingdom, Decennial Reports and periodic supplements have examined mortality in various occupational groupings (Registrar General). The use of census data on occupation allows estimation of a population at risk and therefore calculation of SMRs. A drawback to this approach is that a person included in the numerator as a death may not appear in the denominator, since death and census records are not truly linked for individuals.

Other data bases, such as cancer registries, hospital records and compensation files, and physicians' reports may be utilized for surveillance. The major limitations to these sources of data are lack of comparability in occupational data, lack of coding in machine-readable form, and underreporting. Effective surveillance also requires, of course, that the diseases in question be accurately diagnosed. Failure to recognize occupational disease continues to be a major problem.

An interesting new approach involves the concept of "sentinel health events" (Rutstein, 1983). A sentinel health event is a preventable disease in which the occurrence of perhaps even a single case may signal the need to reexamine preventive practices. Occupational diseases that are clearly linked to specific exposures are all sentinel health events, since most occupational disease is relatively amenable to prevention. The use of an accepted list of sentinel events by epidemiologists will facilitate the recognition of unhealthy workplaces. However, the adoption of an accepted list is not the major obstacle. Some disease, such as coal workers' pneumoconiosis, is inherently occupational, but some, such as lung cancer, may be caused by nonoccupational factors as well. For the diseases that are not inherently occupational, the major obstacle again is the lack of systematically reported and coded data on patients' occupations. To the pathologist, the occupational lung cancer usually looks the same as any other lung cancer. It is left for the epidemiologist, using data on both diagnosed illness and occupation, to quantify and track known occupational diseases and generate hypotheses concerning new ones.

The concept of a sentinel health event may be extended to the search for new occupational health problems. An epidemiologist may scan the data base for groups whose illness may be caused by an environmental agent. For example, the occupations of parents who give birth to more than one child with a congenital defect might be compared with suitable controls in the data base. In this example, the sentinel health event is the birth of a second child with congenital defects to the same set of parents.

Ultimately, surveillance for occupational disease will be conducted routinely through the linkage of large data systems containing occupational history and health outcome information. In Canada, a monitoring system has been established by linking a 10 per cent random sample of the workforce to the national mortality register. The occupation of each member of this cohort was reported annually to the Unemployment Insurance Commission between 1965 and 1971 as part of a larger study. SMRs can then be calculated (Howe and Lindsay, 1983). The value of such a monitoring system increases through time, as the cohort matures and latency periods before the onset of disease elapse. Similar monitoring systems are planned for the United States using census records and the National Death Index.

ENVIRONMENTAL EPIDEMIOLOGY

The study of health effects from exposure in the community or residential environment will only be discussed briefly, since the methods and basic concerns are similar to those encountered in occupational studies. There are some important differences of emphasis, however. When studying environmental exposures, the epidemiologist is usually concerned with doses at concentrations far below those experienced by workers who are directly handling materials. This often requires a larger population for study in order to detect the smaller health effects likely to result. The problem of confounding variables is more serious, since individuals in a study may be scattered and collection of individual data on health status and behavior may be difficult and expensive. Estimation of dose is complicated by the lack of routine data on air or water contamination. In addition, the residential mobility in our society means that even the use of place of residence as a simple surrogate for exposure leads to problems with misclassification. The net result of these problems has been a tendency toward ecologic or correlational studies that require less data on individuals but that rarely suffice for testing hypotheses. Disease rates in residential zones at differing distances from a point source of pollution may be calculated, for example.

Some epidemiologists would argue that the best way to determine the health effects of low-level exposures in the community is to make predictions based on extrapolation from dose-response curves established for workers with higher exposures. This in fact has been done for many problems, such as asbestos exposure resulting from crumbling ceilings in schools. The transfer of findings from the workplace to the community at large raises certain complex questions:

1. A worker will probably be exposed to an agent for 8- to 10-hour periods, punctuated by some degree of removal from exposure, while a resident may be exposed 16 to 24 hours per day.

2. Children, who have different anatomic and physiologic respiratory characteristics from adults, absorb a different amount of an inhaled toxin than do workers exposed to the same ambient level.

3. Insulation of homes for energy conservation purposes may lead to greater accumulation of air contaminants.

4. Residential communities include the ill and elderly, who may be more susceptible to a given exposure.

The increasing urgency to assess health effects in the community from potential pollution sources, such as toxic waste sites and suspect household materials, leads to the belief that epidemiologic resources and techniques coming to bear on these problems will advance rapidly in the future.

SOCIAL POLICY CONSIDERATIONS

The results of epidemiologic studies in occupational and environmental health often have a direct impact on social policies. Epidemiology has become a critical part of the process of regulating health conditions in the workplace and the wider community. Agencies charged with setting standards for permissible levels of exposure must develop "risk assessments" that measure the number of excess cases of disease to be expected at various levels of exposure around the proposed standard level. An important example concerns benzene, which, until 1977 in the United States, had an occupational exposure limit of 10 parts per million (ppm). The United States federal government attempted in 1977 to lower the benzene standard to 1 ppm, on the basis of new epidemiologic evidence linking benzene to leukemia (Aksoy, 1974). The ensuing conflict between government and industry has come before the Supreme Court, while the following questions have been posed to epidemiologists: Can benzene be proved a human carcinogen at low doses? Will reduction of the standard from 10 to 1 ppm save lives? How many? Is there any tolerably safe level of exposure to a human carcinogen?

The need to answer these types of questions will both spur the development and expose the limitations of epidemiology. Already it is perceived that regulatory decisions must often be made in the absence of complete evidence from human populations. Balanced consideration of animal bioassays and short-term laboratory tests (e.g., chromosomal studies and mutagenicity tests in bacteria) in conjunction with epidemiologic evidence will be required. Mathematical modelling of the behavior of carcinogens at extremely low doses and in combination with other chemical exposures will continue to play a role.

The results of epidemiologic studies may also affect the employability of many people in certain industries. The concept of the hypersusceptible worker means that evidence of a greater effect of a toxic substance on a subgroup, compared with the entire population can be used to reduce illness by excluding such subgroups from the workplace. Potential examples include women of childbearing age in the lead industry and persons with alpha-1-antitrypsin deficiencies in industries with pulmonary hazards.

The use of this strategy to prevent illness as opposed to strategies aimed at lowering exposures to all workers will require far more sound laboratory and epidemiologic evidence regarding the nature of hyper-susceptibility than exists at present. Social policy concerns are woven tightly into the entire field of occupational and environmental epidemiology, so that its students and practitioners are constantly reminded of the underlying goal, which is to prevent disease in the fairest way possible.

REFERENCES

Aksoy, M., Erdem, S., and Dincol, G.: Leukemia in shoe-workers exposed chronically to benzene. Blood 44:837, 1974.

Acheson, E. D.: Nasal cancer in the furniture and boot and shoe manufacturing industries. Prev. Med. 5:295–315, 1976.

Axelson, O.: The case-referent (case-control) study in occupational health epidemiology. Scand. J. Work Environ. Health 5:91, 1979.

Blot, W. J., Harrington, J. M., Toledo, A., Hoover, R., Heath, C. W., and Fraumeni, J. F.: Lung cancer after employment in shipyards during World War II. N. Engl. J. Med. 299:620, 1978.

Blot, W. M., and Fraumeni, J. F., Jr.: Geographical patterns of lung cancer: Industrial correlations. Am. J. Epidemiol. 103:539, 1976.

Blot, W. J., Mason, T. J., Hoover, R., and Fraumeni, J. F.: Cancer by county: Etiologic implications. In Hiatt, H. H., Watson, J. D., and Winsten, J. A. (Eds.): Cold Spring Harbor Laboratory, 1977, p. 21.

Cole, P., Hoover, R., and Friedell, G. H.: Occupation and cancer of the lower urinary tract. Cancer 29:1250, 1972.

Covey, L. S., and Wynder, E. L.: Smoking habits and occupational status. J. Occup. Med. 23:537, 1981.

Creech, J. L., and Johnson, M. N.: Angiosarcoma of liver in manufacture of polyvinylchloride. J. Occup. Med. 16:150, 1974.

Enterline, P. E., and Marsh, G. M.: Missing records in occupational disease epidemiology. J. Occup. Med. 24:677, 1982.

Fox, A. J., and Collier, P. F.: Low mortality rates in industrial cohort studies due to selection for work and survival in the industry. Br. J. Prev. Soc. Med. 30:225, 1976.

Frazier, T. M., and Wegman, D. H.: Exploring the use of death certificates as a component of an occupational disease surveillance system. Am. J. Pub. Health 69:718, 1979.

Frost, W. H.: Risk of persons in familial contact with pulmonary tuberculosis. Am. J. Pub. Health 23:426–432, 1933.

Gamble, J., and Spirtas, R.: Job classification and utilization of complete work histories in occupational epidemiology. J. Occup. Med. 18:399, 1976.

Guralnick, L.: Mortality by occupational level and cause of death. Vital Statistics, Special Report, Volume 53(5). United States Department of HEW, Washington, D.C., 1963.

Hoar, S. K.: Epidemiology and occupational classification systems. In Peto, R., and Schneiderman, M. (Eds.): Banbury Report 9: Quantification of Occupational Cancer. Cold Spring Harbor Laboratory, 1981.

Hoover, and Fraumeni, J. F.: Cancer mortality in United States counties with chemical industry. Environ. Res. 9:196, 1975.

Howe, G. R., and Lindsay, J. P.: A follow-up study of a ten percent sample of the Canadian labor force. 1. Cancer mortality in males, 1965–1973. J. Nat. Cancer Inst. 70:37–44, 1983.

An Interim Report to Congress on Occupational Diseases. U.S. Department of Labor, Washington, D.C. June, 1980.

Kurland, L. T., et al.: Minamata disease. World Neurology 1:370, 1960.

Lee, A. M., and Fraumeni, J. F.: Arsenic and respiratory cancer in man: An occupational study. J. Nat. Cancer Inst. 42:1045, 1969.

Lloyd, J. W.: Long-term mortality study of steelworkers: V. Respiratory cancer in coke plant workers. J. Occup. Med. 13:53, 1971.

Mason, T. J., McKay, F. W., Hoover, K., Blot, W. J., and Fraumeni, J. F.: Atlas of cancer mortality for United States counties: 1950–1969. DHEW Publication No. (NIH) 75–780, U.S. Government Printing Office, Washington, D.C., 1975.

McDonald, J. C., Liddell, F. D. K., Gibbs, G. W., Eyssen, G. E., and McDonald, A. D.: Dust exposure and mortality in chrysotile mining 1910–1975. Br. J. Ind. Med. 37:11, 1980.

McMichael, A. J.: Standardized mortality ratios and the "healthy worker effect": Scratching beneath the surface. J. Occup. Med. 18:165, 1976.

Milham, S.: Occupational mortality in Washington State 1950–1971. NIOSH Publ. Nos. 76–175 A, B, and C, U.S. Department of HEW, Washington, D.C., 1976.

Monson, R. R., and Fine, L. J.: Cancer mortality and morbidity among rubber workers. J. Nat. Cancer Inst. 61:1047, 1978.

Morganstern, H.: Uses of ecologic analysis in epidemiologic research. Am. J. Publ. Health 72:1336, 1982.

Musk, H. W., Peters, J. M., and Wegman, D. H.: Lung function in firefighters: A three-year follow-up of active subjects. Am. J. Pub. Health 67:626, 1977.

Redmond, C. K., and Breslin, P. P.: Comparison of methods for assessing occupational hazards. J. Occup. Med. 17:313–317, 1975.

Registrar General's Decennial Supplements, England and Wales, For 1951, 1961, and 1970–72. Occupational Mortality Tables. London, Her Majesty's Stationery Office.

Rogot, E., and Reid, D.: The validity of data from next-of-kin in studies of mortality among migrants. Int. J. Epidemiol. 4/1:51–54, 1975.

Rousch, G. C., Meigs, J. W., Kelly, J., et al.: Sinonasal cancer and occupation: A case-control study. Am. J. Epidemiol. 111:183–193, 1980.

Rutstein, D. D., Mullan, R. J., Frazier, T. M., Halperin, W. E., Melius, J. M., and Sestito, J. P.: Sentinel health events (occupational); A basis for physician recognition and public health surveillance. Am. J. Pub. Health 73:1084, 1983.

Schlesselman, J. J.: Case Control Studies: Design Conduct, Analysis, Oxford University Press, New York, 1982.

Selikoff, I. J., Hammond, E. C., et al.: Asbestos exposure, smoking and neoplasia. J.A.M.A. 204:106, 1968.

Siematycki, J., Day, N. E., Fabry, J., Cooper, J. A.: Discovering carcinogens in the occupational environment: A novel epidemiologic approach. J. Nat. Cancer Inst. 66:217, 1981.

Steenland, K. J., and Beaumont, J.: Accuracy of Occupation and Industry Data on Death Certificates. Personal Communication.

Waxweiler, K. J., Stringer, W., Wagoner, J. K., Jones, J., et al.: Neoplastic risk among workers exposed to vinyl chloride. Ann. N.Y. Acad. Sci. 271:40, 1976.

Wegman, D. H., and Peters, J. M.: Oat cell cancer in selected occupations. J. Occup. Med. 20:793, 1978.

Whorton, D., Krauss, R. M., Marshall, S., and Milby, T. H.: Infertility in male pesticide workers. Lancet 2:1259, 1977.

SELECTED
STATISTICAL
TOPICS

13

Appropriate application of biostatistical tools is essential for valid study design and interpretation. This chapter presents four statistical techniques commonly employed in epidemiologic research. We recognize that it is necessary to study biostatistics in a comprehensive manner in order to properly integrate the methodology with other aspects of research planning and analysis, and we hope that this chapter will motivate students to do so.

SURVIVAL ANALYSIS

Survival analysis is aimed at estimating probability of survival, relapse, death, or any other event that occurs over time in a cohort that is under surveillance for a particular outcome. However, this type of analysis is especially relevant in clinical studies evaluating the efficacy of treatments in humans or animals, and commonly deals with rates of relapse.

In deciding on the analysis strategy, the following points must be taken into consideration:

1. *Do the data, or does the population from which the study sample is drawn, follow a particular mathematical distribution?* In other words, are the data "parametric" or "nonparametric"? If one of the common survival distributions (e.g., exponential, Weibull, lognormal, gamma) fits the data adequately, the parameters of that distribution may be used to describe the pattern of outcomes observed in the sample. In this case, parametric statistical tests would be appropriate. On the other hand, if the distribution of the underlying population is not known, or if no distribution adequately fits the observed data, nonparametric methods of analysis should be employed.

2. *What are the economic and time constraints in conducting the analysis?* In general, nonparametric statistical methods are easier to apply and require less time.

3. *Are the observations censored or uncensored?* When the exact survival times of all subjects are not known, the data are considered censored. Time until the outcome event may not be known, because individuals in the study may be lost to follow-up, patients may drop out of the study, or the event may not have occurred by the time the study period ends.

Figure 13–1 illustrates what commonly occurs in a clinical setting. A study (e.g., a clinical trial) is conducted for a fixed period of time and patients enter and withdraw at various times during the study interval. In the example shown in this figure, of the eight cases in the study, there are six censored observations (two patients lost to follow-up and four withdrawn alive without having relapsed at the end of the study).

4. *What is the size of the sample under study?* Some techniques are more appropriate for small sample sizes. For example, using a nonparametric life table analysis, the Kaplan-Meier Product Limit (PL) method (Kaplan and Meier, 1958) is best when the sample size is less than 30 in any of the patient groups studied, although it may also be used with large sample sizes.

This section will focus on two nonparametric life table approaches to survival analysis, because they are commonly found in the medical literature and may be easily performed by individuals with little or no background in statistics. They are the Kaplan-Meier PL method and the actuarial life table method used when the sample size exceeds 30 in each group.

Both techniques incorporate the survival times contributed by all

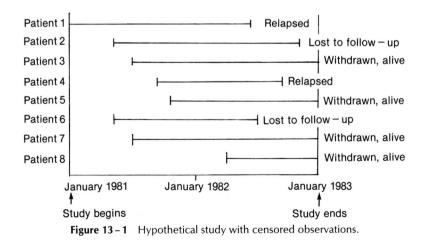

Figure 13–1 Hypothetical study with censored observations.

study subjects regardless of the length of time each patient is followed, i.e., censored as well as uncensored observations. This has the advantage of including individuals with short-term as well as long-term follow-up, resulting in a larger sample size and hence a smaller standard error of the survivorship estimate. The probability of surviving any length of time, t, from the beginning of the study is the product of the cumulative proportion surviving up to the previous time period multiplied by the proportion surviving at time, t.

The Product Limit (PL) Method

The distinctive characteristic of a PL analysis is that the cumulative proportion surviving is calculated at the individual survival time for each patient and there is no grouping of survival times into intervals (see Column 1, Table 13–1). Two important assumptions underlie the validity of this method: (1) that persons withdrawn from the study have a fate similar to those who remain under observation and (2) that the time period during which a person is entered in the study has no independent effect on the risk of the outcome event, i.e., there is no cohort effect.

TABLE 13-1 Method of Calculating Product-Limit Survivorship Estimate

(1) Survival times (t_i) (in months)	(2) Rank	(3) Uncensored Ranks (r_i)	(4) $(n - r)/$ $(n - r + 1)$	(5) $\hat{s}(t)$
3+	1	—	—	—
6	2	2	18/19 = 0.95	0.95
7+	3	—	—	—
7+	4	—	—	—
8	5	5	15/16 = 0.94	0.89
10	6	6	14/15 = 0.93	0.83
11	7	7	13/14 = 0.93	0.77
11+	8	—	—	—
11+	9	—	—	—
12	10	10	10/11 = 0.91	0.70
13	11	11	9/10 = 0.90	0.63
13	12	12	8/9 = 0.89	0.56°
14+	13	—	—	—
16+	14	—	—	—
20+	15	—	—	—
20+	16	—	—	—
22	17	17	3/4 = 0.75	0.42
32	18	18	2/3 = 0.67	0.28
34	19	19	1/2 = 0.50	0.14
36	20	20	0	0

° When there is a tie in survival times, use the most conservative estimate of $\hat{s}(t)$. In this case, $\hat{s}(t)$ at 13 months will be considered to be 0.56.

A practical way to calculate the PL survivorship estimate, as described by Lee (1980), is shown in Table 13–1. This example is based on data published by Pratt et al. (1977), who reported the disease-free intervals (remission times) for 20 osteosarcoma patients who were treated according to a chemotherapy protocol 3 months after amputation:

8 patients relapsed at 6, 8, 10, 11, 12, 13, 13, and 22 months.

11 patients were withdrawn alive at the end of the study, contributing 3, 7, 7, 11, 14, 16, 20, 20, 32, 34, and 36 months of observation.

1 patient refused further therapy after 11 months and withdrew from the study disease free.

On the basis of these data, Table 13–1 would be constructed to calculate the cumulative proportion surviving at any time, t (estimated cumulative survival rate). The five columns are derived as follows:

Column 1 — List all survival times, both censored and uncensored, in order from the smallest to largest. Place a + next to each censored observation. For censored and uncensored observations that have the same survival times, list the uncensored observation first.

Column 2 — List the rank of each observation in Column 1.

Column 3 — List the rank of uncensored observations.

Column 4 — To calculate the proportion of patients surviving through each time interval, let n = the sample size and r = the uncensored rank, and compute $(n - r)/(n - r + 1)$.

Column 5 — To calculate the PL estimate of the cumulative proportion surviving, $\hat{s}(t)$, multiply all values in Column 4 up to and including t for each survival time. If some censored observations are ties, the smallest $\hat{s}(t)$ should be used.

Survival times $[\hat{s}(t)]$ are plotted in Figure 13–2. The value of t at $\hat{s}(t) = 0.50$ (the survival time at the 50th percentile) may be taken as the estimated median survival time. In this instance, the median survival time is approximately 16 months. (To calculate the variance, standard error, and confidence intervals for the PL estimate of the survival rate, see Lee, 1980.)

The Actuarial Life Table Method

The actuarial life table method may be used to estimate prognosis or risk of an outcome event when the study includes a larger number of individuals (at least 30 in each group). Similar to the PL method, the actuarial life table incorporates all survival information, including censored observations (losses to follow-up, withdrawals who are alive) and

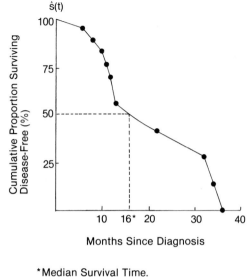

ṡ(t)

Cumulative Proportion Surviving Disease-Free (%)

Months Since Diagnosis

Figure 13–2 Kaplan-Meier survivorship estimate for 20 patients with osteosarcoma.

*Median Survival Time.

complete death data. Survival times are grouped into intervals, the length of the time interval depending on how frequently study subjects experience the condition or event. The intervals chosen need not be equal lengths of time. The lengths of the time intervals depend on one of the primary assumptions underlying the life table technique, i.e., events, withdrawals, and additions occur uniformly over whatever interval is chosen. Note that as a consequence of this assumption, the number at risk of the event in each interval equals the number entering the interval minus one-half the number of withdrawals (losses to follow-up or drop-outs). Two other assumptions in the life table approach shared by the Product Limit method are (1) that persons withdrawn or lost from the study experience the same rate of the outcome event as those who remain under observation and (2) that there is no cohort effect (risk of the outcome event is independent of the time an individual is entered into the study).

Table 13–2 illustrates how a life table is constructed, based on a hypothetical study involving 66 patients who participated in a clinical trial of an experimental drug. Table 13–3 shows the times to relapse, withdrawal, or loss to follow-up for the 66 patients. Although for illustrative purposes 16 of 66 patients in this example are lost to follow-up, this high proportion would cast doubt on the validity of an actual clinical trial. An explanation of the columns in the life table in Table 13–2 and a description of necessary calculations are as follows:

Column 1 — Interval: The interval of time from the starting point of

TABLE 13–2 Method of Constructing an Actuarial Life Table Utilizing Data In Table 13–3

(1) Interval (in months)	(2) Lost to Follow-up	(3) Withdrawn Alive	(4) No. Relapsed	(5) No. Entering Interval	(6) No. Exposed to Risk	(7) Conditional Proportion Relapsing	(8) Conditional Proportion Surviving Disease Free	(9) Cumulative Proportion Surviving Disease Free
0–2	0	0	4	66	66	0.061	0.939	1.000
3–5	0	0	4	62	62	0.065	0.935	0.939
6–8	0	0	4	58	58	0.069	0.931	0.878
9–11	0	0	3	54	54	0.056	0.944	0.817
12–14	0	0	1	51	51	0.020	0.980	0.772
15–17	2	5	2	50	46.5	0.043	0.957	0.756
18–20	1	3	0	41	39	0	1.000	0.724
21–23	1	0	0	37	36.5	0	1.000	0.724
24–26	3	5	0	36	32	0	1.000	0.724
27–29	1	0	1	28	27.5	0.036	0.964	0.724
30–32	1	2	0	26	24.5	0	1.000	0.698
33–35	2	2	0	23	21	0	1.000	0.698
36–38	0	3	0	19	17.5	0	1.000	0.698
39–41	0	3	1	16	14.5	0.069	0.931	0.698
42–44	1	3	0	12	10	0	1.000	0.649
45–47	2	1	0	8	6.5	0	1.000	0.649
48–50	0	3	0	5	3.5	0	1.000	0.649
51–53	2	0	0	2	1	0	1.000	0.649

TABLE 13-3 Experience of 66 Patients Enrolled in a Hypothetical Clinical Trial of an Experimental Drug

Time to Withdrawal (Measured from Date of Diagnosis, in Months)*	No. Patients	Time to Relapse (Measured from Date of Diagnosis, in Months)†	No. Patients
15	3	1	2
16	1	2	2
17	1	3	2
18	1	4	2
19	2	6	1
24	2	7	2
25	1	8	1
26	2	10	2
30	1	11	1
31	1	13	1
34	1	16	1
35	1	17	1
36	1	27	1
37	1	40	1

Time to Withdrawal (cont.)	No. Patients	Time to Loss to Follow-up (Measured from Date of Diagnosis, in Months)‡	No. Patients
38	1	15	1
40	3	16	1
42	1	19	1
43	1	21	1
44	1	24	1
45	1	25	1
49	2	26	1
50	1	28	1
		30	1
		34	1
		35	1
		43	1
		46	2
		52	1
		53	1

* Thirty patients were withdrawn alive (i.e., they had not relapsed during the time they were under observation), and these withdrawals occurred at the designated times.

† Twenty patients relapsed during the study period at the designated times.

‡ Sixteen patients were lost to follow-up at the designated times.

the study, during which events are counted. The length of the interval depends on the frequency and pattern of events and disease-specific considerations. Each interval need not be of identical length.

Column 2—Lost to Follow-Up: The number of individuals lost to follow-up during the interval and whose outcome is unknown.

Column 3 — Withdrawn Alive: The number of individuals alive at the end of the study. The interval in which they are withdrawn is the time between entering the study and the closing date of the study.

Column 4 — Number Relapsed (or Dying): The number of individuals who relapse (or die) during the interval. The time to relapse (relapse-free time, survival time) is the period of time between entering the study and the date of relapse (or death).

Column 5 — Number Entering the Interval: The number entering the first interval is the total number who participated in the study. The number entering other intervals is the number who were present at the beginning of the previous interval minus those in the previous interval who were lost to follow-up, withdrew alive, or relapsed (died).

Column 6 — Number Exposed to Risk: The number exposed to risk of the outcome event (relapse, death, and so on) at the beginning of the interval is equal to the number entering the interval (from Column 5) minus one-half the number lost to follow-up or withdrawn alive during the interval. (See discussion of assumptions of life table method for rationale.)

Column 7 — Conditional Proportion Relapsing: This estimate of the conditional probability of relapsing (dying) during any interval given exposure to risk of relapsing is calculated by

$$\frac{\text{Number relapsing during the interval}}{\text{Number exposed to risk of relapse at the beginning of the interval}}$$

Column 8 — Conditional Proportion Surviving Disease Free: The conditional proportion surviving during the interval is equal to $1 -$ conditional proportion relapsing during the interval ($1 -$ Column 7).

Column 9 — Cumulative Proportion Surviving Disease Free: This proportion is an estimate of the cumulative disease-free survival rate. It is equal to the conditional proportion surviving disease free during the interval times the conditional proportions surviving disease free during the prior intervals. The value for the first interval is always 1.

Comparing Survival Distributions

There are a number of nonparametric tests for studies with and without censoring that are simple to apply, for the comparison of survival distributions. This type of testing is appropriate in a clinical trial to compare efficacy of two or more treatments or in a study of the influence of two preventive strategies on the development of disease in similar groups of individuals.

The log rank test (Peto and Peto, 1972) is one of the most popular of the nonparametric tests. Others commonly employed are Gehan's generalized Wilcoxon test (Gehan, 1965a, 1965b), the Cox-Mantel test (Cox, 1959; Cox, 1972; Mantel, 1966), Peto and Peto's generalized Wilcoxon test (1972), Cox's F-test (1964), and the Mantel-Haenszel chi-square test (1959). All of these tests are described also in Lee, 1980.

To prevent bias in studies of survivorship, it is important to include in the cohort all patients who meet the diagnostic and other criteria for entry. All persons should be enrolled at the time of diagnosis, not at the time treatment is begun. No patient should be excluded because he or she dies shortly after diagnosis, remains untreated, does not respond to therapy, or represents an operative death. Moore (1963), in an article entitled "How to Achieve Surgical Results by Really Trying," has shown that misleading "improvement" in survivorship may be achieved by careful selection of patients for analysis. The bias introduced by excluding nonresponders from analysis has recently been discussed in a paper by Weiss et al. (1983).

The problem of defining a total cohort is particularly crucial in arteriosclerotic heart disease. A number of studies indicate that many patients with myocardial infarction die suddenly, before they can be hospitalized (Kuller, 1976). Studies of prognosis based only on hospitalized patients thus present the survival experience of only a segment of the total number of persons who suffer a myocardial infarction.

Relative Survival

Survival rates that incorporate comparisons with expected survival in a comparable group of individuals in the general population are called *relative survival rates.* A relative survival rate is a ratio of the observed rate in the patient group divided by the expected rate for persons in the general population with the same demographic characteristics, i.e., it is a survival rate that is adjusted for normal life expectancy. Expected survival rates for populations in various age, race, and sex categories may be obtained from life tables published by the National Center for Health Statistics. Figure 13–3 illustrates relative survival rates for breast cancer among white female patients included in the SEER program (Ries et al., 1983). To generate the relative rate, a ratio was formed of the observed survival rate divided by the expected survival for women in the same age-race category in the United States in 1975 for three time periods from diagnosis. It can be seen that the survival experience of women with breast cancer compares increasingly less favorably with that of the general population between 1 year and 5 years from the time of diagnosis. Interestingly, age at diagnosis does not appear to have a significant influence on the relative survival rates.

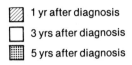

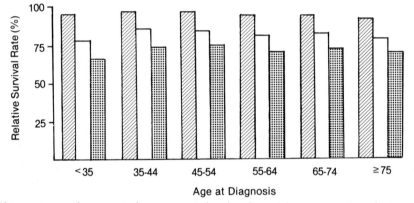

Figure 13–3 Relative survival rates among white females with breast cancer from the SEER* Program by age and time since diagnosis.

ADJUSTMENT OF RATES

Need for Adjusting Rates

Differences in population structure can, by themselves, affect crude rates. For example, in Table 13–4 we see that two populations, A and B, have the same age-specific death rates (Column 4); that is, a person in a specific age group in A is at the same risk of dying as a person of the same age group in B. There is no true difference in risk of death. However, A has relatively more older people, i.e., 30 per cent over 45 years compared with only 10 percent over 45 years in B (Column 3). Because death rates are higher at older ages and because A has more older people, this will lead to a higher crude death rate for the population in A.

The difference in crude death rates for Populations A and B can be explained mathematically as follows: The age-specific death rates (Column 4) multiplied by the number in the population at each age (Column 2) determines the number of deaths in each age group and, therefore, the total deaths (Column 5). The latter divided by the total population gives the crude (average) death rate. The crude rate can also be obtained

TABLE 13–4 Comparison of Death Rates in Two Populations by Age

	Age (years)	Population Number	Population Proportion	Annual Age-specific Death Rate per 1000	Annual Number of Deaths	Crude Death Rate per 1000
	(1)	(2)	(3)	(4)	(5)	(6)
Population A	<15	1500	0.30	2	3	
	15–44	2000	0.40	6	12	
	≥ 45	1500	0.30	20	30	
	All ages	5000	1.00		45	$\dfrac{45}{5000} = 9.0$
Population B	<15	2000	0.40	2	4	
	15–44	2500	0.50	6	15	
	≥ 45	500	0.10	20	10	
	All ages	5000	1.00		29	$\dfrac{29}{5000} = 5.8$

by multiplying each age-specific rate (Column 4) by the corresponding population proportion (Column 3) and summing the resultant number of deaths. The crude death rate is, therefore, really a *weighted average* of the age-specific death rates in which the numbers (or proportions) in each age group are the weights. Since A has a higher proportion (increased weighting) of older persons for whom the age-specific death rates are higher, the crude death rate is higher in A (9.0 per 1000) than B (5.8 per 1000) even though the risk of dying for persons in each age group is the same.

Direct Adjustment of Rates

Table 13–5 shows how this difference in age composition or weighting can be eliminated, thus permitting fair comparison of the two populations. This requires the selection of some population, called a *standard population*, to which the age-specific rates for each population (Columns 2 and 4) can be applied. In this instance, we have arbitrarily chosen the combined populations of A and B as standard (Column 1). Multiplying the standard population by the age-specific rates in A and B yields the number of *expected* deaths in A and B, respectively, as shown in Columns 3 and 5.

Note that the expected deaths in Columns 3 and 5 answer the question: What would be the number of deaths in the standard population (Column 1) if people were dying at the age-specific rates observed in each population (Columns 2 and 4)? The answer is, of course, fictitious. Nevertheless, we see that the number of expected deaths (74)

TABLE 13–5 Computation of Expected Number of Deaths by Direct Method: Example 1: Identical Age-Specific Rates

Age (years)	Standard Population (A and B Combined)	Population A Age-specific Death Rates per 1000	Expected Deaths	Population B Age-specific Death Rates per 1000	Expected Deaths
	(1)	(2)	$(3) = (2) \times (1)$	(4)	$(5) = (4) \times (1)$
<15	3500	2	7	2	7
15–44	4500	6	27	6	27
≥45	2000	20	40	20	40
All ages	10,000		74		74

would be the same for populations A and B. Also, the age-adjusted rates (7.4 per 1000) are the same for A and B. This must be so, since A and B have the same age-specific death rates and population differences have been eliminated by use of the same (standard) population. Thus age-adjustment has demonstrated there is truly no difference between A and B in risk of death.

Let us now assume that the age-specific death rate for age 15 to 44 is *higher* in B than A, 10 versus 6 per 1000 (Columns 2 and 4), as seen in Table 13–6. Multiplying the age-specific death rates in these columns by the standard population now yields more expected deaths for B (Column 5) than for A (Column 3). As a result, the age-adjusted rate is now higher for B than for A, as expected.

Adjusted death rates based on Table 13–6:

$$A = \frac{74}{10,000} = 7.4 \text{ per } 1000$$

$$B = \frac{92}{10,000} = 9.2 \text{ per } 1000$$

TABLE 13–6 Computation of Expected Number of Deaths by Direct Method: Example 2: Different Age-Specific Rates

Age (years)	Standard Population (A and B Combined)	Population A Age-specific Death Rates per 1000	Expected Deaths	Population B Age-specific Death Rates per 1000	Expected Deaths
	(1)	(2)	(3)	(4)	(5)
<15	3500	2	7	2	7
15–44	4500	6	27	10	45
≥45	2000	20	40	20	40
All ages	10,000		74		92

We should point out that the choice of a standard population is arbitrary. In the example above the standard was the **combined** populations of A and B, but **either** one of the two could have been chosen. For comparability among studies it is advantageous that the same standard be used by different investigators. Thus, for many years the United States population of 1940 was widely used as a standard, even when population data for subsequent years were already available. The choice of standard, while affecting the magnitudes of the age-adjusted rates, will usually not affect the relative ranking of the populations unless the standard chosen is grossly different in age distribution from the population or populations under study.

Indirect Adjustment of Rates

There are circumstances in which age-adjustment is required but the procedure just described cannot be applied because the small number of deaths in one group leads to unstable age-specific rates or its age-specific rates may not be known. When this is true, another method is available. This is referred to as *indirect adjustment.*

The indirect method of age-adjustment may be viewed as a mirror image of the direct method. In the direct method just described, an age-adjusted rate is achieved by applying age-specific rates of the population (or populations) of interest (e.g., A or B) to a population of known age structure (e.g., A and B combined) to yield an "expected" number of deaths. The group of known age structure is called the "standard" population.

In the indirect method, standardization is based on age-specific *rates* rather than on age composition. Here the population whose rates form the basis for comparison is referred to as the "standard" population. If two populations are to be compared by the indirect method, the larger of the two is usually chosen as standard because its rates tend to be more stable. However, if a developed and an underdeveloped country are being compared, the developed country would probably be taken as the standard, regardless of comparative size, since age-specific rates might be available only for this country.

The process of indirect adjustment consists of applying the age-specific rates of the standard population to a population of interest (e.g., population A) to yield a number of "expected" deaths. This process is equivalent to asking, what would be the number of deaths (i.e., expected deaths) in population A if people in that population were dying at the same (age-specific) rate as people in the standard population.

A common way of carrying out indirect age-adjustment is to relate the total expected deaths thus obtained to observed deaths through a formula known as the *standardized mortality ratio* (SMR):

TABLE 13-7 Deaths by Age and Pf Reading (Whites) for Three-and-a-Half-Year Observation Period, Muscogee County, Georgia, 1946

Age in 1946 (years)	Negative for Cardiovascular Disease			Suspect for Cardiovascular Disease	
	Population	Number of Deaths	Age-specific death rates per 100	Population	Number of Deaths
15–34	13,681	35	0.25	23	1
35–54	8838	102	1.15	24	5
55 and over	2253	149	6.61	65	14
All ages	24,772	286		112	20
Crude death rate per 100		1.15			17.9

$$SMR = \frac{\text{Total observed deaths in a population}}{\text{Total expected deaths in that population}}$$

If this mortality ratio is greater than 1, it means that more deaths are observed in the smaller or comparison population than would be expected on the basis of rates in the larger (standard) population. If the ratio is less than 1, fewer deaths are observed than expected.*

The use of indirect age-adjustment through calculation of SMR can be illustrated by the Muscogee County, Georgia, study of tuberculosis (Comstock, 1953). In 1946, 70-mm photofluorograms (Pf) were taken primarily for the information they would yield about tuberculosis. However, since they were also read for possible cardiovascular abnormalities, it became possible to compare the subsequent mortality experience of those whose Pf was read as negative with those whose Pf suggested possible cardiovascular disease. Data for three and one-half years of observation are shown in Table 13–7.

The crude death rate for suspects (17.9) is higher than that for the negatives (1.15). However, since the distribution of ages for the two groups is quite dissimilar (Table 13–8), age-adjustment is necessary.

Because the suspect group was small and gave rise to only 20 deaths during the three-and-a-half–year period of observation, the age-specific death rates of this group would be quite unstable. Accordingly, we use the larger group of negatives as the standard population (Table 13–9) and apply the age-specific death rates noted in this group (Column 2) to the suspects (Column 1) in order to determine an expected number of deaths among the suspects (Column 3). The total number of expected deaths among suspects (4.7) is then compared with the number

---

* The SMR is a ratio resulting from a *relative* form of indirect age-adjustment. A more complicated method of indirect adjustment, which yields an *absolute* age-adjusted rate, involves the calculation of an *index death rate* and a *standardizing factor* for each population of interest.

TABLE 13–8 Percentage Distribution by Age of Negatives and Suspects, Muscogee County, Georgia

Age (years)	Negative for Cardiovascular Disease		Suspect for Cardiovascular Disease	
	Number	Percentage of Population	Number	Percentage of Population
15–34	13,681	55.2	23	20.5
35–54	8838	35.7	24	21.4
55 and over	2253	9.1	65	58.0
All ages	24,772	100.0	112	99.9

TABLE 13-9 Calculation of Standardized Mortality Ratio for Suspects Compared with Negatives, Muscogee County, Georgia

Age (years)	Number of "Suspects"	Death Rates per 100 for Persons Negative for Cardiovascular Disease	Expected Deaths among "Suspects" According to Rates for Negatives	Observed Deaths among "Suspects"
	(1)	(2)	(3) = (1) × (2)	(4)
15–34	23	0.25	.1	1
35–54	24	1.15	.3	5
55 and over	65	6.61	4.3	14
All ages			4.7	20

actually observed in this group through the standardized mortality ratio, as shown below.

$$\text{SMR} = \frac{\text{Observed deaths}}{\text{Expected deaths}} = \frac{20}{4.7} = 4.25$$

We see that the SMR is 4.25, indicating that even after age-adjustment the overall death rate is still higher for "suspects" than for "negatives." However, the much larger original ratio of the crude rates, 15.5 (i.e., 17.9 to 1.15) has been much reduced by adjustment.

The indirect method of adjustment does not completely take account of differences in population composition. Therefore, when more than two populations are to be compared, each may be compared with the standard population but not directly to the others.°

COHORT ANALYSIS OF MORTALITY

When the frequency of a disease is changing over time (see page 145), it may be helpful to analyze the data by grouping the patients according to date of birth. The resulting groups are called birth cohorts.

A *cohort* is a group of persons who share a common experience within a defined time period. For example, a *birth cohort* consists of all persons born within a given period of time. A marriage cohort would consist of all persons married within a certain time period. In studies of chronic disease, a cohort of diseased persons (e.g., with stomach cancer or rheumatic fever) could be defined as all whose disease was first diagnosed during a given time period. The advantage of using a cohort

---

° For more detailed discussion of the methods and issues involved in age-adjustment, see Hill, A. B., 1971.

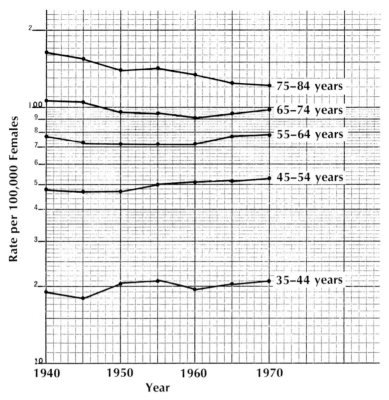

Figure 13–4 Death rates from breast cancer, by age group, white females, United States, 1940–1968 (calendar year on abscissa). (From Grove, R. D., and Hetzel, A. M.: Vital Statistics Rates in the United States, 1940–1960. USPHS Pub. No. 1677, U.S. Govt. Printing Office, Washington, D.C., 1968; National Center for Health Statistics: Vital Statistics of the United States, Vol. IIA. U.S. Govt. Printing Office, Washington, D.C., annual.)

approach to study mortality in a disease of changing frequency was first pointed out for tuberculosis (Frost, 1939).

Information about disease is usually presented as curves of age-specific morbidity or mortality rates for specific calendar years. For example, Figure 13–4 presents age-specific death rates for a disease without a pronounced secular trend, cancer of the breast, over the period 1940 to 1968. A portion of the same information is rearranged in a less usual manner, with age rather than time on the x-axis (Fig. 13–5).

This latter method of presentation can also be applied to a disease of changing frequency, such as tuberculosis. In Figure 13–6 the age-specific death rates from tuberculosis are seen to have declined in each successive time period from 1900 to 1960. In addition, there is an apparent shift in the age pattern. The second peak in rates (following a

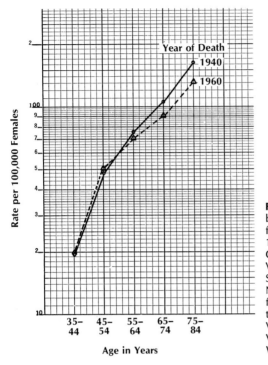

Rate per 100,000 Females

Age in Years

Figure 13-5 Death rates from breast cancer, by age group, white females, United States, 1940 and 1960 (age on abscissa). (From Grove, R. D., and Hetzel, A. M.: Vital Statistics Rates in the United States, 1940–1960. USPHS Pub. No. 1677, U.S. Govt. Printing Office, Washington, D.C., 1968; National Center for Health Statistics: Vital Statistics of the United States, Vol. IIA. U.S. Govt. Printing Office, Washington, D.C., annual.)

peak in early childhood and trough for children of school age) appears to have occurred at successively older ages.

All of the curves presented thus far are called *cross-sectional curves*, because they cut across birth cohorts at a given point in time. They thus provide a "snapshot" of mortality experience at that time. The information on death rates from tuberculosis can also be arranged (Fig. 13–7) so that the lines, instead of connecting age-specific death rates by year of *death*, as in Figure 13–6, connect age-specific death rates by year of *birth*. This creates a family of curves, one for each birth cohort, all of which show a similar age pattern. The peak rate following childhood is reached in early adult life, and there is no longer an apparent trend toward an increase in rates with increasing age. Thus, analysis of the data by birth cohorts indicates that the apparent shift in age seen in cross-sectional curves is essentially an artifact.

The difference between cross-sectional and cohort curves is further clarified in Figure 13–8, which shows how members of one birth cohort enter into different cross-sectional death curves. Two unbroken lines depict cross-sectional death rates from tuberculosis (in 1900 and 1960). The broken line shows the death rates for the birth cohort of 1900.

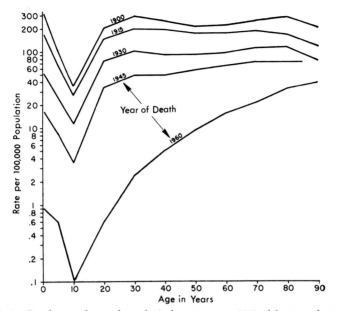

Figure 13-6 Death rates from tuberculosis, by age group, United States, selected years. (Adapted from Doege, T. C.: Tuberculosis mortality in the United States, 1900 to 1960. J.A.M.A., *192*:1045, 1965.)

Members of the 1900 birth cohort who died in infancy are included in the 1900 cross-sectional death curve; those who died at age 60 are included in the 1960 cross-sectional death curve. The same principle would apply to the intervening decades between 1900 and 1960. (We have omitted these curves on the graph but have noted in the cohort curve where the intersections with cross-sectional curves would have occurred.)

Table 13-10, which presents age-specific death rates by decade for 1900 through 1960, further illustrates how the members of one birth cohort enter into different cross-sectional curves. The age-specific death rates for the cohort of 1900 are shown in bold type on the diagonal and correspond to the intersecting points shown in Figure 13-8.

When death rates are decreasing with time, as is true of tuberculosis, the older groups appear to have higher death rates than younger people on cross-sectional curves. This occurs because the elderly come from earlier birth cohorts who are at greater risk. Conversely, when death rates are increasing with time, as is true of lung cancer (Fig. 13-9), cross-sectional curves show apparently decreasing rates with increasing age.

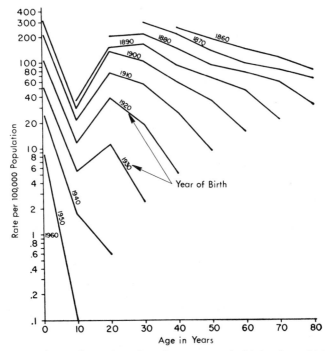

Figure 13–7 Death rates from tuberculosis, by age group, for birth cohorts, United States, 1860–1960. (Adapted from Doege, T. C.: Tuberculosis mortality in the United States, 1900 to 1960. J.A.M.A., *192*:1045, 1965.)

SAMPLE SIZE DETERMINATION

A crucial step in preparing to conduct a study is determination of the number of subjects needed. An adequate number of subjects must be enrolled to answer the question (or questions) posed by the study. In order to calculate the required sample size *before* a study is initiated, the clinician must specify

1. The size of the difference one is interested in detecting (e.g., 25 per cent or 50 per cent reduction in mortality in a clinical trial or a relative risk of, for instance, 2 in a case-control study).

2. The frequency of the outcome in the control group (i.e., current mortality rates for patients treated with standard therapy in a clinical trial or the prevalence of the risk factor of interest among controls in a case-control study. The number of controls likely to be exposed in a case-control or prospective study may be estimated from reliable surveys of the prevalence of exposure in the general population).

3. The level of Type I error (α), or the significance level. That is,

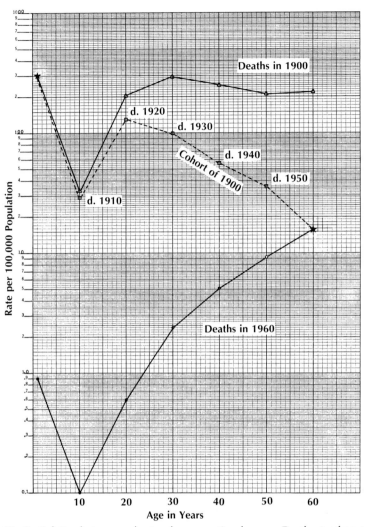

Figure 13 – 8 Relation between cohort and cross-sectional curves. Death rates from tuberculosis, by age group, for 1900 birth cohort and for calendar years 1900 and 1960. (Adapted from table provided through the courtesy of Dr. T. C. Doege.)

the probability of finding a significant difference when none truly exists. Alpha represents the probability that observed significant results have occurred by chance. Significance levels of 0.05 or less are commonly chosen to minimize the probability that the observed results occurred because of sampling fluctuations. Sometimes, however, it may be appropriate to choose an α of 0.1 or greater, to screen for effects that would be worthy of further study. If many associations are to be tested in a single

TABLE 13–10 Death Rates Per 100,000 Population from Tuberculosis, by Age Group, for Selected Years, U.S. Death Registration States°

Year	Age Group							
	under 1	1–4	5–14	15–24	25–34	35–44	45–54	55–64
1900	311.6	101.8	36.2	205.7	294.3	253.6	215.6	223.0
1910	212.9	84.6	29.7	152.0	217.6	214.9	188.1	192.9
1915	168.6	68.0	26.9	146.1	198.0	196.9	176.8	177.0
1920	106.5	45.4	22.4	136.1	164.9	147.4	137.2	141.3
1930	51.6	25.9	11.9	77.3	102.8	92.4	93.2	97.0
1940	24.6	12.3	5.5	38.2	56.3	59.4	66.3	76.1
1945	16.3	8.7	3.6	34.1	49.3	49.8	58.1	66.0
1950	8.5	6.3	1.8	11.3	19.1	26.1	35.9	47.7
1960	.9	.6	.1	.6	2.4	5.1	9.3	15.5

° Adapted from table provided through the courtesy of Dr. T. C. Doege.

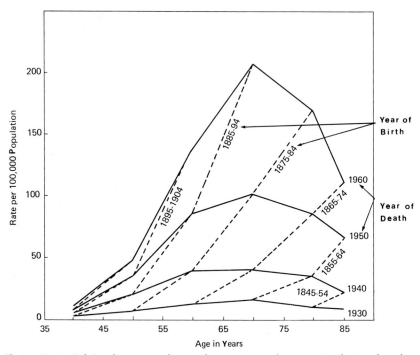

Figure 13–9 Relation between cohort and cross-sectional curves. Death rates from lung cancer, by age, for selected birth cohorts (broken lines) and for selected calendar years (solid lines), white males, 40 years and older, United States. (From NCI Monograph No. 6, 1961; USPHS Pub. No. 113, U.S. Govt. Printing Office, Washington, D.C., 1963.)

analysis, as would occur in initial exploration of a large data set, the cumulative probability of making at least one Type I error is increased. In this case, the significance level should be set at α divided by the number of hypotheses tested.

4. The value of Type II error (β). This refers to the probability of failing to detect a significant difference if one in fact exists. Usually β is chosen to be 4 times the level of significance, so if $\alpha = 0.05$, β will be set at 0.2. 1-β is referred to as the power of the study. *Power* is the probability of rejecting the null hypothesis when it is, in fact, false; otherwise stated, it is the ability to detect and accurately estimate changes in frequency (Bloom, 1981). In choosing α and β, the investigator must weigh the relative disadvantage of falsely rejecting the null hypothesis against missing an effect that is really there. One cannot minimize both α and β simultaneously: as α is decreased, β increases and power declines.

Experts in experimental design have developed procedures that permit investigators to use previously generated data to specify their expectation of types of error and likelihood of various outcomes. There are published formulae and tables one can consult to determine required sample size (Fleiss, 1981; Schlesselman, 1982). In many cases the investigator has a set sample size available and will want to know, given these four specifications, what is the least significant relative risk that

TABLE 13-11 The Relationship Between Frequency of an Outcome in the Control Group, Sample Size of Comparison Groups, and Change in Frequency Detectable with 95% Power

Frequency of the outcome in the group per 100	Sample Size of Comparison Groups	Change in Frequency Detectable with 95% Power[*]
3	50	7.7-fold increase
	100	5.3-fold increase
	250	3.3-fold increase
	300	3.2-fold increase
7	50	4.6-fold increase
	100	3.4-fold increase
	250	2.3-fold increase
	300	2.3-fold increase
15	50	3.0-fold increase
	100	2.4-fold increase
	250	1.8-fold increase
	300	1.7-fold increase

[*] $= 0.10$, two-tailed, or $= 0.05$, one-tailed.

From Bloom, A. D. (ed.): Guidelines for studies of human populations exposed to mutagenic and reproductive hazards. March of Dimes Birth Defects Foundation. White Plains, N.Y., 1981, pp. 45–52.

would be detectable by the study. This will answer the question of whether it would be worthwhile to carry out the study at all (Walter, 1977).

Table 13-11 illustrates the relationship between the frequency of the outcome in the control group, the sample size, and the change in frequency detectable with 95 per cent power. Note that the higher the frequency of the outcome in the control group, the smaller the sample size necessary to detect a comparable change in the study group.

REFERENCES

Bloom, A. D. (ed.): Guidelines for studies of human populations exposed to mutagenic and reproductive hazards. March of Dimes Birth Defects Foundation. White Plains, N.Y., 1981, pp. 45-52.

Comstock, G. W.: Mortality of persons with photofluorograms suggestive of cardiovascular disease. N. Engl. J. Med., 248:1045, 1953.

Cox, D. R.: The analysis of exponentially distributed life-times with two types of failures. J. R. Stat. Soc. (Series B), 21:411, 1959.

Cox, D. R.: Some applications of exponential ordered scores. J. R. Stat. Soc. (Series B), 26:103, 1964.

Cox, D. R.: Regression models and life tables. J. R. Stat. Soc. (Series B), 34:187, 1972.

Fleiss, J. L.: Statistical Methods for Rates and Proportions, 2nd Ed. John Wiley and Sons, New York, 1981, pp. 33-49.

Frost, W. H.: The age selection of mortality from tuberculosis in successive decades. Am. J. Hyg., 30(A):91, 1939.

Gehan, E. A.: A generalized two-sample Wilcoxon Test for comparing arbitrarily singly-censored samples. Biometrika, 52:203, 1965a.

Gehan, E. A.: A generalized two-sample Wilcoxon Test for doubly-censored data. Biometrika, 52:650, 1965b.

Gross, A. J., and Clark, V. A.: Survival Distributions: Reliability Applications in the Biomedical Sciences. John Wiley and Sons, New York, 1975.

Hill, A. B.: Principles of Medical Statistics, 9th Ed. Lancet Ltd., London, 1971, pp. 201-209.

Kaplan, E. L., and Meier, P.: Nonparametric estimation from incomplete observations. JASA, 53:457, 1958.

Kuller, L. H.: Epidemiology of cardiovascular diseases: Current perspectives. Am. J. Epidemiol, 104:425, 1976.

Lee, E. T.: Statistical Methods for Survival Data Analysis. Lifetime Learning Publications, Belmont, California, 1980.

Mantel, N.: Evaluation of survival data and two new rank order statistics arising in its consideration. Cancer Chemother. Rep., 50:163, 1966.

Mantel, N., and Haenszel, W.: Statistical aspects of the analysis of data from retrospective studies of disease. J. Nat. Cancer Inst., 22:719, 1959.

Moore, G. E.: How to achieve surgical results by really trying. Surg. Gynecol. Obstet. 116:497, 1963.

Peto, R., and Peto, J.: Asymptotically efficient rank invariant procedures. J. R. Stat. Soc. (Series A), 135:185, 1972.

Pratt, C., Shanks, E., Hustu, O., Rivera, G., Smith, J., and Kumar, A. P. M.: Adjuvant multiple drug chemotherapy for osteosarcoma of the extremity. Cancer, 39:51, 1977.

Ries, L. G., Pollack, E. S., and Young, J. L.: Cancer patient survival: Surveillance, epidemiology and end results program 1973-1979. J. Nat. Cancer Inst., 70:693, 1983.

Schlesselman, J. J.: Case-Control Studies. Design, Conduct, Analysis. Oxford University Press, New York, 1982, pp. 144-170.

Walter, S. D.: Determination of significant relative risks and optimal sampling procedures in prospective and retrospective comparative studies of various sizes. Am. J. Epidemiol., *105*:387, 1977.

Weiss, G. B., Bunce, H., and Hokanson, J. A.: Comparing survival of responders and nonresponders after treatment: A potential source of confusion in interpreting cancer clinical trials. Control Clin. Trials, *4*:43, 1983.

INDEX

Numbers in *italics* refer to illustrations; numbers followed by (t) refer to tables.